'Simply the best and most authoritative set of articles yet produced on the Covid-19 crisis. Global in scope, and written by top-class academic experts, the book provides an essential source for grasping the impact of the pandemic and what accounts for the huge differences in its impact in different states and regions.'

Anthony Giddens, *Emeritus Professor at the LSE and Fellow of King's College, Cambridge, UK*

'An imaginative collection of uniformly perceptive studies examining how different countries have coped with the havoc caused by the coronavirus. A most valuable contribution to a comparative understanding of a nationally mediated global problem.'

Bhikhu Parekh, *Member of the House of Lords, UK*

COVID-19 AND GOVERNANCE

Covid-19 and Governance focuses on the relationship between governance institutions and approaches to Covid-19 and health outcomes. Bringing together analyses of Covid-19 developments in countries and regions across the world with a wide-angle lens on governance, this volume asks: what works, what hasn't and isn't, and why?

Organized by region, the book is structured to follow the spread of Covid-19 in the course of 2020, through Asia, the Middle East, Europe, the Americas, and Africa. The analyses explore a number of key themes, including public health systems, government capability, and trust in government—as well as underlying variables of social cohesion and inequality. This volume combines governance, policies, and politics to bring wide international scope and analytical depth to the study of the Covid-19 pandemic.

Together the authors represent a diverse and formidable database of experience and understanding. They include sociologists, anthropologists, scholars of development studies and public administration, as well as MD specialists in public health and epidemiology. Engaged and free of jargon, this book speaks to a wide global public—including scholars, students, and policymakers—on a topic that has profound and broad appeal.

Jan Nederveen Pieterse is Suzanne and Duncan Mellichamp Distinguished Professor of Global Studies and Sociology at University of California Santa Barbara, USA.

Haeran Lim is Professor in Political Science and International Relations, Seoul National University, South Korea.

Habibul Khondker, MA (Carleton, Ottawa), PhD (Pittsburgh) is Professor of Social Sciences at Zayed University, Abu Dhabi.

ROUTLEDGE STUDIES IN EMERGING SOCIETIES

Series Editor: Jan Nederveen Pieterse, University of California, Santa Barbara

The baton of driving the world economy is passing to emerging economies. This is not just an economic change, but a social change, with migration flows changing direction towards surplus economies; a political change, as in the shift from the G7 to G20; and over time, cultural changes. This also means that the problems of emerging societies will increasingly become world problems. This series addresses the growing importance of BRIC (Brazil Russia India China) and rising societies such as South Korea, Taiwan, Singapore, Indonesia, South Africa, Turkey, the UAE, and Mexico. It focuses on problems generated by emergence, such as social inequality, cultural change, media, ethnic and religious strife, ecological constraints, relations with advanced and developing societies, and new regionalism, with a particular interest in addressing debates and social reflexivity in emerging societies.

Changing Constellations of Southeast Asia
From Northeast Asia to China
Edited by Jan Nederveen Pieterse, Abdul Rahman Embong, Siew Yean Tham

Eurocentrism and Development in Korea
Kim Jongtae

Social Ontology, Sociocultures and Inequality in the Global South
Edited by Benjamin Baumann and Daniel Bultmann

Covid-19 and Governance
Crisis Reveals
Edited by Jan Nederveen Pieterse, Haeran Lim, and Habibul Khondker

For more information about this series, please visit: www.routledge.com/Routledge-Studies-in-Emerging-Societies/book-series/RSIES

COVID-19 AND GOVERNANCE

Crisis Reveals

Edited by
Jan Nederveen Pieterse, Haeran Lim, and Habibul Khondker

Routledge
Taylor & Francis Group
LONDON AND NEW YORK

First published 2021
by Routledge
2 Park Square, Milton Park, Abingdon, Oxon OX14 4RN

and by Routledge
605 Third Avenue, New York, NY 10158

Routledge is an imprint of the Taylor & Francis Group, an informa business

British Library Cataloguing-in-Publication Data
A catalogue record for this book is available from the British Library

Library of Congress Cataloging-in-Publication Data
A catalog record has been requested for this book

ISBN: 978-0-367-72250-0 (hbk)
ISBN: 978-0-367-72251-7 (pbk)
ISBN: 978-1-003-15403-7 (ebk)

Typeset in Bembo
by Newgen Publishing UK

CONTENTS

FIGURES

TABLES

CONTRIBUTORS

Luciano d'Andrea is Senior Researcher at Knowledge & Innovation (K&I), a Rome-based private social research institute. His research interests have mainly focused on science-society relationships, understood as a privileged observation field to analyze the transformation processes affecting contemporary societies as a whole, especially through European research projects.

Charanpal S. Bal is Lecturer in Political Science and International Relations at the University of Western Australia. He was previously Deputy Head (Global Class) of department at the Bina Nusantara University and Visiting Lecturer at the Parahyangan Catholic University. Charan researches political economy and governance in Southeast Asia with a focus on migration and climate governance.

Nina Callaghan is a researcher at the Centre for Complex Systems in Transition at Stellenbosch University. Her research focuses on governance and State Capture as well as geopolitical influence in Africa. She has co-edited and authored chapters in *Anatomy of State Capture* (provisional title, forthcoming 2020). She has coordinated *South Africa's Energy Transition: The REIPPPP's Potential for Energy Democracy in South Africa* (provisional title, forthcoming 2020). Her MPhil in Sustainable Development at Stellenbosch University focuses on governance dynamics and citizen participation in South Africa's energy transition. In her previous position she was Associate Director for the Children's Radio Foundation, an NGO that partnered with community radio, communities and young people to amplify their voices. She was also a TV journalist at South African broadcaster ENCA for eight years. Nina serves as Board Chair for the Children's Radio Foundation, South Africa, is a board member for Open Streets Cape Town and sits on the advisory council of the Mothertongue Project, an arts organization for and by women and youth.

Adalberto Cardoso holds a PhD in Sociology (University of São Paulo) and is Professor at the Institute of Social and Political Studies of the State University of Rio de Janeiro (IESP-UERJ) and Associate Researcher of the Observatoire Sociologique du Changement (OSC/Sciences Po). Has authored and edited 20 books on political, historical, and economic sociology, including *Middle Classes and Politics in Brazil: 1922–2016* (Rio de Janeiro, FGV, 2020) and *'À beira do abismo: uma sociologia política do bolsonarismo'* (At the edge of the abyss: A political sociology of bolsonarismo), Author's edition, 2020.

Jeanine Condo is Medical Doctor and Adjunct Associate Professor at the School of Public Health (Rwanda) and Tulane University (USA). She is Managing Director and owner of the Center for Impact Innovation and Capacity building for Health Information and Nutrition (CIIC-HIN), a company registered in Rwanda with the aim of equipping health and education professionals with research skills while implementing robust research projects and linking research outputs to evidence-based policies in Rwanda and beyond. Dr Condo held senior government posts at University of Rwanda as Dean of the School of Public Health and Principal of the College of Medicine and Health Sciences. At the Ministry of Health, she was Director General of Rwanda Biomedical Center (RBC) from 2016 to 2019. She currently serves as a member of Evaluation Advisory Committee at GAVI since 2016, a member of the advisory committee of the African Academy of Sciences and a member of Rwanda Academy of Science since 2019. Dr Condo has contributed to research outputs in the country and region and has published more than 40 peer-reviewed articles.

Andrea Declich is Researcher at Knowledge & Innovation (K&I), a private social research institute in Rome. His research experience covers various fields such as urban and rural development, social capital, and SMEs development. In recent years he has been working on Responsible Research and Innovation (RRI) and on energy transitions.

Rwagasore Edson is a medical doctor and field epidemiologist and is currently project coordinator for the Africa Field Epidemiology Network (AFENET) in Rwanda and Field Epidemiology and Laboratory Training Program Coordinator at Rwanda Biomedical Center since 2019. He was appointed by the Ministry of Health as the team leader for the Covid-19 response for the western province in May 2020. He has held positions as Senior Officer for diabetes 2015–2019 and HIV clinical mentor at RBC, 2012–2015. He is an ISPAD fellowship awardee of 2018 for his work on establishing a diabetes registry in Rwanda and has contributed to multiple research outputs in Rwanda.

Wenhao Fan is PhD candidate in the Institute of Global Studies, Shanghai University. His research areas include US-Latin America relations, contemporary history, and social development in Latin America. He has translated several books on Latin America into Chinese.

Frank Fanselow studied anthropology and Middle East Studies at the American University in Cairo before obtaining a PhD from LSE with a dissertation on Muslims in South India. He taught at Yarmouk University in Jordan, The American University in Cairo, University Brunei Darussalam, Zayed University in Abu Dhabi, and the Asian University for Women in Chittagong before joining the Singapore University of Social Sciences. He has also been Visiting Professor at Kyoto University. His current research interests are in the sociology of Muslim societies, specifically Islamicate societies in the Indian Ocean region (Arab Gulf, South India, Sri Lanka, Bangladesh, and Borneo).

Changgang Guo received his BA and MA in history from East China Normal University and PhD from Fudan University, Shanghai. He is Director of the Institute of History at the Shanghai Academy of Social Sciences. His previous positions were Professor of History, Director of Institute of Global Studies, Director of Center for Turkish Studies, and Dean of Graduate School, Shanghai University. He is also Director of the Chinese Association of Religious Studies and Vice Chair of the Shanghai Association of World History. He is a member of the 13th Chinese People's Political Consultative Conference. He has published nine books and is the chief editor of the *Global Studies Review* book series and the *Annual Report on Turkey's National Development*. His recent research interests are global studies, ethnic and religious diversity in the context of globalization, and religion and global politics.

Hyug Baeg Im received his PhD from the University of Chicago and is Professor Emeritus, Korea University and Chaired Professor, Gwangju Institute of Science and Technology (GIST). He was Dean of Graduate School of Policy Studies, Korea University (2008–2012) and Executive Committee member of IPSA (2009–2014). His recent publications include *Democratization and Democracy in South Korea, 1960–Present* (Palgrave Macmillan 2020), *The Possibility of Peace in the Korean Peninsula* (SNU Press 2017), *Authoritarian Developmentalism, Democratic Neo-liberalism, and Economic Growth in Korea* (Routledge 2017), *Globalization, Democracy and Social Polarization in South Korea* (Palgrave Macmillan 2017), *Democratic Development and Authoritarian Development Compared: South Korea* (Routledge 2015), *Political Response to Economic Crisis in 1997 and 2008 South Korea* (Edward Elgar 2014), *Social Welfare, Globalization and Democracy in South Korea* (SNU Press 2014).

Merin Jacob is Research Assistant at the Centre for Complex Systems in Transition, Stellenbosch University, with a background in Mechanical Engineering and Future Studies. She has co-authored the 6th and 7th edition of Bowman's *Africa Insights* series on Urban Development and the Africa Continental Free Trade Agreement.

Prior to this, she worked at the Council for Scientific and Industrial Research (CSIR) and the Integrated Systems Group and was part of a team that used a whole-of-society methodology, addressing problems such as wildlife crime and the rhino poaching, disaster management and food security.

Abbas Jong is PhD candidate in sociology at Humboldt University Berlin. He studied economics, sociology, and philosophy in Iran and Germany. His research focuses on global studies, transnationalism, social philosophy, and political Islam. He is currently conducting research on the politics of transnationalism in modern Iran and a study of Iran globality: configurating new transnational Shiism. He has published articles on Iranian globalization, development, Islamic studies, and transnationalism.

Ahmed Kalebi, MBChB (Nbi) is CEO of Lancet Laboratories, East Africa. He was Director of Pathologists Lancet Kenya, established in 2009, now consolidated in an East Africa Group encompassing Kenya, Tanzania, Uganda, and Rwanda, the largest private laboratory network in the region. He practices in anatomical and clinical pathology. He did his undergraduate and postgraduate studies at University of Nairobi, a fellowship at University of Witwatersrand and training at the University of Toronto and Oxford University. He qualified at the College of Pathologists of South Africa in 2009. His professional affiliations include being Founder Secretary of the East African Division of the International Academy of Pathology, where he is now President-Elect. He is Honorary Lecturer in Human Pathology at University of Nairobi. He is a Founder Trustee of the Haiba Foundation, an education and welfare trust for residents of Kibera. He sits on the board of several hospitals and organizations including the Kenya Healthcare Federation and the Wellness Group. He has received numerous awards.

Wasim Khaled is CEO and co-Founder of Blackbird.AI. He is a serial entrepreneur with a background in computer science and human interface design. He has consulted and advised governments, policy makers, and corporations around the world on the nature of modern disinformation warfare and how these threats can be addressed. He has built companies spanning software engineering, AI, marketing, and ad tech sectors. He has 15 years of experience with Fortune 500 companies, built one of Inc 500's Fastest Growing Companies in America and was awarded Inc. 500's Asian Entrepreneur of the Year.

Ik Ki Kim graduated from Seoul National University (BA), University of South Carolina (MA), and University of Michigan (PhD). His major is sociology, specifically working on population aging in East Asia, urban sociology, and the Korean wave. He was Professor of Sociology at Dongguk University in Korea (1985–2015). Since then he has been teaching at Renmin University of China as a Xin'ao International Outstanding Professor. He was also Visiting Professor at the University of Michigan and Sophia University, Japan.

Habibul Khondker received his MA from Carleton, Ottawa and his PhD from the University of Pittsburgh. He has been Professor of Social Sciences at Zayed University, Abu Dhabi since 2006. He was previously Associate Professor of Sociology at National University of Singapore. He held visiting positions at Institute of Social Studies, The Hague, Columbia University, Cornell University, University of Pittsburgh, Institute of South Asian Studies, National University of Singapore, and United Nations University, Tokyo. He is co-President of the Sociology of Development section of the International Sociological Association. He is co-editor of *Asia and Europe in Globalization* (Brill 2006) with Göran Therborn. He co-authored *Globalization: East/West* with Bryan Turner (Sage 2010). He co-edited with Jan Nederveen Pieterse, *21st Century Globalization: Perspectives from the Gulf* (Zayed University Press 2010).

Sarp Kurgan is a PhD candidate at University of California Santa Barbara, Department of Global Studies. He is working on political theory and intellectual history in the Middle East. He received his BA from the Department of Political Science and International Relations at Boğaziçi University in Istanbul and his MA at Atatürk Institute for Modern Turkish History at the same university. He previously published 'From Discourse to Action: An analysis of securitization policies in Turkey' in *Perspectives on Global Development and Technology*. He is currently based in Istanbul for research.

Rosung Kwak is Professor of International Economics at Dongguk University, Seoul. Previously he was Research Fellow at the Korea Institute of Finance, a member of the Korean Delegation at the Uruguay Round Negotiations, held a Trade Policy Counsel position at the Korean Ministry of Foreign Affairs and Trade and participated in Korea-Chile Free Trade Agreement negotiations. He received his PhD in Economics from University of Texas at Austin and other degrees at Seoul National University. His work includes 41 scholarly articles and 14 books and book chapters.

Wang Hwi Lee received his PhD from the London School of Economics, and is Professor at Ajou University, Suwon, South Korea, where he has taught International Political Economy since 2006. He is co-author of *The Politics of Economic Reform in South Korea: Crony Capitalism after Ten Years* and *Pulling South Korea Away from China's Orbit: The Strategic Implications of the Korea-US Free Trade Agreement*. His research interests focus on the political economy of economic policy and institutions in East Asian countries.

Haeran Lim is Professor in Political Science and International Relations, Seoul National University. She specializes in comparative politics, East Asian and international political economy. She was Vice-president of the Korean Political Science Association, Director of the Institute of Gender Research at SNU, Director of the Institute of Korean Politics at SNU, Visiting Fellow at the Brookings Institute, and has advised Korea's Ministry of Foreign Affairs and Trade (2004–2007). She has published numerous papers and books, including *Revisiting the East Asian Developmental Model, Crisis of Democracy and Economic Reform in Korea, Democratization and Transformation Process of Developmental States*, and *Korea's Growth and Industrial Transformation* (Macmillan).

Rebecca Meckelburg received her PhD from the Asia Research Centre, Murdoch University, and is an academic staff member at the Interdisciplinary Faculty of Satya Wacana Christian University in Salatiga, Indonesia. Rebecca's research interests focus on political and social change, in particular, post-authoritarian experiences of democratization and non-elite forms of political organization.

Mariah Miller is PhD candidate in Global Studies at University of California Santa Barbara. She specializes in global political economy, social economy, and social enterprises. She has studied in the US, the UK, Germany, South Africa, China, India, and Spain. She holds an MA in Global Studies from Albert Ludwigs Universität Freiburg and University of KwaZulu Natal and an MA in Corporate Finance and Law from ESADE, a law school in Barcelona.

Ali Asghar Mosleh is Professor of Philosophy at Allameh Tabaitaba'i University in Iran, the Head of the Iranian Association for Intercultural Philosophy and the Research Institute Director for Contemporary Culture. He was Humboldt Research Fellow at the University of Bonn (2004) and Visiting Researcher at the University of Humboldt Berlin (2018). He is the author of many books and articles on intercultural philosophy, Islamic Sufism, the history of philosophy, and winner of Iran's Book of the Year Award for *The Philosophy of Culture* (2015). His books include *GWF Hegel* (2013), *The Truth of Man: A Comparative Study of Ibn al-Arabiws and Heidegger's Thought* (2016), and *With the Other: Research on Intercultural Thought and the Ethics of Dialogue* (2018).

N.C. Narayanan is Professor at the Centre for Technology Alternatives for Rural Areas, Centre for Policy Studies on Climate Change at the Indian Institute of Technology Bombay, Mumbai, India. He is Visiting Faculty at the Tata Institute of Social Sciences, Mumbai, India (2007–present) and has earlier taught at the Institute of Rural Management, Anand, India. He was a Fulbright-Nehru Academic and Professional Excellence Fellow at the Berkeley Water Centre, UC Berkeley (2016–2017) and Visiting Fellow at Monash University, Australia and University of Lausanne, Switzerland (2011–2012). He was Executive Director of the South Asia Consortium for Interdisciplinary Water Resources Studies, Secunderabad India (2006–2008). He authored/edited *Water Governance and Civil Society Responses in South Asia* (Routledge 2014), *Where to Go from Here? State, Natural Resources Conflicts and Challenges to Governance* (2008), *Against the Grain: The Political Ecology of Land Use in a Kerala Region* (2003) and co-authored *TINA and the Milk: Southern Perspectives on Sustainability in the Netherlands* (Utrecht, 2002).

Jan Nederveen Pieterse is Suzanne and Duncan Mellichamp Distinguished Professor of Global Studies and Sociology at University of California Santa Barbara. He specializes in globalization, development studies, and global political economy. He is the author of many articles and books. Recent books are *Connectivity and Global Studies* (2020), *Multipolar Globalization* (2018), and *Globalization and Culture* (2019, fourth edition).

Ratna Mani Nepal is Lecturer of Rural Development Studies at Tribhuvan University, Kathmandu. His research interests include development perspectives, sustainable economic development, and political economy in the global south. His current research focuses on the changing relations between China and South Asian countries. He has been Visiting Research Fellow in the Department of Global Studies, University of California Santa Barbara. His research articles have been published by Peter Lang Germany, *Global-e* UC Santa Barbara and in research journals in Nepal.

Thiago Peres has a PhD in Sociology from the Institute of Social and Political Studies of the State University of Rio de Janeiro (IESP-UERJ) with the thesis 'From fervor to fever: entrepreneurship, its origins and representations'. Sociologist at the State Center for Statistics, Research and Training of Civil Servants of Rio de Janeiro (CEPERJ). Researcher at the Center for Research and Labor Studies (NUPET-IESP-UERJ) received, in 2017, the Emerging Leaders in the Americas Program (ELAP) award from Global Affairs Canada.

Prabhir Vishnu Poruthiyil is Assistant Professor in the Centre for Policy Studies, International Institute of Technology, IIT Bombay, Mumbai. He teaches social policy usually through the lenses of inequality, sectarianism, and aging in developing societies. His research has appeared in *Business and Society*, *Journal of Social Quality*, *Critical Discourse Studies*, *Economic and Political Weekly*, and the *Journal of Business Ethics*.

Markus S. Schulz is Fellow at the Max Weber Center for Advanced Cultural and Social Studies. He served as the International Sociological Association's Vice-President for Research and President of the Third ISA Forum of Sociology. Schulz taught at the Bauhaus University of Weimar, the New School for Social Research, New York University, University of Illinois, and Virginia Tech. He held Visiting Research appointments in Buenos Aires, Munich, Paris (FMSH) and Oxford. He was awarded the Bielefeld Prize for the Internationalization of Sociology, the Eastern Sociological Society's Candace Rogers Award, Elise Boulding Award, and WSF Award. Schulz co-authored the six-volume book series *Internet and Politics in Latin America*. Among his articles are 'Debating futures: Global trends, alternative visions, and public discourse' (*International Sociology* 31:1) and 'Collective action across borders' (*Sociological Perspectives* 41:3). He edited *Current Sociology* monographs *Values and Culture* (2011) and *Future Moves* (2015). His volume *Global Sociology and*

Struggles for a Better World appeared with Sage (2019). Schulz is founding curator of the Web Forum: The Futures We Want.

Mark Swilling is Distinguished Professor of Sustainable Development in the School of Public Leadership, University of Stellenbosch, and co-director of the Centre for Complex Systems in Transition. His latest book is *The Age of Sustainability: Just Transitions in a Complex World* (Routledge 2020). He co-authored with Eve Annecke, *Just Transitions: Explorations of Sustainability in an Unfair World* (United Nations University Press 2012), co-edited with Adriana Allen and Andreas Lampis *Untamed Urbanism* (Routledge 2016), co-edited with Josephine Musango and Jeremy Wakeford *Greening the South African Economy* (Juta 2016), and was lead author with Ivor Chipkin et al. of *Shadow State: Politics of State Capture* (Johannesburg, WITS Press 2018). He is a member of UNEP's International Resource Panel acting as Coordinator of the Cities Working Group and is on the Board of the Development Bank of Southern Africa. He is co-author of *The Weight of Cities: Resource Requirements of Future Urbanization* (International Resource Panel 2018). He has been Visiting Professor at the Universities of Sheffield and Utrecht and in 2018 was the Edward P. Bass Visiting Environmental Scholar at Yale University.

Kai M. Thaler is Assistant Professor of Global Studies at the University of California, Santa Barbara. His research focuses on political violence, civil conflict, regimes and regime change, and state building, especially in Latin America and Africa. He has conducted research in and on Nicaraguan politics since 2012 and is the author of 'Nicaragua: A return to Caudillismo' (2017, *Journal of Democracy*) and 'Nicaragua is stumbling into Coronavirus disaster' (2020, *Foreign Policy*). His analysis on Nicaragua has been published in *The Washington Post* and *The Conversation*, and he has been interviewed on Nicaraguan politics by the BBC, France 24, and others. He holds a PhD in Government from Harvard University and an MSSc in Sociology from the University of Cape Town.

Roberto Zurbano Torres (San Nicolás de Bari, Cuba) is essayist, editor, and cultural critic specializing in black literature, racial politics, and alternative music. He is an anti-racist activist and a member of the Cuban Writers & Artists Union, the Latin American Studies Association, the Regional Association of Peoples of African Descent (ARAAC) and founder member of the activist collective, el Club del Espendru. He is the author of many books. His work has also been published in the *New York Times*.

Colin Tyler holds a Chair in Social and Political Thought at the University of Hull, UK, where he is also Associate Dean (Research) in the Faculty of Business, Law and Politics. Colin has written extensively on various topics in applied political theory and the history of political thought. He has particular interests in the politics of the common good and British liberal socialism, 1860 to 1939. His most recent monograph is *Common Good Politics: British Idealism and Social Justice in the Contemporary*

World (Palgrave MacMillan, 2017). He is Fellow of both the Academy of Social Sciences and the Royal Historical Society.

Naushad UzZaman is CTO and co-Founder of Blackbird.AI. He has an extensive academic and industrial background representing innovative accomplishments in the area of artificial intelligence. Naushad attended the University of Rochester, where he received his Masters and PhD degrees in computer science. He authored more than 30 peer-reviewed scientific papers and worked in the research divisions of renowned companies such as Microsoft, Yahoo! Research, Nuance, and Bosch and is the recipient of BRAC University Vice Chancellor's Gold Medal.

Chantana (Banpasirichote) Wungaeo is Professor in Political Science. She recently retired and now serves as Adjunct Professor at Faculty of Political Science at Chulalongkorn University, Bangkok. She is also a member of the academic committee at the Peace and Conflict Studies Center of the university. Her recent research interest focuses on crisis of democracy, peace building, nonviolence, and the politics of sustainable development. Her current research is on Youth's Political Platform and Conflict Transformation in Southern Thailand; local self-government; SDGs and sustainability transition; neighborhood history and transformation. She edited books on civil society in the Philippines and Thailand, human security in Southeast Asia, and globalization and democracy in Southeast Asia.

Surichai Wun'Gaeo is Director at the Center for Peace and Conflict Studies, Chulalongkorn University and Director at the Rotary Peace Center at Chulalongkorn University. His expertise is in rural sociology, social movements, democratization and multiculturalism, human security, and social justice. He is Professor Emeritus, Department of Sociology and past Director, Social Research Institute, Chulalongkorn University. He was formerly Joint-Secretary of the National Reconciliation Commission chaired by Mr Anan Panyarachun (2005–2006), former Prime Minister of Thailand. He was Chairperson of the Labor Rights Promotion Network Foundation, and Ecological Alert and Recovery—Thailand (EARTH) and the Maetao Clinic Maesot near the Myanmar border and an Academic Member of the National Health Commission (2013–2019). In 2014, he was designated as Most Distinguished Researcher in Sociology by the National Research Council of Thailand.

ACKNOWLEDGMENTS

I gratefully acknowledge the support of the Seoul National University Asia Center and Hyun-chin Lim, Professor Emeritus of Sociology and Founding Director of Seoul National University Asia Center.

For their advice and support I thank Ian Gordon in Kigali, Sue Herrod in Havana, Boike Rehbein in Berlin, Bhikhu Parekh and Chris Rojek in Britain, and Brett Aho and Giles Gunn in California. We are also indebted to the contributions of Fazal Rizvi, Mouin Rabbani, Tim Rackett, and Vincent Tihon. I thank authors and editors for their collective responsibility. We all 'write with an accent'.

This book is part of the *SNU Asia Center, SNU-Youngone Series in Asian Studies.*

INTRODUCTION

Patterns, confluence, regions

Jan Nederveen Pieterse

Covid-19 is a worldwide test of governance and social resilience. Now with smartphones everyone has comparative data at their fingertips. Everyone does, so to speak, global studies. How do societies deal with the virus, what is the spread of health outcomes? What works and what doesn't? How, according to which criteria do we map, organize and interpret data? Simply by country, by region, or according to patterns of governance?

Data [per early December 2020] indicate that South Korea (11 deaths per million of population), China (3), Taiwan (0.3), Vietnam (0.4), Thailand (0.9), Rwanda (4), Cuba (12), New Zealand (5) have functioned well in preparedness, delivery and health outcomes, several west European countries relatively well (Germany 228), while other countries show high mortality rates (US 870, UK 900, Spain 989, Brazil 830, Peru 1,092, Chile 815).

According to a *Wall Street Journal* headline in October, 'As West Reels, Asia Keeps Coronavirus Cases at Bay'. The report quotes an American public health expert: 'If you can control the virus, you can get 95% of your life back' (Stancati and Yoon 2020). In the words of a Finnish epidemiologist, Pekka Nuorti, 'A pandemic is really a mirror of a whole society's functioning and organization as a whole' (in Milne 2020).

With 4 percent of the world population the US has around 22 percent of the world's Covid-19 deaths. With 17 percent of the world population, Africa has 3.5 percent of Covid deaths (Pilling 2020). How do we explain the wide variation in approaches to the pandemic and in health outcomes?

Two major approaches to Covid-19 are *control the movement of people* (close borders, ban travel, quarantine) for a limited time, and second, *control the movement of the virus* (checkpoints, testing, tracing). Tomas Pueyo calls this the hammer and the dance (2020a, b). The hammer is control movement, close borders, shutdown, methods that go back to ancient times and the Middle Ages. The dance hinges on two movements: pinpoint the virus (testing) and monitor and contain its spread (tracing). The dance is selective, precise and agile. Also the hammer can be pointed and focus on hot zones, if data are available and coordination works. Combine these two phases and it is possible to control the virus spread and gradually resume social and economic activity; thus, societies can coexist with Covid-19.

Societies across the world have adopted these methods with different degrees of success. The hammer and the dance require adequate governance and public health systems. They require competent government, trust in government and effective leadership, which is widely recognized (e.g. Fukuyama 2020). The more chaotic the governance, the longer the virus crisis lasts. The hammer without the dance doesn't work. The dance but no hammer doesn't work either. Another option is no response, no hammer, no dance—deny or trivialize the virus, as many authoritarian and rightwing populist governments do.

When this volume is submitted in early December 2020, it has been in the making since April. In November we enter a second phase of Covid-19 and another round of lockdown in much of Europe. In the US, the spread of Covid-19 reached a new peak with hospitals in many states nearing top capacity and approaching a third of a million Covid deaths. Meanwhile, in most of Asia reopening is working. This introduction presents patterns that seek to organize the avalanche of information. Second, actual responses to Covid-19 stem from a confluence of variables that help or hinder dealing with the virus. Third, regional variation matters as well. This introduction gives an overview of these intersecting strands—patterns, confluence, regions.

Pattern analysis

We would expect public health to function best in societies where public services generally are held in high regard and the public interest is institutionally embedded. In societies that provide services such as universal healthcare, social benefits, affordable mass transit, affordable higher education, public broadcasting and policing as public service, public health too would rank high. In what kind of societies are these conditions likely to exist?

Varieties of market economies provide some orientation. Varieties of capitalism approaches draw distinctions between liberal, coordinated and state-led market economies (Whitley 1999, Hall and Soskice 2001). This approach has been elaborated in institutional analysis, comparative capitalisms, business studies and regional research (Amable 2003, Jackson and Deeg 2008, Fainshmidt et al. 2016, Lim, Pieterse and Hwang 2018). The approach can be further fine-tuned: break state-led market economies (SME) down into developmental, traditional and crony types; add rightwing populism as a category. Varieties of capitalism (VoC) is mostly associated with the differences between liberal and coordinated market economies (LME and CME), the US, UK and continental Europe. I opt for varieties of market economies (VME) as a more comprehensive approach.

TABLE 0.1 Institutions in diverse market economies

Market economies		*Institutions*	*Beneficiaries*	*Examples*
Liberal ME		Deregulation	Corporations, finance	US, UK, Chile
	Populist	Weakening	Cronies, base	Trump, Bolsonaro, Modi
Coordinated		Crucial	Stakeholders, public	EU, Northeast Asia
State-led	Developmental	Crucial	State, legitimacy	China, Singapore, Vietnam
	Traditional	Crucial	State, supporters	Saudi Arabia, Iran, Turkey
	Extractive	Selective	Regime, cronies	Russia, Angola, Cambodia

VME concern the *dominant* institutional pattern that sets the terms for other interactions but is not exclusive (e.g., in China, three forms of capitalism coexist: the state-led sector, the private enterprise sector and public-private partnerships in the states; Nederveen Pieterse 2015). Institutions are keynotes in differentiating types of market economies. Institutions refer to norms and principles that organize economic behavior; they refer to rules of the game rather than the game. Institutions feature in development studies with concerns such as the governance-policy gap (policies can be right but need institutions to back them up) and sustainable development (Rodrik, Subramanian and Trebbi 2004). Table 0.1 is a sketch of institutions in VME.

VME shed light on governance, inequality, populism and regulation of technology (Nederveen Pieterse 2018, 2018b). Are they also relevant in analyzing countries' responses to Covid-19 and public health performance? If we take as key criterion *how governance serves the public interest*, in a schematic fashion we can outline the following *expectations*. 1) We expect public health to function best in market economies where public interest is institutionally anchored in coordinated governance, 2) in *state-led market economies* of a developmental type, public interest ranks high as part of the overall priority of national development. China, Singapore, Vietnam, Rwanda and Cuba match this profile at different development levels, 3) in *liberal market economies*, public interest tends to be defined in terms of growth, jobs and innovation, which are deemed best left to market forces, which prioritize profitability, also in a public health crisis, 4) in SME of a traditional bend, traditional elites hold the front seats, and in extractive SME, the interests of crony elites come well before the public interest and 5) rightwing populist and new authoritarian governments are based on unstable political coalitions, tend to remain in campaign mode and politicize crisis and public health. Table 0.2 outlines types of authoritarian governance.

If we compare Covid-19 containment methods and outcomes in a sample of countries, as in this volume, *do the first two categories mentioned above indeed function better in the crisis*, or do other types of market economies exceed expectations and different variables matter?

TABLE 0.2 Types of authoritarian governance

Types	*Bases*	*Sample*
Conservative	Ethnic or religious elites	Saudi Arabia, Emirates, Brunei, Iran
	Military-monarchy	Thailand, Morocco, Jordan
National security states	Deep state	Israel, Pakistan, N. Korea, Guatemala
	And kleptocracy	Egypt, Syria, Myanmar, Honduras
Developmental states	State-led economies	China, Singapore, Rwanda, Ethiopia, Cuba
	Post-Soviet	Belarus, Turkmenistan, Tajikistan
	Post-communist	Vietnam, Laos
	Post-socialist	Nicaragua, Venezuela
Extractivist-oligarchic	Kleptocracy	Russia, DRC, Angola, Kazakhstan, Afghanistan
New authoritarianism	Unstable coalitions	Turkey, AKP; India, BJP; Brazil, Bolsonaro; Philippines, Duterte

Two chapters also discuss analytical frameworks to address approaches to Covid-19. Nina Callaghan and co-authors discuss varieties of institutional systems (Fainshmidt et al. 2016) which overlap with VME; applying these to developing and emerging economies and Africa is work in progress (Chapter 21). Adalberto Cardoso and Thiago Peres compare eight South American countries, four of which adopt *collective responsibility* in relation to Covid-19 (Uruguay, Argentina, Colombia, Bolivia) and four treat Covid-19 as a matter of *individual responsibility* (Brazil, Chile, Peru, Ecuador). Covid-19 cases and mortality in the first category are much lower than in the second (Chapter 16). The differences were significant but faded later when most countries (not Uruguay) began to relax social distancing under economic and political pressure. Collective responsibility implies proactive states while individual responsibility in effect means state abdication.

Does this pattern correlate with VME? Coordinated and developmental state-led market economies tend towards collective responsibility. CME prioritize public interests—though how they actually perform also depends on other variables. In Northeast Asia, experience with infectious diseases, capacious states, focused leadership and island nations (several), all work in tandem.

LME lean towards individual responsibility, materially because the state has been eviscerated and isn't up to the job; morally because individual responsibility (bootstraps) is a general credo; ideologically because of anti-big government ideology. More important than public health is that the economy stays open. Narratives paper over the gap—'it will magically disappear' (Trump), 'just sniffles' (Bolsonaro). The idea of herd immunity has been toyed with (in the UK, US and Sweden), which epidemiological experts widely reject (Alwan et al. 2020). Liberal market economies that have bet on corporations for decades, defunded state agencies and pooh-poohed society, Republicans in the US, Tories in the UK, arrive empty handed at a public health crisis. The siren call of rightwing populists—'deconstruct the administrative state' (Steve Bannon), bypass the civil service (Dominic Cummings)—leaves them empty handed. Neoliberalism and rightwing populism are fair weather stories and when crisis arrives—financial, economic, natural or viral—tax payers are supposed to be delighted to bail out.

Crony state-led market economies shirk responsibility—'all is under control', according to Putin, while abdicating responsibility to the penniless states. The spread of virus in the US, Brazil, India and Russia has been greater than anywhere else: because of false narratives there is no containment. Authoritarian regimes such as Belarus, Kazakhstan and Cambodia follow a similar route. Thaler provides an in-depth discussion of authoritarian indifference in Nicaragua (Chapter 18). Without the hammer and the dance, economies cannot open without major mortality.

VME concern fundamentals of collective organization that resonate widely. How do VME relate to *social inequality*? The pattern of inequality trends in the same direction as public health. Inequality tends to be lower in coordinated and developmental state-led market economies and higher in liberal and crony market economies (Nederveen Pieterse 2018). In LME, a high Gini index comes with resistance to ameliorating the lot of the less well-off. The higher the Gini index, the lower the capacity to contain risk and the greater the risk of infection. Social inequality itself is a risk factor and among advanced economies is most pronounced in the US. The US' Gini index is .48 in 2020 (compare Nordic Europe around .30; Northeast Asia slightly higher). The Gini index of Manhattan is .59, at the same level as Brazil, Haiti and South Africa.

A substantial literature shows that high inequality is detrimental to public health (e.g., Wilkinson and Pickett 2009). The precariat include the poor who survive on day labor and with closure there is no work; the homeless who are to shelter in place but have no place, to stay clean but where can they wash, to keep distance but how in slums, camps and prisons? More vulnerable still are refugees and migrants in zones of war and crisis such as Yemen, Syria, Afghanistan, Gaza and Lebanon. Also 'Xinjiang battles scores of infections' (Yang and Shepherd 2020). Every crisis is also a *distribution crisis* (Rasmus 2020). In the UK, 'coronavirus is a class issue' ('the hardest hit include taxi drivers, bus drivers, security guards, chefs and care workers') and also matches ethnic divides (Jones 2020). In the US, black Americans are 'dying of Covid-19 at three times the rate of white people' (Pilkington 2020).

Inequality as a spreader includes migrant workers (Sammadar 2020). Headlines such as this have been common: 'Kerala reels as migrants return to India. Pandemic exposes economic weakness of state that relies of remittances' (Parkin and Singh 2020). Migrant workers and undocumented migrants escaped the hammer and produced virus surges in Singapore, Borneo, Kerala, Nepal and the Emirates, as Narayanan and Vishnu Poruthiyil, Ratna Nepal, and Habib Khondker discuss (Chapters 4, 5, 22).

Many religious gatherings escaped the hammer such as evangelical megachurches in the US, churches in Korea and Tabliq Jamaat gatherings in Delhi and Kuala Lumpur. Large gatherings have been virus spreaders such as carnival in Germany, Mardi Gras in New Orleans, football matches in Bergamo and Valencia, concerts, weddings, funerals, street and student parties and election rallies in the US (Chapter 15).

VME also shape the character of *federalism* and center-periphery relations. In coordinated and developmental state-led market economies, the center and the states tend to share a common purpose. Federal states with national economic strategies tend to function well—such as China and Germany (Chapters 1, 12). Federal states without national cohesion where decentralization means fragmentation and local elite capture, don't do well in crisis. Governance dysfunction in tandem with decentralization plays a part in Indonesia and Kenya (as Meckelburg/Bal and Kalebi discuss, Chapters 6, 20). In liberal and crony market economies, provinces or states replicate divisions at the center. In the US, states are to fend for themselves and compete for frontline basics such as personal protective equipment (PPE) and ventilators; each state and cities within states follow different approaches, often along party lines (Chapters 14, 15).

Indigenous communities across the world have applied the hammer and the dance; they have barred entry and exit, have applied traditional medicines and selective outside engagement, with uneven outcomes.

Confluence

What does Covid-19 reveal about the quality of institutions? This volume presents country analyses. Institutions derive from history, their backdrop is structural change, whereas politics is situational (Chapters 4, 14, all). *Governance* arises from a confluence of institutions and politics. Do institutions, politics and policies align or clash? Upon a change in government, institutions and politics may be out of whack. A public health emergency reveals the dynamics at play.

How the Covid-19 crisis intersects with other crises and reveals underlying social organization or disorganization is a theme that runs through all chapters. Cuba is the target of 60 years of American hostility and embargo; Iran suffers American sanctions; China is the target of an American trade and propaganda war; in each of these, institutional synergies buffer the impact (Chapters 17, 8, 1). India and Brazil are political economies in transition. The UK is experiencing the Brexit process, as Colin Tyler discusses (Chapter 10). Turkey is experiencing economic crisis (Chapter 14). Spain is recovering from years of corrupt Popular Party government (1989–2018).

Governance is not all about government, also in a public health crisis. Martin Wolf notes, 'Covid exposes society's dysfunctions' (2020). Yet crisis also catalyzes social resources and resilience; across the world, community organizations step up, in spite of or against the grain of state dysfunction. Examples discussed in this book are China, Kerala, Indonesia, Thailand and Rwanda (Chapters 1, 4, 6, 7 and 19). In Spain, cooperatives, nonprofits, and small business and local government partnerships provided relief in the wake of the economic crisis of 2008 as well as in the Covid crisis, which Mariah Miller takes up (Chapter 11).

Varieties of market economies are a pattern with radar functions, but the map is not the territory. Schemas lack granularity and how they are used can carry bias. One risk is reproducing or producing stereotypes of countries: pardon shorthand labeling in this introduction; this section adds qualifications. VME function not only at the level of countries but also in part of countries.

Responses to Covid-19 and its economic ramifications are a *confluence* of many variables in different combinations in different countries and parts of countries and at different times. Lines of causality are opaque and the combinations are so many that they cannot be modeled. Covid-19 is a moving target, a pandemic in flux, knowledge about the virus is incomplete (how does it mutate, what are side-effects) and countries and parts of countries are at different stages of spread curves. In Kerala, India's majority Christian, socialist-led state, public services and public health performance stand out (Chowdhury and Jomo 2020; Tharoor 2020; Chapter 4). States in India, north and south, east and west differ widely. What is also at issue in India is a gap between state and society that goes back to colonial times.

Perplexities of governance yield perplexities of dealing with Covid-19. Ultra-orthodox Haredim in West Jerusalem resist social distancing and masks (as they do in Brooklyn). When their stance is referred to Israel's Rabbinical Court, it is not condemned because Haredi parties are a crucial part of Netanyahu's Likud coalition.

> One of the drivers for the Haredi alliance with the right is the perception that the left wants to secularize them and instill progressive universal values ... It is clearest in the left's harsh criticism of the Haredi community's treatment of women, its views on homosexuality, and the number of children they have.
>
> *(Kalev 2019)*

Not just *what* is done matters (hammer and dance) but also *how* it is done. Unlike neighboring countries, Japan skipped lockdown, just as Sweden's approach deviated from other Scandinavian countries, but Japan came with a masking culture. Sweden saw its case numbers and deaths per million soar (698) but Japan did not (18) and was able to contain surges (Chapter 3).

Speed and timing also matter. China (after a delay), South Korea, Singapore, Rwanda, Cuba, Nepal and other countries applied the hammer swiftly (Noor and Jomo 2020), though later faced virus surges. 'Go hard and fast' was Jacinda Ardern's motto in New Zealand. Several chapters discuss timing (1, 2, 3 and 5).

Culture, collective conditioning and learning over time informs governance and policy. In cultures of low trust in government (weak society-state relations or anti-government ideology), the same policies (hammer and dance, vaccines) work out differently than in high trust settings.

Experience matters as part of collective learning. In East Asia public health preparedness has been at a high level after the SARS and MERS outbreaks (Chapters 2, 3). In Africa, after HIV and Ebola (Chapters 19, 21). As a dynastic monarchy Saudi governance may be less effective, yet as Frank Fanselow shows, as a world custodian of vast religious gatherings (hajj, Umrah) it is thoroughly experienced in matters of public health, prudent and efficient (170 deaths per million; Chapter 9). Saudi Arabia is also in the process of turning into an entrepreneurial state.

Is there a relationship between VME and *data and science*? Power and knowledge tend to move in tandem. In liberal market economies, science is a profit center. Data points organize accumulation. In developmental state-led market economies, science serves national development and is a source of pride, as Roberto Zurbano discusses in Cuba (Chapter 17). In coordinated market economies, science is a public good, which also competes in budget battles and in the crisis attention economy (Chapter 23). In traditional state-led market economies, science coexists with religious authority, as in Iran and Saudi Arabia (Chapters 8, 9). In rightwing populism, science is politicized. The US is experiencing a clash of narratives and a 'coronavirus data crisis' (Warzel 2020; Chapters 15, 24). In authoritarian regimes, data and science are censored and under political camouflage (as in Nicaragua, Chapter 19).

The *reliability of Covid-19 data* and mortality figures varies considerably. Data for several countries are unreliable under counts (such as Belarus 128, Indonesia 65, Myanmar 39, India 101, Venezuela 32, Brazil 830). For Cambodia there are no Worldometer data. As the World Health Organization (WHO) notes, this is also a global infodemic. Extensive research by BlackBird.AI shows that 40–60 percent of social media content, clustered around key narratives (reopen economy, medical misinformation, Covid) is manipulated through a combination of propagandists, conspiracy theorists and bots seeding networks from where disinformation spreads to mainstream media (Khaled 2020). Khaled and UzZaman discuss organizational patterns in disinformation (Chapter 24).

In a public health crisis, science emerges not as product (validated, chiseled to precision) but as process, with a higher level of uncertainty and ambiguity than publics associate with science. People are used to science as product, not as ongoing experiment balancing many variables as part of a political arena. Luciano d'Andrea and Andrea Declich discuss science and politics in the setting of Italy (Chapter 23).

In this volume the key standard of measurement are *Worldometer* data (Covid deaths/per million of population, etc.), which are readily available and readers can easily verify and update. This introduction uses Worldometer data per early December 2020.

Regions

In November we enter a second phase in much of Europe. In the US cases reached a new peak. In most of Asia reopening is working. In China and Northeast Asia, the hammer and the dance have worked well. Economic recovery is way ahead of other regions. Because South Korea, Taiwan, Singapore, Hong Kong and Japan are island nations or nations where entry is easily controlled, the hammer was light and easy to apply. Experience was on their side. Public health preparedness has been at a high level after the SARS and MERS outbreaks. Masking culture is common. Capable states, leadership and trust in government prevail. Shanghai scholars Guo and Fan attribute China's success to swift, effective organization and people's commitment (Chapter 1). Korean scholars Lee, Kim and Kwak also refer to cultural legacies of Confucianism (Chapters 2, 3). Hyug Baeg Im draws a comparison between US and South Korean governance institutions in relation to Covid-19 (Chapter 14). 'South Korea had a strategy from the very start—called "TRUST", the action plan was spelled out by the acronym: "Transparency; Robust screening and quarantine; Unique but universally applicable testing; Strict control; and Treatment"' (Seung-Youn 2020; Noor and Jomo 2020).

Pattern variations in Southeast and South Asia tend to match VME—effective in developmental SME (Singapore five deaths per million of population, Vietnam 0.4); less effective in crony market economies (Indonesia 65, Myanmar 39, India 101, Nepal 54, Philippines 78). Thailand (0.9) and Malaysia (12) show remarkably low scores; in a public health crisis they function as CME.

In West Europe, austerity after the 2008 crisis cut social services alongside 'creeping liberalization' (Streeck 2011). LME (US, UK) and societies undermined by austerity and institutional decay (Italy, Spain) underperform because of the erosion of public services: no slack, no health care surge capacity, dysfunctional agencies, lack of coordination, low trust in government. Besides, is a society a surplus or a deficit economy? Differences between Nordic and Mediterranean Europe played a part in the aftermath of the 2008 crisis and continue to play a part (Royo 2014, Sánchez 2020; Chapters 10, 11, 15, 23).

In Europe, the hammer stopped in July because of summer travel and again in September because of returning holiday travelers. Amsterdam, a city of 880,000 saw an inflow of 110,000 students in September. Belgium counted suspected, but not confirmed Covid-19 deaths in nursing homes as Covid deaths. Either Belgium over counted or all other counties under counted (Bergeron 2020). Yet overall high Covid mortality over time (1,486 deaths per million) indicates more is going on: 'One reason Belgium is suffering so badly is its long history of weak central government and deep regional divisions … "That's Belgian politics— it's a real lasagna"' (Peel 2020).

Specific conditions affect each country. Since summer the Netherlands government recommended but did not require mask wearing in public places (according to the prime minister, because the Dutch are adults they don't need rules). By end October Covid cases went through the roof, the Dutch were among the hardest hit in Europe (565 deaths per million) and lockdown is back in effect since fall (Erdbrink 2020). Angela Merkel noted, 'The virus punishes half-heartedness' (Chazan 2020).

This volume brings together analyses of Covid-19 developments in countries and regions with a wide-angle lens on governance. What works, what hasn't and isn't, and why? Features of the book are wide international scope and analytical depth, combining institutions, policies and politics. Together the authors represent a diverse and formidable database of experience and understanding. They include sociologists, anthropologists, scholars of development studies and public administration, and MD specialists in public health. The book is engaged, without jargon and speaks to a wide international public on a topic that has deep and broad appeal.

References

Alwan, Nisreen A. et al., 2020 Scientific consensus on the Covid-19 pandemic: We need to act now, *The Lancet*, October 15, DOI: https://doi.org/10.1016/S0140-6736(20)32153-X.

Amable, Bruno 2003 *The diversity of modern capitalism*. London: Oxford University Press.

Bergeron, Jonathan 2020 Responses to Covid-19 in different market economies, University of California Santa Barbara course paper, spring.

Chazan, Guy 2020 Merkel appeals for national effort on Covid, *Financial Times*, November 3.

Chowdhury, Anis and Jomo Kwame Sundaram 2020 Kerala Covid-19 response: Model for emulation, IPS, April 9, www.ipsnews.net/2020/04/kerala-covid-19-response-model-emulation/.

Erdbrink, Thomas 2020 As Coronavirus surges, chastened Dutch wonder, 'What Happened to Us?' New York Times, October 29.

Ezrow, Natasha, Erica Frantz and Andrea Kendall-Taylor 2016 *Development and the state in the 21st century*. London: Palgrave Macmillan.

Fainshmidt, S., Judge, W.Q., Aguilera, R.V. and Smith, A. 2016 Varieties of institutional systems: A contextual taxonomy of understudied countries, *Journal of World Business*, 53, 3: 307–322.

Fukuyama, Francis 2020 The pandemic and political order: It takes a state, *Foreign Affairs*, 99, 4: 26–32, July/August.

Gurtov, Mel 2020 The 'end of poverty' illusion: Global and East Asian realities in the Covid-19 pandemic, *The Asia-Pacific Journal*, 18, 17(5): 1–7.

Hall, Peter A. and David Soskice, eds. 2001 *Varieties of capitalism: The institutional foundations of comparative advantage*. Oxford: Oxford University Press.

Jackson, Gregory and Richard Deeg 2008 Comparing capitalisms: Understanding institutional diversity and its implications for international business, *Journal of International Business Studies*, 39: 540–561.

Jones, Owen 2020 Boris Johnson's message to the working class: good luck out there, *The Guardian*, May 12.

Kalev, Gol 2019 The ultra-orthodox will determine Israel's political future, *Foreign Policy*, April 17.

Khaled, Wasim 2020 The disinformation olympics: The Covid-19 infodemic has just begun, April, www.blackbird.ai.

Lim, Hyun-chin, J. Nederveen Pieterse and Sukman Hwang, eds. 2018 *Capitalism and capitalisms in Asia*. Seoul: Seoul National University Press.

Milne, R. 2020 Precise planning helps Finland contain Covid-19, *Financial Times*, September 28.

Nederveen Pieterse, J. 2015 China's contingencies and globalization, *Third World Quarterly*, 36: 11.

——— 2018 *Multipolar globalization*. London: Routledge.

——— 2018b Populism is a distraction, *New Global Studies* 12, 3: 377–386 | https://doi.org/10.1515/ngs-2018-0020.

——— 2021 *Connectivity and global studies*. London, Palgrave Macmillan.

Noor, Nazihah Muhamad and Jomo Kwame Sundaram 2020 East Asian lessons for controlling Covid-19, IPS, March 26, www.ipsnews.net/2020/03/east-asian-lessons-controlling-covid-19/.

Parkin, B. and J. Singh, Kerala reels as migrants return to India, Financial Times, August 3.
Peel, M. 2020 Belgium's fight against Covid hindered by regional rivalries, *Financial Times*, November 3.
Pilkington, Ed 2020 Black Americans dying of Covid-19 at three times the rate of white people, *The Guardian*, May 20.
Pilling, David 2020 How Africa fought the pandemic, *Financial Times*, October 26.
Pueyo, Tomas 2020a Coronavirus: The hammer and the dance, *Medium,* March 1.
——— 2020b To stop the pandemic, build a fence, *New York Times,* September 20: 6–7.
Rasmus, Jack 2020 Covid-19 and the working class, *Counterpunch*, March 9.
Rodrik, D., A. Subramanian and F. Trebbi 2004 Institutions rule: The primacy of institutions over geography and integration in economic development, *Journal of Economic Growth*, 9, 2: 131–165.
Royo, Sebastián 2014 Institutional degeneration and the economic crisis in Spain, *American Behavioral Scientist*, 58, 12: 1568–1591.
Samaddar, Ranabir, ed. 2020 Burdens of an epidemic: A policy perspective on Covid-19 and migrant labour. Kolkata: Calcutta Research Group.
Sánchez, Pedro 2020 Europe's future is at stake in this war against coronavirus, *The Guardian*, April 5.
Seung-Youn Oh 2020 South Korea's success against Covid-19, *The Regulatory Review*, Pennsylvania University, May 14.
Stancati, M. and D. Yoon 2020 As West reels, Asia keeps Coronavirus cases at bay, *Wall Street Journal*, October 21.
Streeck, Wolfgang 2011 The crises of democratic capitalism, *New Left Review*, 71: 5–29.
Tharoor, Shashi 2020 The Kerala Model, *Project Syndicate*, May 11.
Warzel, Charlie 2020 The Coronavirus misinformation war, *New York Times*, April 15.
Whitley, Richard 1999 *Divergent capitalisms: The social structuring and change of business systems*. Oxford: Oxford University Press.
Wilkinson, Richard and Kate Pickett 2009 *The spirit level: Why more equal societies almost always do better.* London: Allen Lane.
Wolf, Martin 2020 Covid exposes society's dysfunctions, *Financial Times*, July 15.
Yang, Y. and C. Shepherd 2020 Xinjiang battles scores of infections, *Financial Times*, October 27.

Asia

1

CHINA'S FIGHT AGAINST COVID-19

Domestic and external implications

Changgang Guo and Wenhao Fan

China is the first country in the world to report cases of Covid-19, and it is also one of the first countries to successfully control the epidemic. The outbreak of the Covid-19 coincided with the most important festival in China—the Spring Festival. The government carried out the most comprehensive, strict and thorough prevention and control measures in Chinese history. It caused vast social dissatisfaction and posed great challenges to Chinese Communist Party's (CCP) national governance capacity. With the initial epidemic turning into a global pandemic, there has been international propaganda accusing China of being responsible for the pandemic. The sudden changes in the international environment makes Chinese society re-examine the government's anti-epidemic policy and even the whole system of China, and, to some extent, helps to subvert the rosy expectations and worship of Western society and Western media of Chinese society. There are so many voices in the world about China's Covid-19 campaign. Attacks and accusations on China can be seen everywhere. But what is the reaction of mainstream Chinese society? This chapter will try to provide a Chinese perspective on China's anti-epidemic campaign.

Measures to fight the epidemic

We can roughly say that China's anti-epidemic campaign already ended at the end of April. According to the information released by National Health Commission, on March 18, there were no new local confirmed cases in China for the first time. By April 26, Wuhan City, the original Covid-19 epicenter, had all the hospitalized cases of Covid-19 cleared. On April 27, the Central Steering Group[1] left Hubei and returned to Beijing, marking decisive victory in fighting Covid-19 in Wuhan as well as in other cities of Hubei Province. This also marks the significant strategic achievements in national epidemic prevention and control.[2]

TABLE 1.1 Covid-19 data of mainland China as of 24:00 April 28, 2020

Cumulative confirmed	*Existing confirmed*	*Suspected*	*Cumulative cure*	*Cumulative deaths*
82,858	647	10	77,578	4,633

TABLE 1.2 Covid-19 data for Hubei Province and Wuhan City as of 24:00 April 28, 2020

	Cumulative confirmed	*Existing confirmed*	*Suspected*	*Cumulative cure*	*Cumulative deaths*
Hubei	68,128	0	0	63,616	4,512
Wuhann	50,333	0	0	46,464	3,869

After that, a 'new round' of Covid-19 cases began to take place in Beijing on June 11, but the so-called 'second wave' turned out to be just a leaper, and it was soon successfully controlled after only 21 days.[3] As Chinese netizens ridiculed, Beijing was 'doing homework again' to show it to some countries who believe that China's anti-epidemic campaign is Draconian-style based on China's 'special' political and social system, which cannot be copied in other places and cannot be used for reference by other countries. (See Tables 1.1 and 1.2)

On June 7, China's State Council Information Office published a white paper titled 'Fighting Covid-19: China in Action', which divides China's anti-epidemic response into five stages:

- Stage I: Swift Response to the Public Health Emergency (December 27, 2019–January 19, 2020);
- Stage II: Initial Progress in Containing the Virus (January 20–February 20, 2020);
- Stage III: Newly Confirmed Domestic Cases on the Chinese Mainland Drop to Single Digits (February 21–March 17, 2020);
- Stage IV: Wuhan and Hubei—An Initial Victory in a Critical Battle (March 18–April 28, 2020);
- Stage V: Ongoing Prevention and Control (Since April 29, 2020).

Summarizing China's anti-epidemic measures, the following aspects deserve special attention.

1) *The establishment of a centralized and efficient national-level command.* China's top leadership responded to the epidemic very quickly. As early as January 7, when Xi Jinping presided over the meeting of the Politburo Standing Committee, he put forward requirements for the prevention and control of the epidemic. China's anti-epidemic policy in the initial phase was marked by three meetings of the Politburo Standing Committee (PSC), which were held on January 25, February 3,

and February 12. Three consecutive meetings of PSC during such a short period is unprecedented in history. Especially the one on January 25, it was the day of the most important festival in China – the New Year's Day of the Spring Festival, which was supposed to be the day for family reunion to celebrate the New Year. These three meetings formulated corresponding policies for the initial stage.

The Chinese government established the 'Central Leading Group for Epidemic Prevention' (January 25, the lunar New Year's Day of China), headed by Premier Li Keqiang. A Central Steering Group was set up (January 27) with Vice Premier Sun Chunlan as the leader, it was responsible for guiding Hubei Province and Wuhan City to strengthen prevention and control work. Besides this, the central government built a government-level coordination platform named 'Joint Prevention and Control Mechanism of the State Council' (JPCMSC, January 20). It was used to hold regular meetings to track and analyze the epidemic situation, strengthen the dispatch of medical personnel and medical materials, and adjust prevention and control strategies and key tasks according to the development and changes of the epidemic.

The State Council also set up the 'Working Mechanism for Resumption of Production', strengthened the overall guidance and coordination services for resumption of production, opened up the industrial chain and supply chain blocking points, and enhanced the kinetic energy of collaborative resumption of work and resumption of production. All provinces, cities, and counties across the country set up emergency command mechanisms headed by party and government leaders, and built an emergency decision-making command system with unified command, frontline guidance, and coordination and cooperation from top to bottom. For example, on January 20, Shanghai set up a leading group for epidemic prevention and control with the party secretary and the mayor as double leaders.

2) *Effective coping strategies.* In terms of specific coping strategies, the following series of 'four' plans have played a vital role. The first is the 'four early', that is early detection, early reporting, early isolation, and early treatment. Then there is the 'four musts', which literally requires that local governments must take in all the infected, cure all the patients, test all the suspected, and isolate all in need. Another one is the 'four concentrations', which means the concentration of patients, doctors, resources, and treatment. Under this circumstance, the Huoshenshan Hospital, Leishenshan Hospital,[4] and 16 temporary treatment centers were built.

3) *Mobilize the whole country.* At the beginning of the anti-epidemic campaign, when the Chinese government decided to lock down Wuhan, a megacity with a population of 10 million, it actually made clear the national anti-epidemic strategy. That is, to contain the epidemic situation in Wuhan and Hubei as much as possible, to avoid the spread of the virus to other provinces, and then to fight the virus in Hubei and Wuhan with the concentrated strength of the whole country.

So we saw all-round support for Hubei Province and Wuhan City nationwide. It was the largest medical support action since the founding of the People's Republic of China (PRC) in 1949. From January 24 New Year's Eve to March 8, the government mobilized 346 national medical teams, 42,600 medical personnel, and more than 900 public health personnel to aid Hubei to carry out the 'one province helps one city' project. All supporting teams were assembled and dispatched to Hubei within 24 hours after receiving the order. The reason why Huoshenshan Hospital, Leishenshan Hospital and 16 temporary treatment centers could be built in just over 10 days is this kind of general mobilization of the whole country.

Large-scale and powerful medical support actions have effectively guaranteed the treatment of patients in Hubei Province and Wuhan City, and greatly relieved the severe shortage of medical resources in the hardest hit areas. The WHO chief Dr Tedros Adhanom fully affirmed the Chinese government's anti-epidemic efforts:

> the high speed and massive scale of China's moves are rarely seen in the world; it showed China's efficiency and the advantages of China's system. China's measures are not only protecting its people, but also protecting the people in the whole world.[5]

4) *Legislation for Epidemic Prevention and Control.* On February 5, 2020, the Commission for Comprehensive Law-based Governance of the Communist Party of China (CPC) Central Committee held a meeting, stressing that efforts should be made in various aspects such as legislation, law enforcement, judicature, and law compliance, so as to improve the ability of prevention and control according to law and provide a strong legal guarantee for epidemic prevention and control. The government listed Covid-19 as a Class B infectious disease in the Law of the People's Republic of China on Prevention and Treatment of Infectious Diseases, while addressing it with measures applicable to a Class A infectious disease.[6] It also applied control and quarantine measures under the Frontier Health and Quarantine Law of the People's Republic of China in cohesion with relevant provisions of international law and other domestic laws.

Some prefecture-level governments also enacted urgent legislation, authorizing local governments to stipulate temporary emergency administrative measures in health care and epidemic prevention management. For example, on February 7, Shanghai issued the Decision of the Standing Committee of Shanghai Municipal People's Congress on Managing to Prevent and Control the Current Coronavirus Pneumonia Epidemic, which was implemented on the same day, provided legal guarantee for the government to implement the strictest epidemic prevention and control measures, and provided legal compliance for resuming production. The Shanghai Municipal People's Congress translated the Decision into ten different foreign languages, contributing to the prevention of imported cases in Shanghai.

Law and order and market supervision have been strengthened. Price gouging, hoarding and profiteering, production and sales of counterfeit or sub-standard products, and any other crimes impeding response efforts have been punished by law. Quality and price control of anti-epidemic supplies has been reinforced, and stronger measures have been taken against deceptive and illegal advertising, ensuring social order and stability.

Strengthen the supervision of administrative law enforcement during epidemic prevention and control, strictly regulate law enforcement, enforce the law fairly and in a civilized manner, resolve legal disputes related to the epidemic according to law, and provide legal protection and services for epidemic prevention and control and enterprises to resume work and resume production. Strengthen the publicity of legal popularization and guide the public to act according to law.

Supervision on administrative law enforcement has been intensified during epidemic control to ensure that the law is enforced in a strict, impartial, procedure-based, and non-abusive way. Legal disputes associated with the epidemic have been resolved in accordance with the law, and legal guarantees and services have been provided to respond to Covid-19 and for businesses returning to normal. The government has also made greater efforts to raise public legal awareness and guide people to act within the parameters of the law.

Challenges to China's social governance

The impact of Covid-19 on China has been all-encompassing, ranging from political, economic, social, and cultural values, work and life style, and even attitudes towards life. It is not possible to discuss all these dimensions; we would like to consider the impact on the socio-political level.

At the beginning of the outbreak, the economic blow had not yet fully showed itself. People were locked up at home, unable to go out, and were afraid of virus infection. At the time it was the Spring Festival season, the most important holiday in China. It was a time to visit friends and go out (at home and abroad) for sightseeing. Then everything was forced to stop, so there was all kinds of dissatisfaction among the public.

On November 17, 2016, at the Third World Internet Conference in Wuzhen, Li Bin, then director of the National Health and Family Planning Commission,[7] said that in the field of public health, China has built the world's largest direct reporting network system for infectious diseases and public health emergencies. With the help of this system, the time from the discovery of symptom of a trend at the grassroots level to the reception of the report by the Chinese Center for Disease Control and Prevention has been shortened from five days to four hours, creating a 'tight encirclement' for quickly catching the epidemic information.[8] Given such an elaborately woven system, why did the SARS tragedy of 2003 repeat itself?

Therefore, the public wanted to know whether these epidemics were natural calamities or man-made misfortunes. This was also the focus of the press and social media at the beginning of the epidemic. Unfortunately, this questioning just became the real problem. This problem is most likely to cause doubt and dissatisfaction among people with the administrative system, and this kind of doubt and dissatisfaction bears the most serious political sensitivity.

There are two reasons that deepened people's doubts and stimulated their dissatisfaction. First, some leading officials in Hubei Province and Wuhan City were too indolent and sloppy to perform their duties, and lacked ability in the face of the epidemic. On January 26, the Governor of Hubei Province was confused about the number and production capacity of masks at a press conference. On the evening of January 30, the Secretary of Hubei Party Committee (the de facto highest political officer in this jurisdiction) gave irrelevant answers to questions from the press and just bowed his head to read the manuscript.

The main government leaders in Wuhan chose to wait for the approval of their superiors instead of taking the initiative on their own. On January 29, the Central Steering Group sent an inspection team to Huanggang City for inspection and verification. The director of the local Health Commission was not clear about the hospital's treatment capacity and was not able to provide the data of nucleic acid detection capacity. Huanggang was then the second highest epidemic area in Hubei Province after Wuhan.

These were manifestations of the shortcomings of China's governance structures. The new virus had been detected in Wuhan some weeks before the beginning of the outbreak, yet the bureaucracies at several levels did not raise the alarm and the authorities did not maintain sharp vigilance. Given the formidable scale of governance in China, the centralization of authority inevitably introduces a separation between policymaking at the center and policy implementation at local levels.[9]

Second is the 'supervision' of public opinion. It is widely rumored in social media that doctors who first sent out the warning of the epidemic, such as Li Wenliang of Wuhan Central Hospital, were admonished by the police as 'rumor spreaders'. During the 'two sessions' (National People's Congress (NPC) and the Chinese People's Political Consultative Conferene (CPPCC)) in Wuhan and Hubei (January 6–18), local official media stopped reporting the development of the epidemic, and people could not get the facts.[10]

Some foreign media began to use these rumors on social media to distort the truth and discredit China. Since the founding of PRC in 1949, Western media have antagonized China's social and political system and ideology. Although the United States began to adopt the policy of engagement with China since 1970s, the purpose of this engagement is to change China, turn China into a Westernized state, follow the Western development path and finally adopt the Western system. However, China has always adhered to its own development path. Secretary of State Pompeo's speech at the Nixon Library on July 23 was evidence of this. Pompeo thought it was time for the United States to abandon its policy of cooperating with China since the Nixon era.[11]

The main focus of the Western attacks on China's social system is that China does not have a Western-style democracy; there is no freedom in China, and speech and the media are heavily controlled. Therefore, the incompetence and bureaucracy of local officials in Wuhan and Hubei and the Li Wenliang incident in the early stage of the epidemic, if not properly handled, could easily—in fact already had been—used by Western media to point to problems in China's social system. The central government attaches great importance to this trend. On February 3, at the Standing Committee of the Political Bureau of the Central Committee specially held to deal with the epidemic situation, President Xi Jinping demanded that 'We should resolutely oppose formalism and bureaucracy in the epidemic prevention and control work' and 'all cadres should be investigated and identified in the practice'.

Since then, media and think tanks have conducted nationwide special questionnaires on anti-formalism and anti-bureaucracy. On February 13, the Central Committee removed the Hubei Provincial Party Committee Secretary and Wuhan Municipal Party Committee Secretary who failed to cope with the epidemic situation, and appointed Ying Yong and Wang Zhonglin to replace them. The public hailed this quick and decisive act. According to statistics, as of mid-April, Hubei has punished more than 3,000 officials of different levels because of dereliction.

As for the Li Wenliang incident, on February 7 the Central Committee sent an investigation team to Wuhan to conduct a comprehensive investigation, and finally Li Wenliang was awarded the title of 'martyr' and 'hero in the anti-epidemic campaign'. Meanwhile, the Chinese press is also discussing how to face problems directly and convey the truth, and at the same time how to better participate in social governance through constructive news. According to the investigation, Dr. Li Wenliang was not a so-called 'whistle blower', he just spread inaccurate information about a then unexplained pneumonia. The earliest whistleblower was Ms. Zhang Jixian, a respiratory doctor of Hubei Hospital of Integrated Traditional Chinese and Western Medicine. Her 'whistling' was not only transmitted to government departments in time, but the government also took quick action according to her report.

Another challenge of the epidemic is China's grassroots social governance capacity. International public opinion generally believes that China has a big government and a small society, and China lacks NGOs, so the ability of self-governance of Chinese society is quite weak. This is basically a shared view of so-called dissidents. This epidemic just tested China's grassroots social governance ability.

Communities are cells of a society and the basic units of urban governance. In this anti-epidemic campaign, community is the key line of defense for joint prevention and control of epidemic situation. To control the spread of virus, the most effective means is to restrict the flow of people, implement physical isolation, and block the channels of virus transmission. After the outbreak, nationwide local communities acted quickly and adopted unconventional measures such as closed management.

Civil servants and volunteers worked hard to carry out the registration of personnel and vehicles, and set up posts at the entrance and exit of every neighborhood to measure body temperature. They take turns on duty day and night, strictly prohibiting outsiders from entering; they go from house to house to identify infected people, suspected cases, and those who have close contact with the infected people; they report suspected cases immediately, and then do isolation and transshipment; they clean up community garbage on time, disinfect public areas, do community health work well, and so on. Therefore, it is really a people's war with full participation of the whole society.

Some people in Western societies think that this community management mode in China was Draconian and was done at the sacrifice of 'freedom'. But human rights are, first and foremost, the right to life. Chinese culture puts emphasis on life of this world instead of heaven, and Chinese medicine is almost synonymous with keeping in good health and seeking longevity. Therefore, strict community management not only caused social protests, just as Chinese people would not protest about wearing masks, but everyone actively participated, looked out for each other and jointly maintained the safety of the community.

According to a joint study conducted by Yale University and Jinan University in China, as of February 29, the public health measures implemented in China on the national and provincial level may have avoided more than 1.4 million infections and 56,000 deaths outside Hubei Province. In addition, the basic reproduction number (R0) reflecting the spread of virus dropped rapidly from 2.99 at the end of January to 1.24 in the epicenter of Hubei at the end of February, and to 0.61 outside Hubei.[12]

Millions of deliverymen (of food and online shopping packages), sanitation workers, truck drivers, volunteers and so on constituted another beautiful sight. During the epidemic, thousands of households had their doors closed, and millions of delivery men braved the wind, snow and epidemic, rushing around in cities and villages, bringing supplies to the people. The country's 1.8 million sanitation workers got up early and worked tirelessly, doing sanitary cleaning, disinfection and sterilization, centralizing the treatment of medical waste, and garbage cleaning and transportation to high standards.

Tens of millions of transport employees stuck to their posts, and taxi drivers in many cities did not stop working, which effectively guaranteed epidemic prevention and control, transportation of production and living materials and resumption of production. Many ordinary people devoted themselves to frontline volunteer service. According to incomplete statistics, as of May 31, there were 8.81 million registered volunteers participating in epidemic prevention and control in China, with more than 460,000 volunteer service projects and recorded volunteer service time exceeding 290 million hours.[13]

On March 16, US President Trump tweeted that coronavirus was a 'Chinese virus', which marked China's anti-epidemic as entering another 'inflection point': from fighting the coronavirus to fighting the 'ideological virus'. Facing the epidemic was a complete disaster for some Western countries, such as the fall of many nursing homes and the huge death toll, but their media are full of deep-rooted prejudice. It was even disclosed that the US Republican Party has a road map to discrediting China.[14] This 57-page memorandum, dated April 17, 2020, suggests that when asked 'Isn't this the fault of President Trump?' the answer should be 'Don't defend Trump but point the finger at China'.

Ironically, the smearing of China by some US politicians and Trump's herd-immunity style of fighting Covid-19 make Chinese people become 'herd immune' to American democracy, freedom, and ideology.[15] According to the poll report of American think tank the Eurasia Group Foundation (EGF), Chinese people's affection for American democracy dropped sharply. Chinese respondents increasingly dislike the American democratic system. The report said:

> From last year to this year, we have observed great changes in our views on the United States and its government and political and cultural forms. The biggest drop was in China, where respondents' positive views on America and American democracy decreased by 20% and 15% respectively. Half of Chinese respondents believe that the influence of the United States has made the world worse.[16]

The report emphasized that the Covid-19 epidemic had not yet spread all over the world when the survey was conducted, and the Trump administration's response to the epidemic may affect the trajectory of this trend in the report.[17]

In short, the anti-epidemic performance of Western societies has taught Chinese society a lesson: 'the epidemic sweeping across the world has made us see three Western truths clearly: the incompetence of the government, the selfishness of the so-called "civilization", and the instrumental nature of media in the name of freedom' (Song, 2020). Covid-19 held a mirror to Western democracy and civilization. This should also be a major impact of the pandemic on Chinese society: the Trump administration together with the virus have enhanced China's social solidarity and political identity.

Covid-19 and 'eventful' global China

The World Health Organization called the Covid-19 outbreak 'the most serious health crisis in human history'. China received great assistance from many countries across the world in the early stages. After getting the epidemic under control, with gratitude and enthusiasm for taking on international responsibilities, China began to support countries suffering from the epidemic.

With regard to the impact of the epidemic on international relations, scholars generally believe that the epidemic will have a fundamental impact on the international pattern; as former US Secretary of State Henry Kissinger recently warned, 'the coronavirus epidemic will forever alter the world order'. From China's perspective Covid-19 and the change in the international pattern is reflected in the following aspects:

First of all, in the early stage of China's anti-epidemic campaign, the international community gave China great support, which the Chinese people and the Chinese government expressed their appreciation of and stated they would never forget it. As of March 2, 62 countries and seven international organizations pledged epidemic prevention and control supplies to China.[18]

In the early stage of the anti-epidemic campaign, Chinese society and people were flustered by the sudden epidemic. Many medical staff had to take risks to work on the frontline without personal protective equipment (PPE). At this time, overseas aid greatly eased the difficulties of Chinese medical personnel and improved their working environment. Overseas aid played a great role in helping China's victory against the epidemic. Such a huge and timely assistance is the embodiment of international humanitarian spirit, which shows that the international community has a high sense of responsibility and mutual aid spirit, and also shows that the concept of 'community of shared future' is deeply rooted in the hearts of the people across the world.

Second, with the alleviation of the epidemic, China has consistently provided support to the international community and has become the world's 'anti-epidemic factory':

(1) From March 1 to May 31, China exported protective materials to 200 countries and regions, which included more than 70.6 billion masks, 340 million protective suits, 115 million pairs of goggles, 96,700 ventilators, 225 million test kits, and 40.29 million infrared thermometers;
(2) As of May 31, China had sent 29 medical expert teams to 27 countries, and offered assistance to 150 countries and four international organizations. China has instructed its medical teams stationed in 56 countries to support the local fight, and provide counseling and health information to local people and overseas Chinese;
(3) On May 18, President Xi Jinping addressed the opening of the 73rd World Health Assembly, calling for a joint effort on the part of all countries to overcome the virus and build a global community of health for all. He also announced a series of major measures that China would take in supporting the global fight, including US$2 billion of international aid over two years, the establishment of a global humanitarian response depot and hub in China in cooperation with the United Nations. 'This is the largest global emergency humanitarian operation in the history of PRC'.[19]

On June 17, President Xi Jinping presided over the China-Africa Summit on Solidarity against Covid-19 and delivered a keynote speech entitled 'Uniting against the Epidemic and Overcoming the Difficulties Together'. China will work with G20 members to implement the debt relief initiative. China is willing to cooperate with the United Nations, WHO, and other partners in aiding Africa and fighting epidemics on the basis of respecting the wishes of Africa.[20]

On July 23, foreign ministers of China and of Latin American and Caribbean (LAC) countries held a special video conference on Covid-19. Chinese State Councilor and Foreign Minister Wang Yi and Mexican Foreign Minister Ebrard co-chaired the meeting. Experts from many Latin American countries believe that this meeting provided a new platform and created new opportunities for strengthening international cooperation against epidemic diseases and coping with epidemic challenges together.[21]

Third, facing the smearing of China by the United States and the so-called new Cold War, President Xi Jinping stressed the importance of bottom-line thinking of 'preparing for a long time to cope with changes in the external environment'.[22]

Moreover, China has shifted to a 'dual circulation' development strategy. The concept was first raised at a high-profile meeting on May 14. At the meeting, President Xi Jinping urged the nation to 'fully bring out the advantage of its super-large market scale and the potential of domestic demand to establish a new development pattern featuring domestic and international dual circulations that complement each other'.[23]

Some foreign politicians and media accused China of deliberately concealing and delaying a response to the epidemic. Actually, the Chinese government responded promptly after receiving the information of the disease and doctors in Wuhan were on high alert. On December 26, 2019, Dr. Zhang Jixian of Hubei Hospital of Integrated Traditional Chinese and Western Medicine detected four cases of 'pneumonia of unknown cause'; she reported her unusual findings to Wuhan CDC through official channels the next day. On 28 and 29, three more similar cases were found. Wuhan CDC began to conduct epidemiologic investigation on December 29. The National Health Commission sent a team of experts immediately after receiving the alert. These experts arrived in Wuhan on December 31. On the same day, the WHO office in China was informed of these cases.[24] On January 3, China informed the US about the pneumonia of unknown cause. 'China has been acting in an open, transparent and responsible manner, earnestly implementing its duties and obligations under the IHR, and timely sharing Covid-19 information with the WHO and relevant countries'.[25] On May 9, China's Foreign Ministry issued an announcement titled 'Reality Check of US Allegations against China on Covid-19', refuting all kinds of incredible lies fabricated by some American politicians and media.[26]

People across the world, including the Chinese, tend to believe the US could easily get the epidemic under control with its rich resources and most powerful medical team, which would set an example for other countries, and then start to aid other countries. However, it seemed that the US fundamentally failed both itself and the international community in ways that were hard to imagine. What it displayed to the world is inaction and ineptitude. Even with its own people floundering in the inferno, Trump and some media continued to smear China and its efforts and contribution in the fight against Covid-19.

Michael Spence, Nobel laureate in economics, believed that the epidemic had provided a new opportunity for China to better demonstrate its good will to play a role in the international arena. 'Against the background of the epidemic, China was willing to help other countries, whether developed or developing, which will enhance the impression of the international community on China'. Many other international observers also think highly of China's Covid-19 fight.[27]

The pandemic highlights the differences in cooperation, tolerance, ideology, and multilateral cooperation values among countries. In addition, it may widen the gap between Eastern and Western societies, developing countries and developed countries. After the pandemic, countries need to build a more inclusive global development framework and a more balanced global system that can better reflect the changes in contemporary international relations through comprehensive cooperation.

Covid-19 poses more challenges to human development, and all countries face urgent tasks in promoting global governance innovation. In response to the epidemic, China's pragmatic, efficient, robust, and powerful national governance system has been further consolidated and improved, which shows that China has the strength to play more leading roles in global governance. Therefore, it should actively communicate with the world and propose a plan of global governance reform that can bridge the global gap and imbalance.

Conclusion

As the first country with concentrated outbreaks, China fought the first battles of the worldwide anti-epidemic campaign. After suffering great pains, the epidemic was finally successfully contained in China. As time goes on, the severity of the epidemic varies greatly among countries. There are many reasons for this, such as differences in social response and the medical system, but in the final analysis, anti-epidemic performance is a comprehensive manifestation of a country's governance capacity, especially at a critical stage.

The Covid-19 epidemic can be seen as a major test of China's governance capacity. It has exposed China's weaknesses, such as excessive bureaucracy and unnecessary formality within the system, incompetence in response to public opinion, and inadequacy of news coverage, especially in international media coverage and guiding public opinion. Moreover, China is yet to improve its national emergency management and national reserve systems, hence the need for enhancing its reserve efficiency and emergency response capabilities to handle urgent and dangerous situations as well as optimizing the production capacity of essential supplies.

On the other hand, the Covid-19 epidemic has highlighted China's strengths. First of all, the Communist Party of China has a well-established organizational structure and operating mechanisms so that an across-the-board crisis response can be set up in a short time, mobilizing all parties down to the community level to follow national instructions to rally against the epidemic. In addition, the epidemic has witnessed the social cohesion of Chinese society—the sense of community and the volunteer spirit of the ordinary Chinese.

The Covid-19 outbreak is a truly global crisis and it has dealt a serious blow to all countries. The Chinese character for 'crisis' (WEI JI) is composed of two characters 'WEI' (danger) and 'JI' (opportunity), symbolizing the coexistence of the danger and opportunity in crisis situations. For China, the institutional failure of the United States and some other Western societies in terms of a crisis response serves as an unexpected opportunity to knock themselves off the pedestals of liberty and civilization. As a result, the ideological propaganda of the West no longer poses a major danger for the Chinese government as it did before; instead, it has turned into an opportunity to boost China's confidence in the socialist system with Chinese characteristics during the epidemic crisis.

Notes

1 The Central Steering Group has worked proactively in Wuhan and other places to direct the work on the ground. This group is the administrative body of the Central Leading Group for Novel Coronavirus Prevention and Control which was established on January 25, headed by Premier Li Keqiang.
2 China white paper on fight against Covid-19 (retrieved from http://en.nhc.gov.cn/2020-06/08/c_80724.html).
3 China Appears to Have Tamed a Second Wave of Coronavirus in Just 21 Days with No Deaths (retrieved from https://time.com/5862482/china-beijing-coronavirus-second-wave-covid19-xinfadi/).
4 Huoshenshan Hospital ('Mount Fire God Hospital') is an emergency specialty field hospital, built between January 23 and February 2, 2020, in response to the Covid-19 pandemic. It accommodates 1,000 beds. In traditional Chinese medicine, the metal element governs the lung. As fire overcomes metal, the hospital's name conveys the hope that the hospital will overcome the respiratory infection caused by SARS-CoV-2. The name of Leishenshan Hospital conveys basically the same meaning, which accommodates 1,500 beds.
5 China Focus: Xi voices full confidence in winning the battle against novel coronavirus (retrieved from www.xinhuanet.com/english/2020-01/28/c_138739962.html).
6 According to China's CDC, infectious diseases are divided into three categories, A, B and C, with a total of 40 species. It also includes other infectious diseases designated by the National Health Commission to be included in the management of Class B and Class C infectious diseases, and other serious infectious diseases which ought to be reported by emergency monitoring as Class A infectious diseases. Class A includes only pestis and cholera.
7 This institution was replaced by National Health Commission in 2018.
8 www.china.com.cn/top/2016-11/17/content_39725017.htm
9 Coronavirus Crisis Exposes Fundamental Tension in Governing China, Says Stanford Sociologist and China Expert Xueguang Zhou (retrieved from https://fsi.stanford.edu/news/coronavirus-crisis-exposes-fundamental-tension-governing-china-says-stanford-sociologist-and).
10 The Chinese government CDC started the official daily report of Covid-19 cases on January 21. People do not doubt the official data, as every province has specific hospitals to treat Covid-19 patients, and all cases are noted. It is impossible for the government to hide the cases.
11 Event Recap: Secretary Pompeo at the Nixon Library (retrieved from www.nixonfoundation.org/2020/07/event-recap-secretary-pompeo-nixon-library-2/).
12 Strong Public Health Response in China Slowed Coronavirus Transmission, YSPH Study Finds (retrieved from https://medicine.yale.edu/news-article/25007/).
13 China publishes white paper on fight against Covid-19 (retrieved from http://en.nhc.gov.cn/2020-06/08/c_80724.htm).
14 GOP memo urges anti-China assault over coronavirus (retrieved from www.politico.com/news/2020/04/24/gop-memo-anti-china-coronavirus-207244).
15 As Eli Sweet, a US citizen who is vice-chair of the American Chamber of Commerce of southwest China, stated in an interview, 'People in the western society would imagine China to be politically oppressive and authoritarian … this pandemic and the stay in China has made me look at the US politics differently, the political conflict is higher than in China recent years, I thought I was a huge believer in the value of democracy … the

US polity is poorly served by the democratic system' (retrieved from www.wvxu.org/post/china-dream-new-silk-road-begins-home#stream/0).

16 Survey: Chinese Report Less Favorable Views of US Democracy (retrieved from https://thediplomat.com/2020/04/survey-chinese-report-less-favorable-views-of-us-democracy/).

17 Survey: Chinese Report Less Favorable Views of US Democracy (retrieved from https://thediplomat.com/2020/04/survey-chinese-report-less-favorable-views-of-us-democracy/).

18 Foreign Ministry Spokesperson Zhao Lijian's Regular Press Conference March 3, 2020 (retrieved from www.fmprc.gov.cn/mfa_eng/xwfw_665399/s2510_665401/t1751740.shtml).

19 State Councilor and Foreign Minister Wang Yi Meets the Press (retrieved from www.fmprc.gov.cn/mfa_eng/zxxx_662805/t1782262.shtml)

20 China's commitment to cooperation, solidarity with Africa displayed in their anti-epidemic fight, experts say (retrieved from www.xinhuanet.com/english/2020-06/18/c_139149026.htm).

21 China and Latin American and Caribbean Countries Hold Special Video Conference of Foreign Ministers on Covid-19 (retrieved from www.fmprc.gov.cn/mfa_eng/zxxx_662805/t1800563.shtml).

22 Update-Xi Focus: Xi chairs leadership meeting on regular epidemic control, work resumption (retrieved from www.xinhuanet.com/english/2020-04/08/c_138958796.htm).

23 'Dual circulation', a new mode for development (retrieved from www.chinadaily.com.cn/a/202008/14/WS5f35eff9a310834817260521.html).

24 Novel Coronavirus (2019-nCoV) – World Health Organization (retrieved from www.who.int/docs/default-source/coronaviruse/situation-reports/20200121-sitrep-1-2019-ncov.pdf).

25 Foreign Ministry Spokesperson Zhao Lijian's Regular Press Conference on July 6, 2020 (retrieved from www.fmprc.gov.cn/mfa_eng/xwfw_665399/s2510_665401/t1795337.shtml).

26 www.xinhuanet.com/english/2020-05/10/c_139044103.html

27 The book *China's Fight against the Covid-19 Epidemic: Its Contribution and Implications in the Eyes of Foreigners* (Contemporary China Publishing House, 2020) includes interviews with more than 20 politicians, experts, and scholars from all over the world and their reflections on China's Covid-19 fight.

Reference

Song Zhenlu (2020) 'China was Taught a Severe Lesson by the Western Media', https://m.guancha.cn/SongLuZheng/2020_04_25_548198.shtml, accessed August 2020.

2

SOUTH KOREA, TAIWAN, HONG KONG, SINGAPORE AND COVID-19

Wang Hwi Lee

Hong Kong, Singapore, South Korea and Taiwan (collectively known as the Asian Tigers) have attracted international attention because their management of the coronavirus pandemic has been more effective than that of any other region worldwide. In terms of numbers of pandemic infections and deaths, the Tigers have been in good shape compared to European and North American countries (Pew Research 2020). In the early stage of the pandemic, Korea and Taiwan emerged as role models for infection control. US Assistant Secretary for Health Brett P. Giroir said, 'Everyone talks about South Korea being the standard' (White House 2020). Taiwan's response to the pandemic is the envy of many nations (Rowen 2020).

The Asian Tigers' success is widely attributed to institutional capacity, governance structure and cooperation between the state and civil society (Cha 2020a; Kennedy and Tan 2020). The legacy of the developmental state has been instrumental in mobilizing medical/human resources and implementing social distancing measures. Well before the crisis, the public healthcare system had developed to the level of advanced countries. Furthermore, policy making is largely orchestrated by expert-led government agencies (the Centers for Disease Control or the equivalent thereof) rather than politicians with little expertise in epidemiology and immunology. These countries' experiences with severe acute respiratory syndrome (SARS) in 2002 and Middle East respiratory syndrome (MERS) in 2015 played a crucial role in building institutional capability. Failures to manage those two epidemics led the governments of these countries to establish new agencies that are intended to function as a control tower in times of crisis. The collective memory of the epidemics also helped citizens to tolerate some constraints on private privacy and individual liberty. In this regard, the role of the state in the Tigers has significant implications for varieties of capitalism (Acemoglu 2020; Fukuyama 2020; Mazzucato and Quaggiotto 2020; ; Rajan 2020).

A closer look reveals both similarities and differences among these nations. The Asian Tigers are densely populated and geographically close to China, which could have made it very difficult for them to cope with the crisis (von Carnap, Drinhausen and Shi-Kupfer 2020). At a very early stage, however, all of them managed to flatten the curve through a combination of widespread testing, aggressive contact tracing and effective treatment. After the outbreak of the second wave, it seems that the four countries have split into two tracks. Only Taiwan has consistently brought the virus under control. Hong Kong, Korea and Singapore have seen triple-digit growth in the number of infections, although their death rates have not increased sharply.

It also should be noted that the crisis management in these countries has been far from perfect. Repeated resurgences of the pandemic have exposed and widened the political, economic and social cleavages that had been masked by the success of early responses. The impacts of the pandemic have been uneven, hitting vulnerable groups such as the unemployed and foreign migrants especially hard. Discrimination against ethnic minorities, religious sects and LGBTQ individuals have also emerged in the process of social distancing. The blame game between neighboring countries over the pandemic has obstructed effective international cooperation. Rigorous and comprehensive contact tracing measures have also raised the question of how much privacy can be breached for the sake of public health.

This chapter investigates the responses to the pandemic in Hong Kong, Korea, Singapore and Taiwan from an institutional perspective. The chapter is organized into four parts. The first part examines how the four countries have managed the pandemic and why their experiences have earned high praise from the rest of the world. The next compares their policy responses and institutional frameworks in greater detail. Then, problems caused by social distancing are analyzed. The final part discusses the lessons and implications of these East Asian cases.

Another East Asian model?

In terms of responses to the Covid-19 pandemic, China, Germany, Korea, Taiwan and Sweden have drawn interest from the world. Except for Sweden, which pursued a herd immunity strategy, the rest flattened the curve at an early stage and the number of deaths remained relatively low. China, the first epicenter of the pandemic, imposed a very strict lockdown, restricting all non-essential internal movement, on Wuhan and neighboring cities in Hubei Province for more than two months. The city-wide lockdown was quite helpful in stopping the spread of the virus, but its economic, social and psychological costs cannot be underestimated. For this reason, social distancing has been viewed as a better option. The problem is that few countries have controlled the contagion of the pandemic with social distancing. Even Germany, one of the best performers in Europe, used nationwide restrictions to address the pandemic. As Figure 2.1 shows, the Asian Tigers are a rare success story, although Singapore introduced heavy lockdown measures just after the eruption of the second wave in April 2020.

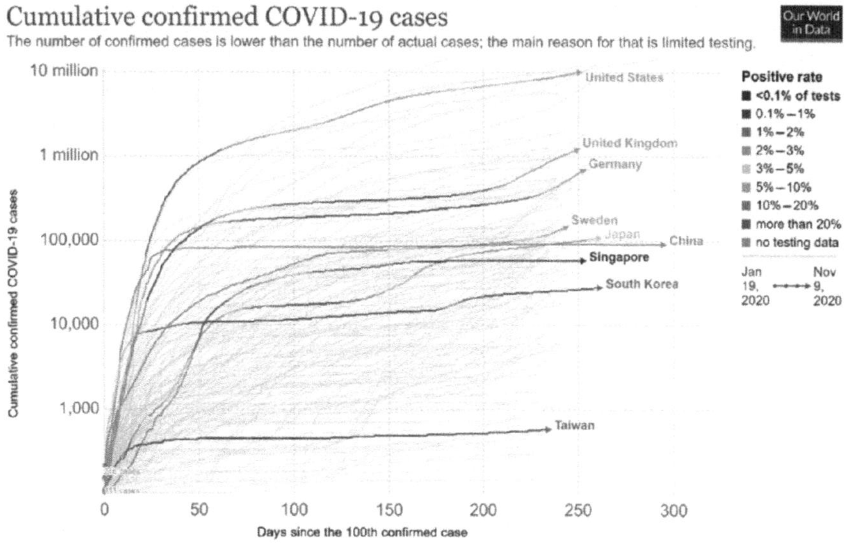

FIGURE 2.1 Total confirmed cases in Asian Tigers

Source: Our World in Data (https://ourworldindata.org/covid-cases?country=CHN~JPN~HKG~SGP~KOR~TWN~USA~SWE~DEU~GBR; accessed December 5, 2020).

The main achievement of the Asian Tigers is a relatively low death rate. In terms of the number of infections per one million population, as Table 2.1 demonstrates, Singapore is slightly higher than the US, the country with the highest number of cases and one of the worst victims of the pandemic. Surprisingly, Korea and Hong Kong have more infections per million population than China, although the credibility of Chinese statistics has been questioned. In East Asia, Taiwan is the only country that has performed better than China.

Responses to the pandemic: similarities and differences

From January to March 2020, the Asian Tigers successfully managed to contain the initial spread of the pandemic without a nationwide lockdown. Just after the outbreak of the pandemic in Wuhan, China, all of them quickly deployed preventive measures including travel restrictions, border control, mandatory quarantines, and social distancing. At the same time they developed and produced test kits even before the pandemic spread throughout the countries. Medication and medical gear (face masks, hand sanitizers, ventilators, etc.) were also stockpiled to meet potential demand. After the first wave hit the countries, high levels of social distancing were imposed to slow the spread of the virus. All these efforts made it possible for the Tigers to flatten the curve without a nationwide lockdown. The numbers of

TABLE 2.1 Covid-19 pandemic

Country	*Total*			*One million population*		
	Cases	*Deaths*	*Tests*	*Cases*	*Deaths*	*Tests*
Korea	36,915	540	3,180,496	720	11	62,012
Taiwan	693	7	112,412	29	0.3	4,716
Hong Kong	6,803	112	4,382,709	904	15	582,578
Singapore	58,255	29	4,658,858	9,924	5	793,673
China	86,601	4,634	160,000,000	60	3	111,163
Japan	155,232	2,240	3,675,244	1,229	18	29,097
USA	14,775,308	285,668	203,887,324	44,526	861	614.427
UK	1,690,432	60,617	44,812,139	24,845	891	658,627
Germany	1,152,283	18,691	29,141,172	13,734	223	347,337
Sweden	278,912	7,067	3,457,247	27,544	698	341,416
World	66,362,745	1,527,219		8,514	195.9	

Source: Worldometer, Covid-19 Pandemic (www.worldometers.info/coronavirus/?utm_campaign=homeAdvegas1? accessed December 5, 2020).

confirmed cases and deaths were relatively low, and adverse economic and social impacts were less severe.

After the second wave took place in Singapore in April, the extent and damage of the pandemic began to vary considerably from country to country. As of November 10, 2020, the best performer is Taiwan, with just 578 confirmed cases and seven deaths. Unlike its peers, the country has not suffered a big resurgence so far. The number of active cases peaked in late March and early April. Since April 12, there has been no domestically transmitted case of the disease.

Outside China, Taiwan was the first country to perceive the danger of the pandemic in late December 2019. After finding out that a cluster of patients with pneumonia of an unknown cause suddenly increased in Wuhan, the Taiwan Centers for Disease Control started monitoring all travelers from Wuhan on January 5, 2020. Two weeks later, the Central Epidemic Command Center was activated and immediately coordinated policy responses across government agencies.

Taiwan's response has been both decisive and comprehensive. In January, the government mobilized face mask and sanitary alcohol production facilities and temporarily banned the export of face masks. In February, a face mask rationing system was introduced, and the opening of primary and secondary schools was postponed. In March, at-home quarantine for 14 days became mandatory for travelers from countries with a high risk of infection. All passengers on public transport were required to wear face masks. Successful crisis management allowed the government to lift the export controls on face masks and to donate masks to foreign countries in April. The professional baseball league resumed its regular-season play in empty stadiums (Ministry of Foreign Affairs 2020).

In many ways, Korea's early responses were very similar to Taiwan's. As of December 5, 2020, the total number of confirmed cases amounts to 36, 915 with 540 deaths. Travel bans, self-quarantines and mandatory face mask wearing on public transportation were orchestrated by the Korea Centers for Disease Control and Prevention (KCDC) in January. As a result, the spread of the pandemic was brought under control by mid-February. However, after a large cluster of infections, most of which occurred among participants in a gathering at a Shincheonji Church of Jesus the Temple of the Tabernacle of the Testimony church in Daegu, were discovered in late February, Korea became the second worst-hit country after China. Its daily number of new confirmed cases soared to almost 1,000 at the end of February.

To deal with the surge of infected cases, the KCDC intensified their efforts. One of the most important innovations was aggressive contact tracing measures, which 'objectively verify the patient's claims (medical facility records, Global Positioning System, card transactions, and closed-circuit television)' (Korea Centers for Disease Control & Prevention 2020: 60). Another is drive-through testing sites where patients be tested in their vehicles. This method substantially contributed to increasing mass testing outside the hospital facilities. In addition, training institutes and dormitories of business organizations, including Samsung and LG, were temporarily converted into treatment centers for patients with no or minimal symptoms. These novel methods played a crucial role in the sharp decline of confirmed cases in mid-March. At that moment, Korea's reputation suddenly tuned from bad to good, especially in contrast with Italy, which was on the other side of the curve (Ahn 2020; Cha 2020a; Martin and Yoon 2020; Parodi et al. 2020).

In early May, a new cluster surfaced in nightclubs in Itaewon, Seoul. The Seoul Metropolitan Government stopped the spread of this outbreak to other provinces with a combination of rigorous contact tracing and strong quarantines. Thanks to the rapid response, the country managed to avoid a second wave of infections (National Assembly Research Service 2020).

As the daily number of new confirmed cases reached 400 in mid-August, Seoul (the capital city) is likely to become an epicenter of the pandemic. On National Liberation Day (August 15), more than 10,000 people gathered in the heart of the city to protest the Moon administration. The anti-government rally was organized by Reverend Jeon Kwang-hoon, who criticized the prohibition of church worship as part of social distancing. Because participants came from all parts of the country, the possibility of nationwide contagion associated with this event was very high. By the end of August, the number of new confirmed cases jumped up to almost 400 a day.

Singapore's experience has similarities with that of Korea. As December 5, 2020, the total number of confirmed cases jumped to 58,255, with 29 deaths. The number of deaths per one million population in Singapore is just five, lower than Korea's. Just one day before the first case was confirmed in late January, the government established a multi-ministerial committee that did not hesitate to implement a policy package of travel restrictions, self-quarantine and social distancing. The initial responses were so preemptive and effective that the city-state controlled the spread of the pandemic until late March. However, massive outbreaks in dormitories for foreign workers forced the government to impose a near-total lockdown in early April. At the same time, 20,000 migrant workers in two dormitories were under mandatory quarantine. Among them, patients with mild symptoms were transferred to private hospitals, the Singapore Expo and the Changi Exhibition Center. This so-called 'circuit breaker' continued until early August, when the number of confirmed cases clearly fell below 100 (Tay and Chen 2020).

Since the pandemic was first confirmed in late January, Hong Kong has gone through ups and downs. As of December 5, 2020, the total number of confirmed cases was 6,803, with 112 deaths. Due to its geographical proximity to mainland China, news about the outbreak in Wuhan quickly reached the city. In late January the government swiftly suspended high-speed rail and ferry services between the city and China. The number of flights from China was drastically decreased and all borders except three control points were closed. Social distancing and wearing face masks were also instrumental in slowing down the contagion of the pandemic. In early February, the shortage of face masks and sanitary alcohol caused social unrest. Nonetheless, the pandemic remained under control until mid-July when the number of daily new confirmed cases jumped to three digits. Although there were fears of political interference, the government asked their Chinese counterparts to send medical staff who could help testing and treating patients. Notably, Hong Kong has fared worse than China in terms of the number of confirmed cases and deaths per one million population.

Institutional capacity for social distancing

What enabled the Asian Tigers to weather the pandemic better than many other countries? An emerging consensus is that the Tigers were well-prepared to deal with the pandemic. As Scott Kennedy and Shining Tan pointed out, 'the general data on government capacity are far from definitive' (Kennedy and Tan 2020). The worldwide governance indicators compiled by the World Bank suggest that the Asian Tigers are slightly better than North American and Western European countries only in terms of government effectiveness (World Bank 2020).

However, the public health systems of these the four countries are not far behind those of advanced countries (Maizland and Felter 2020). Table 2.2 illustrates that Korea and Singapore have developed very good public health systems. In terms of infectious diseases and service capacity, the two countries ranked only second to the US and Japan. Hong Kong and Taiwan are believed to have similar systems, although the WHO does not compile their statistics because neither are member states.

Table 2.3 shows similar results. Korea ranked 9th in the world, much higher than Japan (21st) and Singapore (24th). The country earned good marks in detection, reporting and rapid response. Singapore's rank was comparatively low because its compliance with international norms was much below average.

TABLE 2.2 Healthcare indicators in Asian Tigers and selected countries

Country	*UHC Service Coverage Index*	*Infectious diseases*	*Service capacity and access*		
		At least basic sanitation	*Hospital bed density*	*Health worker density*	*International Health Regulations core capacity index*
Korea	86	100	100	100	98
Taiwan					
Hong Kong					
Singapore	86	100	100	100	99
China	79	85	100	100	100
Japan	83	100	100	100	100
USA	86	100	100	100	100
UK	87	99	100	100	89
Germany	83	99	100	100	96
Sweden	86	99	100	100	93

Source: World Health Organization (2019: 108–112).

TABLE 2.3 Global Health Security (GHS) Index (Ranking)

Country	*Overall*	*Prevention*	*Detection and reporting*	*Rapid response*	*Health system*	*Compliance with international norms*	*Risk environment*
Korea	70.2 (9)	57.3 (19)	91.2 (5)	71.5 (6)	58.7 (13)	64.3 (23)	74.1 (27)
Taiwan							
Hong Kong							
Singapore	58.7 (24)	56.2 (23)	64.5 (40)	64.6 (11)	41.4 (38)	47.3 (101)	80.9 (15)
China	48.2 (51)	45.0 (50)	48.5 (64)	48.6 (47)	45.7 (30)	40.3 (141)	64.4 (58)
Japan	59.8 (21)	49.3 (40)	70.1 (35)	53.6 (31)	46.6 (25)	70.0 (13)	71.7 (34)
USA	83.5 (1)	83.1 (1)	98.2 (1)	79.7 (2)	78.3 (1)	85.3 (1)	72.9 (19)
UK	77.9 (2)	68.3 (10)	87.3 (6)	91.9 (1)	59.8 (11)	82.2 (2)	74.7 (26)
Germany	66.0 (12)	66.5 (13)	84.6 (10)	54.8 (28)	48.2 (22)	61.9 (29)	82.3 (11)
France	68.2 (11)	71.2 (6)	75.3 (21)	62.9 (13)	60.9 (8)	58.6 (44)	83.0 (9)

Source: Nuclear Threat Initiative and Johns Hopkins Center for Health Security (2019: 20–29).

In the Asian Tigers, the Centers for Disease Control and Prevention or equivalent agencies have served as the control tower and orchestrated social distancing measures. These agencies have played a crucial role in designing and implementing detailed guidelines on social distancing measures. The dominance of medical experts has left very little room for politicians and bureaucrats to manipulate the

TABLE 2.4 Summary of probable SARS cases

Country	*Total*			*Date of onset*	
	Cases	*Deaths*	*Case fatality rate (%)*	*First probable case*	*Last probable case*
Korea	3	0	0	25-Apr-03	10-May-03
Taiwan	346	37	11	25-Feb-03	15-Jun-03
Hong Kong	1,755	299	17	15-Feb-03	31-May-03
Singapore	238	33	14	25-Feb-03	5-May-03
China	5,327	349	7	16-Nov-02	3-Jun-03
Japan					
USA	27			24-Feb-03	13-Jul-03
UK	4	0	0	1-Mar-03	1-Apr-03
World	8,096	774	9.6		

Source: World Health Organization (2004).

situation to their advantage. As a result, a high priority has been placed on public health, rather than political considerations and economic impacts.

Expert-initiated approaches originated in previous epidemics, especially those of SARS and the MERS. As Table 2.4 shows, in 2003, Hong Kong, Taiwan and Singapore were among the worst victims of the SARS outside China. Hong Kong's case fatality rate was 17 per cent, more than twice than that of China. Only Korea was not seriously affected by the virus.

In the aftermath of the SARS outbreak, Taiwan, Hong Kong and Singapore expanded and upgraded their public health systems to prepare for a future pandemic. After a government-led investigation into the pandemic in 2004, Hong Kong launched the Centre for Health Protection, which is exclusively responsible for disease prevention and control. In Singapore, the pandemic gave rise to the establishment of public health control measures involving cross-sectional inter-ministerial collaboration and coordination (Ooi and Phua 2009). In Taiwan, the National Health Command Center established the Central Epidemic Command Center in 2005. This center has been activated twice: just after the outbreak of the 2009 swine flu pandemic and the Covid-19 pandemic. Vice President Chen Chien-Jen (2016–2020), took charge of managing the SARS crisis in 2003 and oversaw the policy responses in the early stage (Hernández and Horton 2020).

In Korea, a comprehensive upgrade of the public health system was prompted by the MERS outbreak in 2015. As of July 21, 2017, the number of confirmed cases reached 185. Korea's infections were much worse than those of the United Arab Emirates, Jordan and Qatar, which share borders with Saudi Arabia, the epicenter of the epidemic (see Figure 2.2). There were no infections among its East Asian neighbors. In 2016, the Center for Public Health Emergency Preparedness and Response was created as part of the KCDC.

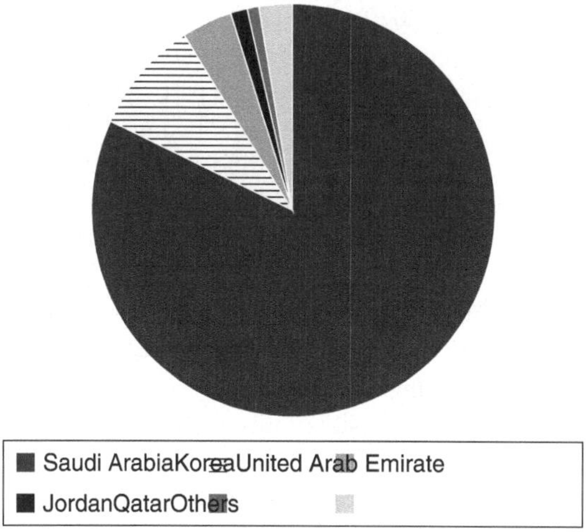

FIGURE 2.2 Summary of probable MERS cases

Source: World Health Organization (2017: 3).

The dark side of state-led social distancing

As far as the first wave of the pandemic is concerned, there is little doubt that the Asian Tigers handled the pandemic better than their neighboring countries. That does not mean that their responses were perfect. The 'test, trace, and isolate' approach was very effective in flattening the curve in the early stage. New forms of surveillance based on high-tech devices and apps as well as an immense expansion of state regulations have made it much easier for governments to track and control the movement of citizens and foreigners. However, this approach has a dark side. There are growing concerns about privacy breaches. Particularly in Korea, the authorities have extensively accessed and shared patients' private information including medical facility records, global positioning system data, credit card transactions and CCTV footage. Moreover, some information on places where patients visited were both displayed on public notice boards and alerted by mobile text messages (Klingner 2020). Despite pervasive violations of privacy, this approach has remained largely undisputed, not because privacy infringement is regarded as legitimate and lawful, but because there is no better alternative to tracing chains of contagion.

The pandemic has laid bare many political, economic and social cleavages, which have hindered government agencies from enforcing social distancing measures in more decisive ways. In Taiwan, the escalation of diplomatic confrontations with China has distracted the government from managing the pandemic. China has consistently blocked Taiwan's participation in WHO meetings on the basis that Taiwan is not a member country. As a result, the country has been largely excluded by international cooperation, despite donating medical equipment to many countries

(Lu and Chung 2020; Wong 2020). The Universal Community Testing Program (UCTP) conducted by the government in September was successful. 1,783,000 citizens (a quarter of the population) voluntarily participated in the UCTP and 42 new infections was identified (Wong, Low and Cheung 2020).

Hong Kong has a similar problem with a different cause. Under the one country, two systems doctrine, Hong Kong has been a special administrative region of China since 1997. Political controversies provoked by the 2019 extradition bill and the 2020 national security law have made it very difficult for government agencies to collaborate with their Chinese counterparts. To ramp up testing capacity, the government invited Chinese medical staff in July 2020, but Hong Kong experts were reluctant to collaborate with them. The Hong Kong Liaison Office of the Chinese government maintained that politically motivated resistance would threaten public health and safety (Cheng, Choy and Low 2020).

Religious and gender discrimination has emerged as a result of the unexpected consequences of social distancing in Korea. Several large clusters were identified among Protestant churches that stubbornly oppose online worship services. The first major outbreak in mid-February was initiated by the Shincheonji Church, and a resurgence in confirmed cases in mid-August was linked to Reverend Jeon's Sarang Jeil Church. The pandemic rapidly spread all over the country just after the church mobilized a conservative demonstration against the Moon administration in central Seoul that drew more than 10,000 participants (Choe 2020). In addition, the role of the LGBT community in the Itaewon club infections has been debated. To avoid disclosing their identity, many club goers did not voluntarily get tested. Compared with Western democracies, tolerance for and protection of gender minorities are limited in Korea. To address charges of discrimination, the authorities introduced a diagnostic test protocol that only required patients to fill in their phone number (i.e., without an identity card number) (Park 2020).

Criticism of the Singapore government concentrated on the lack of attention to 32,000 foreign workers, most of whom are poorly paid and live in overcrowded dormitories on the outskirts of city center. Even after their accommodations became a new epicenter of the pandemic, it took a few weeks for all the workers to be tested, isolated, and treated (Toh 2020; Palma 2020).

Conclusion

The Asian Tigers have managed the pandemic effectively. However, this assessment is tentative and partial. Success in the first wave does not guarantee success in a possible second wave. Until the development of medication and a vaccine for Covid-19, premature lifting of social distancing can wipe out early achievements in a very short period. A good example is the resurgence that Korea experienced in late August.

Without addressing problems of privacy and discrimination, it is highly unlikely that the responses of these countries can serve as a model for other countries to follow. Irrespective of their effectiveness, surveillance-based social distancing methods would be very difficult to replicate in Western democracies (Kluth 2020; Wright 2020). Furthermore, it is too early to conclude whether these approaches will withstand the test of a possible second and third wave of infections in the coming months. Until the pandemic is effectively controlled, it is an exaggeration to claim that the responses to the pandemic by the four Asian Tigers will be regarded as another East Asian miracle.

References

Acemoglu, Daron 2020 The Post-Covid State, *Project Syndicate*, June 5.

Ahn, Michael J. 2020. *Combating Covid-19: Lessons from South Korea*, Washington, DC: Brookings Institution.

Cha, Victor. 2020a South Korea Offers a Lesson in Best Practices: The United States May Be Left with Only the Most Invasive of Them, *Foreign Affairs*, April 10.

Cha, Victor. 2020b Asia's Covid-19 Lessons for the West: Public Goods, Privacy, and Social Tagging, *Washington Quarterly* 43, 2: 1–18.

Cheng, Lilian, Gigi Choy and Zoe Low 2020 Hong Kong Third Wave: Officials to Prioritise Next Round of Testing for Covid-19 as First Experts from Mainland China Arrive to Help with Fight, *South China Morning Post*, August 2.

Choe, Sang-Hun 2020 In South Korea's New Covid-19 Outbreak, Religion and Politics Collide, *New York Times*, August 20.

Fukuyama, Francis 2020 The Pandemic and Political Order: It Takes a State, *Foreign Affairs* 99, 4: 26–32.

Hernández, Javier C. and Chris Horton 2020 Taiwan's Weapon against Coronavirus: An Epidemiologist as Vice President, *New York Times*, May 21.

Kennedy, Scott and Shining Tan 2020 *Better Governance, Better Outcomes: East Asian Experiences Tackling Covid-19*, Washington, DC: CSIS.

Klingner, Bruce 2020 *South Korea Provides Lessons, Good and Bad, on Coronavirus Response*. Commentary, Heritage Foundation.

Kluth, Andreas 2020 If We Must Build a Surveillance State, Let's Do It Properly, *Bloomberg*, April 21.

Korea Centers for Disease Control & Prevention 2020 Contact Transmission of Covid-19 in South Korea: Novel Investigation Techniques for Tracing Contacts, *Osong Public Health and Research Perspectives* 11, 1: 60–63.

Lu, Yi-hsuan and Jake Chung. 2020. Virus Outbreak: Allies Urge Taiwan's Inclusion in WHA. *Taipei Times*, May 15.

Maizland, Lindsay and Claire Felter 2020 *Comparing Six Health-Care Systems in a Pandemic*, New York: Backgrounder, Council on Foreign Relations.

Martin, Timothy W. and Dasl Yoon 2020 How South Korea Successfully Managed Coronavirus, *Wall Street Journal*, September 25.

Mazzucato, Mariana and Giulio Quaggiotto 2020. The Big Failure of Small Government. *Project Syndicate*, May 19.

Ministry of Foreign Affairs 2020 The Taiwan Model for Combating Covid-19 (www.mofa.gov.tw/en/theme.aspx?n=B13D460AE0B33449&s=9C13959F19F93B2F&sms=BCDE19B435833080, accessed December 5, 2020).

National Assembly Research Service 2020 *Covid-19: How We Are Handling the Outbreak*. Second edition. Seoul (in Korean).

Nuclear Threat Initiative and Johns Hopkins Center for Health Security 2019 *Global Health Security (GHS) Index 2019*.

Ooi, Giok Ling and Kai Hong Phua 2009 SARS in Singapore: Challenges of a Global Health Threat to Local Institutions, *Natural Hazards*, 48: 317–327.

Palma, Stefania 2020 Surge in Covid Cases Shows up Singapore's Blind Spots over Migrant Workers, *Financial Times*, June 4.

Park, Han-na 2020 Seoul Scales up Tracing and Testing amid Specter of Second Wave, *Korea Herald*, May 13.

Parodi, Emilio, Stephen Jewkes, Sangmi Cha and Ju-min Park 2020 Italy and South Korea Virus Outbreaks Reveal Disparity in Deaths and Tactics, *Reuters*, March 12.

Pew Research 2020 Americans Give Higher Ratings to South Korea and Germany than US for Dealing with Coronavirus, May 21.

Rajan, Raghuram G. 2020. Which Post-Pandemic Government? Project Syndicate (www.project-syndicate.org/commentary/covid19-decentralized-vs-centralized-government-by-raghuram-rajan-2020-05?barrier=accesspaylog, accessed May 22, 2020).

Rowen, Ian 2020 Crafting the Taiwan Model for Covid-19: An Exceptional State in Pandemic Territory, *Asia-Pacific Journal: Japan Focus* 18, 9: 1–13.

Tay, Simon and Kevin Chen 2020 *Singapore and Covid-19: Strengths, Shifts and Limits of National Response*, New York: Council on Foreign Relations.

Toh, Ting Wei 2020 Most Migrant Workers Expected to be Cleared of Coronavirus by End July, *Strait Times*, June 26.

Von Carnap, Kai, Katja Drinhausen and Kristin Shi-Kupfer 2020 *Tracing, Testing, Tweaking: Approaches to Data-driven Covid-19 Management in China*, Berlin: MERICS.

White House 2020 Remarks by President Trump in a Press Briefing on Covid-19 Testing (https://trumpwhitehouse.archives.gov/briefings-statements/remarks-president-trump-press-briefing-covid-19-testing/, accessed May 11, 2020).

Wong, Chun Han 2020 Taiwan's Success in Coronavirus Fight Poses Challenge to China, *Wall Street Journal*, April 11.

Wong, Natalie, Zoe Low and Elizabeth Cheung 2020 Hong Kong's Mass Coronavirus Testing Cost Taxpayers HK$530 Million, Leader Labels Scheme a Success. *South China Morning Post*, September 15.

World Bank 2020 Worldwide Governance Indicators (https://databank.worldbank.org/source/worldwide-governance-indicators, accessed December 5, 2020).

World Health Organization 2004 Summary of Probable SARS Cases with Onset of Illness from 1 November 2002 to 31 July 2003 (www.who.int/csr/sars/country/table2004_04_21/en/, accessed December 5, 2020).

World Health Organization 2017 *WHO MERS-CoV Global Summary and Assessment of Risk*.

World Health Organization 2019 *Universal Health Coverage Report 2019*.

Wright, Nicholas 2020 Coronavirus and the Future of Surveillance Democracies Must Offer an Alternative to Authoritarian Solutions, *Foreign Affairs*, April 6.

Webpages

Hong Kong: Centre for Health Protection (www.chp.gov.hk/en/index.html / www.coronavirus.gov.hk/eng/index.html).

Korea: Center for Disease Control and Prevention (www.cdc.go.kr/cdc_eng/).

Singapore: Ministry of Health (www.moh.gov.sg/covid-19 / www.gov.sg/features/covid-19).

Taiwan: Centers for Disease Control (www.cdc.gov.tw/En).

Our World in Data: Covid-19 database – Coronavirus Pandemic (Covid-19) (https://ourworldindata.org/coronavirus).

3

CHINA, KOREA, JAPAN AND COVID-19

Ik Ki Kim and Rosung Kwak

Coronavirus disease 2019 (Covid-19), which emerged in China, first spread to neighboring countries like Korea and Japan, and then to the whole world. By mid-February 2020 China and Korea showed the world's highest numbers of Covid-19 infections and deaths. Globally, the numbers of confirmed cases and deaths have consistently increased day by day. The worldwide number of confirmed cases exceeded 66.3 million, including 1,527,219 deaths as of December 5, 2020 (Worldometer 2020). The number reached 10 million in the first six months since the initial outbreak in China, and then increased by another 10 million in 43 days (Chosun Daily 2020.8.11). The pace of the increase in the number of confirmed cases has accelerated. However, responses to Covid-19 have varied from country to country.

China, Korea and Japan share many sociocultural similarities, but have shown somewhat different patterns of responses to Covid-19. These three countries are geographically located in close proximity in East Asia, and have several sociocultural factors in common (Sodei 1996). First, they belong to the Confucian cultural sphere. Confucianism, which originated in China about 2,500 years ago, was imported through Korea and then to Japan in Sui and Tang dynasties. Although the effects of Confucianism differ from country to country, the Confucian tradition is still prevalent, even with trends of globalization. Second, these three countries have experienced the demographic transition from high birth and death rates to low birth and death rates in a very short period of time, which has led to rapid population aging. Third, these countries also achieved economic development in a very short period of time.

Despite similarities in their processes of economic growth, Japan and Korea are coordinated market economies, while China is a state-led market economy (Nederveen Pieterse 2015: 2). In addition, there are other relevant differences among these countries. Korea and China were invaded by Japan. Japan as a defeated nation regarded its pre-war tradition as a 'remaining feudalistic' system and was enthusiastic about abolishing the patriarchal family system (Sodei 1996). In contrast to Japan, Korea has maintained the traditional family system and China, as a socialist country, did not make serious attempts to break its traditional family system.

The welfare policies adopted by China are different from those of Korea and Japan. Korea has followed almost the same course as Japan in the implementation of a national pension system and health insurance system. However, China with its huge population and substantial regional differences has not yet established a unified nationwide welfare system (Kim and Chung, 2018). Differences in the responses of these three nations to the Covid-19 have also been shaped by different experiences with the severe acute respiratory syndrome (SARS) in 2002 and Middle East respiratory syndrome (MERS) in 2015 outbreaks: China experienced a serious impact from SARS, Korea experienced a weak impact from SARS and was seriously affected by MERS, and Japan did not have any experience of these coronavirus diseases.

This chapter will introduce and compare important factors influencing different responses to the Covid-19 pandemic in China, Korea and Japan. More specifically, this chapter will focus on the onset and spread of the Covid-19 and will analyze the number of confirmed cases and deaths by age group in each country. Then, this chapter will elucidate different responses to Covid-19, plausible factors affecting control measures and the effects of the control measures in fighting the disease. The chapter concludes by illustrating the socioeconomic impact of Covid-19 in each country.

Onset and spread of Covid-19

The outbreak of the Covid-19 pandemic took place in Wuhan, China. The first confirmed patient of Covid-19 was reported to have symptoms on December 1, 2019 in Wuhan. The Wuhan Center for Disease Control (CDC) determined that there was a cluster of pneumonia cases with an unknown cause related to Huanan Seafood Market in Wuhan. The Chinese CDC reported this situation to the World Health Organization (WHO) on December 31. The new coronavirus was identified as the cause of the pneumonia on January 8, 2020. The outbreak of the new coronavirus was formally recognized after more than a month of delay.

The first confirmed case of Covid-19 in Korea was identified as a 35-year-old Chinese woman who came to Korea from Wuhan on January 20, 2020 (Kim 2020). The first Korean national to be infected was a 55-year-old man who worked in Wuhan and returned for a checkup with flu symptoms. In Japan, a resident of Kanagawa Prefecture in his 30s who had previously traveled to Wuhan developed a fever and subsequently returned to Japan on January 6. Since then, the Covid-19 pandemic rapidly spread to throughout Japan. Overall, the initial cases of Covid-19 in all three countries were directly linked to Wuhan, China.

Interestingly, a common feature in the spread of Covid-19 in these three countries is that a certain city in each country was the major source of a large spark in the number of confirmed cases in the early stage: Wuhan in China, Daegu in Korea, and Tokyo in Japan (Daum Portal 2020.7.5). As of May 4, 2020, the proportion of the confirmed cases of each city to the confirmed cases of the total population was 56 percent for Wuhan, 64 percent for Daegu and 30 percent for Tokyo. The proportion of deaths from Covid-19 in each city to the total number of Covid-19 deaths in each country is 84 percent for Wuhan, 69 percent for Daegu and 25 percent for Tokyo. It may be worthwhile to explore the reason why one city in each country has been the major source of mass infection.

In China, delayed and controversial responses by Wuhan and Hubei authorities failed to contain the outbreak in its early stage. In addition, a company that did not acknowledge the seriousness of the coronavirus held a large party for 40,000 families in Wuhan on January 18 (Daum Portal 2020. 1.20). This may have triggered the rapid spread of the disease in Wuhan. Then, it spread to the whole of China.

In Korea, the daily number of confirmed cases increased by 20 on February 19, and then by 58 on February 20, giving a total of 346 confirmed cases. The sudden jump of the cases in Korea was mostly attributed to 'Patient No. 31', who attended a mass gathering at Shincheonji Church of Jesus in Daegu (Maeil Daily 2020.2.20). The Shincheonji Church of Jesus in Daegu became the main source of the mass infection in Korea. The Shincheonji Church is a cult, which claims that their founder Lee is the second coming of Jesus Christ and the disease spread among Shincheonji's members and thousands of others in Daegu.

In Japan, the Covid-19 pandemic can be divided into two waves based on genomic sequencing of Covid-19 virus samples obtained from Japanese patients (Yomiuri Newspaper, 2020.4.20). The Japanese National Institute of Infectious Diseases (NIID) indicated that the first wave of Covid-19 was derived from the Wuhan type. After entering Japan in January through travelers and returnees from China, the virus resulted in numerous infection clusters across the country. The first wave was followed by a second one that originated from a Covid-19 variant of the European type that was traced back to early patients from European countries. The NIID has established that majority of viral strains spreading in Japan since March is the European type.

Table 3.1 compares the selected statistics of Covid-19 in three countries. In terms of number of tests for Covid-19, China is much ahead of the two other East Asian countries. Even controlling for the size of the population, the same pattern is found. The number of tests per million in China (111,163) is much greater than the corresponding figures for Korea (62,012) and Japan (29,097). Strikingly, the number of tests in Japan is substantially smaller than those in China and Korea. This fact may imply that the efforts of Japan in controlling Covid-19 have fallen far behind those of China and Korea. Despite the smaller number of tests, however, the number of confirmed patients in Japan is much greater than in Korea. Korea also has markedly fewer deaths, both in absolute terms and per capita, than China and Japan.

Table 3.2 shows the proportions of confirmed patients and deaths by age group in China, Korea and Japan. This table indicates that the highest proportion of confirmed patients in China and Japan is among people aged 50–59, whereas the

TABLE 3.1 Comparison of selected statistics of Covid-19 in China, Korea and Japan

Country	*Number of tests*	*Number of tests per 1 million*	*Confirmed cases*	*Deaths*	*Death rate (%)*
China	160,000,000	111,163	86,601	4,634	5.35
Korea	3,180,496	25,864	36,915	540	1.46
Japan	3, 675,244	29,097	155,232	2,240	1.44

Source: www.worldometers.info/coronavirus/ (December 5, 2020).

Note: Death rate = Number of deaths/confirmed cases × 100 (%).

TABLE 3.2 Confirmed patients and deaths by age group in China, Korea and Japan (%)

Age group	*Confirmed patients*			*Deaths*		
	China	*Korea*	*Japan*	*China*	*Korea*	*Japan*
80+	3.2	4.2	10.0	20.3	50.5	56.6
70–79	8.8	8.1	9.7	30.5	32.6	25.3
60–69	19.2	15.9	11.3	30.2	10.7	10.9
50–59	22.4	18.4	16.6	12.7	4.8	4.0
40–49	19.2	13.3	15.9	3.7	0.9	2.0
30–39	17.0	12.3	14.7	1.8	0.5	0.5
20–29	8.1	19.8	16.0	0.7	0.0	0.0
10–19	1.2	5.5	2.3	0.1	0.0	0.0
0–9	0.9	2.5	1.6		0.0	0.0
Total	100.0 (44,672)	100.0 (24,988)	98.1 (15,382)	100.0 (1,023)	100.0 (4,39)	99.3 (557)

Sources: China: The Novel Coronavirus Pneumonia Emergency Response Epidemiology Team. The epidemiological characteristics of an outbreak of 2019 novel coronavirus diseases (Covid-19) in China. China CDC Weekly 2020. 2(8), 113–122; Korea: Korea Disease Control and Prevention Agency. Updates of Covid-19 in Korea, October 15, 2020; Japan: Ministry of Health, Labour and Welfare. Updates of Covid-19 in Japan, May 8, 2020.

proportion in Korea is highest among people aged 20–29. This statistic illustrates that Covid-19 does not follow the common-sense perception that older people are more vulnerable to contracting pneumonia-related disease. However, the death rates show a consistent pattern, as consistently increases with age with the small exception of that in China, the highest death rate is found among people aged 70–79 instead those aged 80 and over.

Control measures and factors affecting responses to Covid-19

Control measures for Covid-19 have differed substantially across the three countries. China took measures to block whole cities, including Wuhan and Beijing, and did not permit the entry of people from countries with active infections. The policy of a complete blockade of entire cities could be the most effective control measure for preventing the spread of the disease. The Korean government, however, did not ban the entry of people from China, the main source of the coronavirus, leading to the outbreaks that occurred in religious groups, logistics centers, clubs catering to foreigners in Itaewon, and so on. Nevertheless, the disease was relatively well controlled through a range of measures, especially the three T's (testing, tracking, and treatment) (Kwak 2020).

Japan refused the disembarking of infected travelers on a foreign cruise ship that was docked in Yokohama, and delayed the quarantine, because of concerns over the Tokyo Olympics, which were scheduled to be held in July 2020. In addition, as of April 7, Japan had only taken temporary emergency measures in seven metropolitan cities, including Tokyo, in the initial stage. On July 22, the Japanese government launched the 'Go Travel' campaign, a travel incentive policy aimed at supporting tourism, food, event industries and shops in order to recover from Covid-19, resulting in a secondary wave of mass infections, particularly among young people.

People tend to have different behavioral patterns in relation to accepting containment and mitigation polices for Covid-19. Several factors may explain the response patterns towards Covid-19 in East Asia. First, Confucianism as a way of life seems to have affected patterns of responding to Covid-19. Kang (2010: 91) stated:

> China as a hegemon- and its main philosophy, Confucianism, had a powerful effect on the rest of East Asian domestic and international politics, even while what it meant to be Chinese and how best to organize society and government was continually modified and debated within China itself.

Confucianism has emphasized group benefits more than individual interest and has been practiced as a way of life among Chinese people for more than 2,000 years. Confucianism spread to several Asian countries, including Korea and Japan. The degree to which the Confucian framework has been preserved, however, is different from country to country. In addition, the effects of Confucianism on the everyday life of the common people have somewhat changed in the process of the modernization in each country.

In mainland China, the Communist revolution may have weakened the influence of Confucianism on the people's character. In controlling Covid-19, the Chinese Communist regime adopted a complete lockdown policy in several cities. Complete lockdwon may be the most effective control measure for preventing the spread of Covid-19, but this approach may be permissible only in a Communist system. The Chinese Communist Party's strong leadership, which can transcend human rights issues, enabled the full blockade and control of social activities (Kwak 2020). Thus, the Communist regime may have played a bigger role than Confucianism in controlling Covid-19 in China.

Korea is perceived to have been relatively successful in controlling Covid-19 without a full-scale lockdown. This may be partially explained by the fact that

Confucian traditions remain strong in Korea. The Confucian emphasis on group benefits seems to have effectively worked in the three T's in Korea. However, in Japan, which has the weakest tradition of maintaining Confucian traditions in East Asia, the idea of pursuing group benefits did not seem to work in shaping the public response to Covid-19.

The next possible factor influencing the pattern of responses are institutional characteristics. In reviewing the salient institutional characteristics of each country, we may note that China has kept a system of party-oriented Sinocentrism, while Koreans have sought democratic collectivism through a series of political turmoil, and Japanese have practiced a 'manual culture' (without a manual, people do not act) and the *nemawashi* tradition (pre-negotiation system). Sinocentrism made it possible for Chinese leaders to conceal the Covid-19 outbreak in its early stage and delay of epidemic confirmation enabled its spread. Political actions, including the case of Li Wenliang, who was a whistleblower warned by Wuhan police, indicate the Chinese government's intention to conceal the Covid-19 outbreak. This led to international concern regarding China's responsibility for the spread of Covid-19.

As Korea has a coordinated market economy system (Lim 2018), the central government was able to establish close coordination among central and local governments as well as public-private cooperation and commitments by medical staff to implement pandemic prevention, detection and treatment. Korea's democratic collectivism also served as a basis for people following the rules of wearing masks and keeping physical distance. Even the general election in the middle of April in Korea went well without any problems. In Korea, members of the KCDC, not political leaders, took the main responsibility for directing control measures.

In Japan, the traditions of 'manual culture' and *nemawashi* hindered the Japanese people from quickly responding to the Covid-19 crisis. In Japan, political leaders interested in economic achievements approached the question of implementing quarantine measures based on the principle of allowing economic activity, and thus the Japanese people, who are obedient to their leadership and accustomed to a 'follow me', top-down, collectivistic culture, could not prevent the massive spread of the infection (Mizubayashi 2020). The Olympic Games were originally scheduled for August 2020 and it was vitally important to decide whether to hold this important event as scheduled or to postpone. The Abe government hesitated to make the decision, and thus Covid-19 began to quickly spead throughout Japan. In addition, Prime Minister Abe, instead of officials of the national public health authorities, tried to direct most of the control policies. The attitudes of governmental leadership towards Covid-19 turned out to be an important factor shaping the mitigation policies.

Other factors that affected responses to Covid-19 include medical systems and health insurance, the preparedness of public services and public awareness of Covid-19, given previous experiences with SARS and MERS. (SARS, a diserase caused by another coronavirus that in 2002 resulted in 5,317 patients and 349 deaths in mainland China.) Since the outbreak of SARS, Chinese government has reformed and continued to develop its medical security system (Kim and Chung 2018). MERS is a viral respiratory infection caused by the MERS-coronavirus. By June 27, 2015, 19 people in Korea died from this disease, with 184 confirmed cases of infection. Since the outbreak of MERS in Korea, the Korean quarantine system has been enhanced. In addition, KCDC concluded a memorandum of understanding with KSID (Korean Society of Infectious Diseases) in 2018 in order to improve the quarantine system, especially for preventing coronavirus diseases (KCDC Portal 2020.7.30). The experiences of SARS and MERS in China and Korea enabled those countries to respond promptly to Covid-19.

Population composition may be another important factor influencing the spread of Covid-19 and responses to the disease because the elderly are more vulnerable to the coronavirus. The proportion of the elderly population (aged 65 or older) in 2019 was 11.5 percent in China, 14.9 percent in Korea, and 28.0 percent in Japan (KNSO 2020). As shown in Table 3.2, Japan's high death rate (5 percent) may be partially explained by the high proportion of the elderly population. However, China's high mortality rate is difficult to explain given the low proportion of the elderly population. It seems that China's medical system has not yet developed sufficiently. Nonetheless, the relatively large number of tests in China may be explained by the high level of governance in the quarantine system.

Socioeconomic impacts of Covid-19

The Covid-19 pandemic has had far-reaching consequences beyond the spread of the disease itself. First of all, the impact on personal gatherings has been strong and local authorities often issued stay-at-home orders to prevent gatherings of any size in order to maintain physical distance. Conferences and events across the domains of technology, fashion and sports have also been canceled or postponed. Such gatherings have sometimes been replaced by teleconferencing, or with unconventional attempts to implement activities in a way that maintains physical distance.

The pandemic has affected educational systems worldwide, leading to widespread school closures. Religious activities have also been affected. Many churches and temples in Korea were forced to close because of Covid-19. Religious activities have been a strong focus of control measures by the Korean government because of the mass infection linked to the Shincheonji Church in Daegu at the beginning of the spread of the Covid-19. Many churches and temples have offered worship services through livestreams amidst the pandemic.

Economically, Covid-19 has caused a simultaneous shock of supply and demand. The closure of factories because of Covid-19 has induced supply shortages and reduced employment. Demand falls with less income and with constraints on shopping activities. With complex global value chains, world production fell sharply after the closure of factories in China.

The three East Asian countries, which have open economic systems with a heavy dependence on trade with foreign countries, greatly suffered from the pandemic (KDI 2020). Korea's industrial production index showed drastic changes: in the first quarter of 2020 it increased by 5.1 percent, while in the second quarter it fell by 5.1 percent year-on-year. The pattern was somewhat different in Japan and China. While Japan's industrial production in the first and second quarter of 2020 decreased by 4.4 percent and 19.7 percent respectively, that of China in the first quarter of 2020 fell by 7.6 percent but increased by 4.4 percent in the second quarter. In terms of exports, Korea's exports in the first and second quarter of 2020 fell by 1.4 percent and 20.3 percent year-on-year, while China's exports in the first half of 2020 fell by 24.3 percent and Japan's by 15.3 percent.

The unemployment rate also rose in the three countries because of factory closures and shorter operations. In Korea, the unemployment rate increased by 4.2 percent year-on-year in the second quarter of 2020, while that in Japan increased by 2.6 percent, and that in China by 6.4 percent year-on-year in the first half of 2020. According to the OECD's forecast, the projected 2020 growth rate is -1.2 percent for Korea, -2.6 percent for China and -6.0 percent for Japan (Kyungin Daily 2020.8.11).

During the period of the pandemic and even after that, the 'untact' (no-contact) economy will be normalized globally. Moreover, family ties will be strengthened as more work will be done at home and thus the time spent with family members will be longer. At the same time, domestic discord between spouses and among family members might also become worse than before the pandemic. Online delivery services such as Amazon will thrive. Society will thus be less open and less free.

Conclusion

This chapter compared response patterns to Covid-19 in China, Korea and Japan. It analyzed several factors affecting responses to Covid-19 as follows: Confucianism, institutional characteristics, medical systems, the preparedness of public services and public awareness of Covid-19, given previous experiences with SARS and MERS. Population composition is another important factor influencing patterns of infections and deaths from Covid-19. All the factors in this chapter may have complementary effects in shaping responses to Covid-19. Without a sophisticated method such as multiple regression analysis, it may not be possible to conclusively analyze the relative importance of each factor. Covid-19 is an extremely serious pandemic. The initial failure to block the entry of people from China is thought to be the biggest reason for the wide spread of Covid-19 in East Asia. Mass infections in religious organizations and nursing homes have been a major factor in increasing the number of infections. The outbreak of Covid-19 teaches us that a moment's carelessness can spark flare-ups of the disease.

This pandemic has already had a serious impact on the entire world. This situation may lead to a 'new normal', which we have never expected or experienced before. With border closings and tight control of the entry of people from other countries, the world may plunge into a 'dark age', as with the Black Death in the 14th century. Furthermore, the decoupling of financial markets from the real economy following major governments' increases in money supply and historically low interest rates will produce a bubble economy, where asset prices, including real estate, shoot up but the real sectors of the economy stagnate. This may lead to stagflation, as in the 1970s.

In Japan, there has been an explosive increase in the number of secondary infections. Since the beginning of August 2020, more than 1,000 patients have been diagnosed every day in Japan (Joongang Daily 2020.8.8). Other countries also have the latent possibility of secondary and tertiary infections of Covid-19. To prevent the further spread of the disease, and eventually to eliminate it, international cooperation is urgently needed, especially in East Asia.

References

Chosun Daily, Korea, 2020. 8.11.

Daum Portal, 2020.7.5.

Joongang Daily, Korea, 2020.8.8.

Kang, David, C. 'Civilization and state formation in the shadow of China,' in P. J. Katzenstein (ed.), *Civilizations in World Politics*. London: Routledge, 2010.

KDI Monthly Economic Trends, Korea Development Institute, August 2020.

Kim, B. C. and K. Chung. Social Security System in China (Korean). Seoul: Nanam Publishing Co., 2018.

Kim, Ik Ki. 'The Covid-19 and medical security system in China'. (Korean). *Philosophy and Reality* 125: 34–49, 2020.

KNSO (Korean national statistical Office) portal, Retrieved July 30, 2020.

Kwak, Rosung. Korea, China and Japan in the Corona 19 Prevention: Institutional Differences and the Effects (Korean), Column, E-Today Daily, June 1, 2020.

Kyungin Daily, Korea, 2020.8.11.

Lim, Hyun-Chin. 'How to Study Capitalism in Asia? A Theoretical and Methodological Consideration,' *Asia Review*, 7(2): 3–32, 2018.

Maeil Daily, Korea, 2020.2.20.

Nederveen Pieterse, Jan. 'Capitalism in East and West: A Comparative Perspective,' Paper presented at International Conference on 'Capitalism and Capitalisms in Asia: Origin, Commonality, and Diversity,' Seoul National University Asia Center, Seoul, Korea, October 22–23, 2015.

Sodei, Tamaki. 'Introduction', in T. Sodei and I. Kim (eds). Decline of Fertility and Population Aging in East Asia. Tokyo: International Longevity Center. 1996.

Worldometer. www.worldometers.info/coronavirus/country, December 5, 2020.

Yomiuri Newspaper, 2020.4.20.

4

INDIA, KERALA AND COVID-19

N.C. Narayanan and Prabhir Vishnu Poruthiyil

Deeply unequal societies fare low on most social parameters that matter to societal wellbeing. Covid-19 has shown that they do worse under pandemics. Existing inequalities are being aggravated while the situation of the vulnerable is rendered even more precarious. In societies where inequalities are compounded by the rise of far-right populism, the pandemic has become an opportunity to weaken or bypass the remaining institutions of democracy.

India is a multi-party polity with a federal system of governance with responsibilities distributed and overlapping between the national and provincial governments (henceforth Center and State). Health and law enforcement, for instance, are under the States' purview but which have to work under the guidelines set by the Center. The federal system in India was designed to provide unity of purpose at the level of national developmental goals while acknowledging the diversity of a large population spread over different geographies. In times of crises, however, the Center assumes the primary role. The signals that the Center sends are crucial when responding to national emergencies as key organizations such as the Ministry of Health and the Indian Council of Medical Research, National Disaster Mitigation Center (NMDC), Indian Railways, Airports Authority of India, are crucial to the management of crises like the pandemic.

In what follows we will describe the policy responses to Covid-19 by the Government of India run by a far-right and neoliberal coalition, the National Democratic Alliance (NDA). Using a comparative approach, we contrast the national policy response with one province, the South Western state of Kerala governed by a center-left coalition, the Left Democratic Front (LDF). The responses to the pandemic at national and sub-national levels are contrasted using three criteria – readiness, sensitivity to inequality and transparency in governance.

Such a comparison is methodologically viable as institutions of both the Center and the State are, on the one hand, embedded in constitutional constraints and consequences of a neoliberal political economy such as high inequality, privatization of essential services like health care, lack of welfare protections (Skocpol and Somers, 1980; Snyder, 2001). On the other, institutions are embedded in contexts with different socio-cultural histories, distinct combination of interest groups and unsynchronized electoral cycles. The political dimensions at the time of pandemic are also in stark contrast – while both coalitions have comfortable majorities, the NDA has four more years (having been re-elected in 2019) while the LDF is heading into elections (in 2021). After discussing the national and Kerala governance responses, the discussion section will analyze and compare the two experiences. Reversing decades of the trend towards decentralization of governance, the ascension of the NDA in 2014 had set in a process of centralization of power by the Center. The pandemic has accelerated this trend towards further concentration of powers at the center.

National policy response

Three features of policy response of the Center to the pandemic observed were its lack of (1) readiness, (2) sensitivity to inequalities and (3) transparency in governance. Each of these reveals a key feature of the Indian state. Only the first is a response to the pandemic. The others were already part of a neoliberal-authoritarian agenda; the pandemic merely provided an opportunity to push them through without the political resistance of normal times. The contrast between the delayed and ad-hoc nature of response to the pandemic, without considering the consequences for the poor, with the efficiency with which the neoliberal and authoritarian policies were made, when it benefited elite interests, is stark.

Readiness

Even acknowledging the unprecedented nature of the pandemic and the size of the country, the Center's response was delayed, uncoordinated and insufficient. Though the first cases were reported January, the lockdown was issued only by the end of March. During this period it took a number of U-turns on export of safety gear essential for health workers and different government ministries were giving conflicting signals on the seriousness of the pandemic (*The Caravan*, 2020). Even as the infectious nature of the virus was being reported, the Center went ahead with hosting a visit of the American President Donald Trump in February that involved huge crowds. When the decision to impose a lockdown was taken on March 24, it was sudden – with four hours' notice, the Center imposed a lockdown that was harsh in comparison to many other countries.

It appears that no consideration was given to the consequences for the poorer sections of the society – what studies of India's development trajectory had called is ugly 'underbelly' (Corbridge and Shah, 2013). Informality in Indian employment is well known to be as high as 90 percent. It is also known that most of these jobs are done by migrants from rural areas living on daily wages and staying in crammed conditions (Iyer, 2020). In one stroke, the Center shut off their sources of daily wages without providing any safety net, pushing many families into hunger and destitution (Center for Sustainable Employment, 2020). In India, economic inequality is compounded by ascripted identities that suffer graded discriminations. Even among the poor, the lowest socioeconomic and most discriminated categories – the uneducated, Muslims, underprivileged caste groups – suffered more (Bhalotia, Dhingra and Kondirolli, 2020).

The States where these migrants were located were as unprepared as the migrants. As migrants are not voters (their votes in their hometowns), local political parties and the administrative bureaucracy were under no pressure to respond to the catastrophe right under their noses. The better-off areas in the cities were either unconcerned with the suffering or were scared of getting infected if they ventured out to help. Many seasoned observers predicted food riots (Thapar, 2020). Facing starvation and mistreatment by the police, millions of urban migrants started making plans to return to their villages (Ellis-Peterson and Rahman, 2020). With the transport system not working, migrants chose to walk, cycle and hitch rides in trucks to villages hundreds of miles away from the cities. This phase is now called the 'migrant exodus'. The media reported gruesome experiences of migrants and clamor by civil rights groups forced their hand. The Center started special trains for inter-state movement of migrants, doubled food rations for the poor, made cash transfers to the poor and allocated more funds to employment guarantee schemes. Even this late response was cruelly insufficient, poorly delivered and a fraction of what was required (Ghosh, 2020, Lahoti et al, 2020).

Entrenching neoliberalism

While unable to foresee the suffering of migrants, the Center was alert to the concerns of corporate sector. Moratoriums of bank loans and payments were put in place before the lockdown (Vaishnav, 2020). A slew of privatization reforms followed for major sectors such as coal, power distribution and even defense and space, in addition to removing existing restrictions on market entry into the agriculture sector and removal of labor protections.

The government dismantled a number of protections of farmers and workers from the vagaries of market forces (*Scroll.in*, 2020b). The minimum support prices that allowed farmers leverage when negotiating prices with large corporate buyers were removed along with controls on hoarding of essential commodities by large corporations with huge warehouses (EPW Editorial, 2020a). A set of labor policies made strikes near impossible and allowed more companies to hire and fire workers without government approval (Madhavan, 2020).

The draft Environmental Impact Assessment (EIA) 2020 notification has attempted to dilute the existing provisions and failed to uphold either the State's constitutional duty or the citizen's fundamental right to a healthy environment (EPW Editorial 2020b). It freed many categories of projects from scrutiny, diluted the information needed for granting clearance, and limited the scope of the most important element to instill transparency-public engagement. The proposed change dilutes the rigors of many such requirements and reduces them to mere paper formalities. This would systemically weaken the decision-making framework and irreversibly threaten fragile ecosystems and the broader ecological balance (Dhar, 2020), but help 'growth' depleting nature and related livelihoods. New policies expand social security to informal workers (also acknowledging gig workers for the first time), but the overall policy goal is unmistakable in this statement: 'The ultimate goal of the government is to see India figure in top 10 nations in ease of doing business index of World Bank with completion of long-pending labour reforms' (quoted in *The Economic Times*, 2020).

Inhibiting transparency

When the parliament met after 174 days, the new rules did away with the 'question hour' when tough questions could be posed to the government (Roy, 2020). The pandemic was the ostensible reason given by the government, denying the opposition the venue to expose the mishandling of the crisis. Both the farm and labor policies were passed when the opposition was protesting outside the parliament against its undemocratic stance. The government has argued that there is nothing illegal about the procedures of either the suspension of opposition MPs or ignoring the boycott. For observers, the NDA's lack of concern for democratic propriety is an alarming disrespect for the opposition (EPW Editorial, 2020a).

Policies with far-reaching implications for the republic were rammed through parliament during the pandemic. Policies that severely curtail the work of civil society organizations in the country were enacted. The new laws limit administrative expenses to 20 percent. This upper limit is a death knell for policy-oriented think-tanks that employ professionals. The reason the government has given is corruption and misuse of funds among civil society organizations. But there are prevailing laws in the country to deal with corruption. The more plausible intention is to snuff out another source of dissent.

A fund called Prime Minister's Citizen Assistance and Relief in Emergency Situations (PM Cares) was created in the midst of the migrant exodus ostensibly to reduce the suffering of the poor. To date it has received close to USD300 million dollars from both public and private sectors (*Scroll.in*, 2020a). These include the corporate sector donations, public sector enterprises and salaries of government officials, including employees of public-funded universities. However, the Center, with the help of an increasingly subservient judiciary, has successfully kept the fund out of the purview of the Right to Information Act that ensures transparency.

To summarize, in the early stages, the Center was grappling with dysfunction and with multiple agencies often working at cross purposes. The indecision in the early stages was in striking contrast to the efficiency with which neoliberal and authoritarian policies were implemented in the later stages.

Kerala's welfare-oriented governance in response to Covid-19

Kerala's achievement of high human development in spite of low per capita incomes has received global recognition. This was a result of conscious interventions of resource redistribution, investments in welfare programs especially above the national average allocation on health and education with progressive political participation. Earlier studies summarized the mechanics, historical process and cultural specificities that resulted in concerted public action that made welfare a central concern of public policy. It was made possible by policies in education, especially female education, health care, universal immunization, family planning, land reform, competitive polity, public action and so on (Franke and Chasin, 1993; Isaac and Tharakan, 1995; Parayil, 1996; Dreze and Sen, 1997; George, 1998). The major argument put forward in this section is that Kerala's governance during the time of tackling the pandemic was based on normative ideas of compassion and care. Three features of Kerala's response to Covid-19 were Proactive, Sensitive, and Transparent.

Proactive

Kerala initiated preventive action by alerting district administration as early as late-January, soon after the World Health Organization issued warnings about the dangers of the pandemic. The government readied health officials in every district to be alert. Guidelines for laboratory tests, treatment, clinical observation, awareness campaigns and training of health professionals were prepared in collaboration with a panel of experts and shared with local officials (Government of Kerala, 2020a).

A unique advantage Kerala enjoys in comparison with other States in India is strong decentralized governance units at the lowest level of governance (Heller, 2020; Issac and Sadanandan, 2020). This is reflected in the public health care system with major focus on ensuring adequate infrastructure and personnel at the lowest level of governance. The LDF government that was elected in 2016 added 5,289 posts of hospital workers and doubled the investments from Rupees (Rs) 6290 million in 2014–15 to Rs 14190 million in 2018–19 through budgetary resources with an additional amount of Rs 22660 million raised through a special purpose vehicle to improve hospital infrastructure, leading to a dramatic rise in the use of government facilities, from 34 percent in 2014 to 48 percent in 2018 (Isaac and Sadanandan, 2020).

As a result, in spite of constraints on resources, Kerala adopted an aggressive testing, monitoring and surveillance strategy. Kerala has the highest population density (people per sq. km) in India and the inflow of residents of Kerala facing job losses from the Middle East and from other less managed hotspots in the rest of India has led to a surge in the number of cases. In spite of these conditions, the virus transmission rate Kerala's was 0.4 while the national rate was 2.6 (Issac, 2020). The State also reaped the benefits of decades of investments described above; recovery and mortality rates in Kerala were 0.5 percent, while the national averages were 11 and 2.6 percent (ibid.). Global media and other State administrations took note and recognized Kerala's response in these early months of pandemic as exemplary (Spinney, 2020).

Sensitive: ensuring governance with care and compassion

Political language can influence policy goals (Schneider and Ingram, 1993). The government's use of the label 'guest workers' had significant influence on commitments of the administration to ensure the welfare of migrant workers. The State administration, trade unions, NGOs, contractors, builders and Welfare Fund Board and local community groups coordinated the smooth delivery of food and ensured there were no evictions or other forms of harassment that migrants face in other parts of India. To enroll in camps and avail rations, guest workers did not have to show official unique identification number (UID, Aadhaar) or ration cards, but only provide their mobile phone number and a self-declaration. In a few instances, migrants raised grievances about inadequacies in camps. This has to be compared with the plight of migrant workers in other parts of India who, in the absence of supportive measures from the State, had to walk hundreds of kilometers to reach their homes, braving the consequences of 'illegality' of movement. Community kitchens were set up in the State under the aegis of Local Self-Government with the help of the wide network women self-help group *Kudumbasree* with a vision that no one should stay hungry. A total of 426 community kitchens have been functioning in 249 panchayats across 14 districts of the State with the funds to run them allocated to respective local self-governments. Another intervention with care was the government delivering midday meals to older persons living alone and underprivileged children in the 3-6 year age group who cannot get to preschools (*anganwadis*) at their home amidst lockdown (Sebastian, 2020).

Dealing with trauma during the pandemic: Perceiving that the new norms of life amidst pandemic can have huge repercussions in the mental health of people, a Psychological Support Team was instituted in the State. Counseling services were given to mentally ill patients, children with special needs, guest workers, senior citizens living alone and to alleviate stress of personnel working in corona outbreak control activities. Coordination with community-based de-addiction centers are made to support alcoholics (Government of Kerala, 2020b). Relief centers were established to rehabilitate destitute and homeless people in the State, benefitting 3,766 people. Kerala alone accounted for 68 percent of relief camps set up in India during lockdown, indicating how the crisis was handled through governance with care and compassion. Prisons set up special wards to isolate inmates showing symptoms.

A welfare package of Rs 200000 million was announced for economic revival that was highly inclusive as its primary focus is to provide relief to poor and vulnerable sections. The bulk of the financial package was frontloading the State's Financial Year 2021 spending to the initial three months, anticipating a severe demand slowdown in the immediate period after the Covid-19 outbreak. The emphasis was to immediately put cash in the hands of the people to revive the

State's economy, especially the rural economy, by implementing rural employment guarantee schemes. The loans provided through *Kudumbasree* ensured handing over money to the women to enable them to better control spending. The question that comes up here is the sustainability of such interventions in a State such as Kerala facing dire financial crisis compounded by a hostile central government (Isaac and Sadanandan, 2020).

Transparency and participation

The concerted efforts for disseminating information, maintaining transparency from the highest tier of the government, helped to instill credibility and trust in governance. Senior politicians gave daily press conferences to inform the public on the progression of the pandemic and the State response. These briefings were carried live on 6 pm prime time news by TV channels. Measures taken by the government that day and new issues raised by the media ensuring accountability and transparency in governance were discussed. These briefings helped generate trust in the administration and in turn facilitated voluntary compliance by the public to the lockdown norm. Participation was deepened by the involvement of a semi-formal network of accredited social health activist (ASHA) workers and the women's self-help group *Kudumbasree* with presence in each ward and neighborhood. Large groups of volunteers brought not only numbers but also functioned as an effective accountability mechanism of the local State and bureaucracy because of the involvement of people belonging to all political affiliations.

Such expectations of transparency did not emerge from a vacuum. Decades of building public consciousness and democratization of polity with a fiercely competitive political culture and vigilant media have contributed to conditioning the government to display a commitment to transparency. In Kerala there is a consensus on welfare among both leftist and centrist political coalitions in the State. The dominant political groups have contributed almost equally to the long struggles and public action that led to Kerala's development trajectory. As a result the welfare consensus could not be disrupted by a blatant neoliberal agenda.

Comparing policy responses

At the national level the weakening of the Indian National Congress (henceforth Congress) that had led the independence struggle created a growing political vacuum. Since the 1990s, the dominant trend was the rise of regional parties that helped to decenter power to the States. Since 2014, the rise of the right-leaning Bharatiya Janata Party (BJP), the main party of the NDA, the trend reversed towards the central government once again. Neoliberalization of India in its early stages was facilitated using 'stealth' (Jenkins, 2007). Political parties until recently were forced at least to pretend to care for the poor and for democratic norms. The muted and sporadic objection, and indeed the support for these policies among a significant section of the public is proof of the popularity of the blend of neoliberalism and far-right agendas. In implementing its neoliberal and authoritarian agenda, the Center's policymaking has been strikingly efficient.

As the virus was spreading, the government went ahead with a pre-planned visit of President Donald Trump at the end of February ('Namaste Trump'). During the event in a stadium with 10,000 people, Prime Minster Narendra Modi and Trump reasserted their strategic relations. Trump said: 'America loves India, America respects India and America will always be faithful and loyal friends to the Indian people' and boasted of defense deals worth USD3 billion. Within a few days after Trump's visit, public gatherings were to be avoided and compulsory screening of all international passengers was initiated. Opponents of the regime have alleged that the delayed response to the pandemic was to accommodate Trump's visit. If this is indeed the case, as political commentators suggested, this event reveals the similarities of two far-right populists who value spectacle above public health (Mudde, 2019).

The Center is culpable for not considering in advance the consequences of its decisions on the poorer sections of the society. Then it took more than a month of unnecessary suffering of the poor for a response to the consequences of its harsh and unplanned lockdown. Even this late response was cruelly insufficient and poorly targeted (Ghosh, 2020). To give an example, the amount the Center transferred was 500 rupees per month, which translates to four rupees per day, while the poverty line is 50 rupees per person per day in rural areas and 73 rupees in urban areas (Lahoti et al., 2020).

The enthusiasm with which pro-market goals were maintained even in the midst of the pandemic is clear evidence of the deep-seated commitment to neoliberalism. In addition to making it easier for the corporate sector to exploit farmers and workers, the extent of foreign investments even in defense projects was raised from 49 to 74 percent; quite remarkable for a political group that seeks to portray itself as the sole guardian of nationalist interests. In normal times, vociferous opposition may have created troublesome hurdles in parliament and on the streets. The pandemic created an opportunity so these policies were rammed through parliament without resistance.

The PM Cares fund that concentrated an astronomical fund for the Center has to be understood in the context of the newly implemented tax regime that reduces the independence of States to raise independent taxes to a few products (alcohol was one). The States are therefore far more dependent on the Center's approval for spending decisions. Borrowing limits are set by the Reserve Bank of India (with independence severely curtailed under the NDA), so are decisions to receive foreign funds for relief efforts (Dhaniyal, 2020). A basis for the State's agreeing to give up control under the new regime was the assurance that yearly shortfalls would be met by the Center. However, the pandemic led to massive reductions in tax collection as economic activity came to a standstill. When the States, reeling from additional expenses, demanded compensation due to them, the Center refused, claiming it was helpless against an 'act of god' and suggested the States borrow from the Reserve Bank of India instead (Ghosh, 2020). Furthermore, the Center placed additional restrictions on the corporate sector from contributing to the State government's response while receiving huge funds into the PM Cares fund (*Scroll.in.*, 2020a). This has to be contrasted with the resounding success of Kerala in the first three months of the pandemic. The State's response to citizen demands and proactive pursuit of a welfare agenda in an era of unfettered neo liberal governance is remarkable. The sensitive identification of vulnerable sections, devising mechanisms to cater to their needs, building institutional capacities within and outside the government system, were key welfare interventions.

In the fall of 2020, Kerala's government encountered a serious threat to its credibility when its senior officials were linked to illegal smuggling of gold into the country. And elections are around the corner. The opposition is alarmed by the public approval of the State in dealing with the pandemic. For the Hindu nationalist NDA ruling the Center, Kerala is the only province in the country without an elected representative. As many as six national investigating agencies are now focusing on the state government for involvement in the smuggling.

The entire opposition has pounced on this issue and is waging regular street battles and protests marches, ignoring social distancing norms. The media, driven by corporate interests, are fueling antagonisms; representatives of different parties hurling accusations against each other offer more profitable spectacles for prime-time TV than dour reporting on the progression of the pandemic. This leads to loosening the vigilance created earlier and affects the morale of health workers and volunteers. Fatigue from continuous work pressure and an increasing number of cases are adding to fragility of the State's response. Despite these challenges, the mortality rate in Kerala remains the lowest in the country. It is doubtful whether Kerala's 'care and compassionate-oriented governance' can be sustained much longer: because of central fiscal policies. Whether the existing infrastructure that is struggling to cope can meet the demand when the pandemic peaks is uncertain. The financial burden is mounting; the State resorted to opening alcohol outlets as it is one of the few remaining sources of taxes over which Center has limited control. Without central government assistance or permissions to borrow, it will be difficult to sustain the scale of interventions.

The comparison above points to the need for an urgent rethink of the neoliberal understanding of health services as a commodity in the context of inequalities. The experience of Kerala shows how even in the peak of economic reform in India, it is possible to keep and deepen healthcare as a public good.

References

Bhalotia, S., Swati Dhingra, S., and Kondirolli, F. (2020). City of Dreams no More: The Impact of Covid-19 on Urban Workers in India, Center for Economic Performance, https://cep.lse.ac.uk/pubs/download/cepcovid-19-008.pd (accessed August 2020).

Center for Sustainable Employment (2020), Covid-19 Livelihoods Survey, https://cse.azimpremjiuniversity.edu.in/wp-content/uploads/2020/06/Compilation-of-findings-APU-Covid-19-Livelihoods-Survey_Final.pdf (accessed August 2020).

Corbridge, S. & Shah, A. (2013). Introduction: The Underbelly of the Indian Boom. *Economy and Society*, 42(3), 335–347.

Dhaniyal, S. (2020). What Does the Covid-19 Crisis Tell Us About GST's defects? *Scroll.in*, https://scroll.in/article/print/965718 (accessed August 2020).

Dhar, Preeta (2020). Draft EIA Notification, 2020: Institutionalising Information Blind spots. *Economic and Political Weekly*, 55(28–29), 20.

Dreze, J. and A. Sen (1997) *Indian Development: Selected Regional Perspectives*. UNU/WIDER Studies in Development Economics, Delhi: Oxford University Press.

Economic Times, (2020). Labour Reforms Intend to Put India among Top 10 Nations in Ease of Doing Business, https://economictimes.indiatimes.com/news/economy/policy/labour-reforms-intend-to-put-india-among-top-10-nations-in-ease-of-doing-business/articleshow/78257939.cms?utm_source=contentofinterest&utm_medium=text&utm_campaign=cppst (accessed September 2020).

Ellis-Petersen, H. and Rahman, S.A. (2020). 'I just Want to Go Home': The Desperate Millions Hit by Modi's Brutal Lockdown, *The Guardian*. www.theguardian.com/world/2020/apr/04/i-just-want-to-go-home-the-desperate-millions-hit-by-modis-brutal-lockdown (accessed August 2020).

EPW Editorial (2020a), Bills of Contention. *Economic and Political Weekly*, 55(39), 26 September.

EPW Editorial (2020b), Review of EIA Notification, *Economic and Political Weekly*, 55(25), 20 June.

Franke, R.W. and B.H. Chasin (1993) *Life is a Little Better: Redistribution as a Development Strategy in Nadur Village Kerala*. Boulder: Westview Press.

George, K.K. (1998). 'The Kerala Model of Development: A Debate (Part 2)', *Bulletin of Concerned Asian Scholars*, 30(4), 35–40.

Ghosh, J. (2020) Indian Economy Was Rolling Down a Hill: With Covid-19, it's Falling Off a Cliff. QZ. https://qz.com/india/1830822/coronavirus-may-push-indias-struggling-economy-off-the-cliff/ (accessed September 2020).

Ghosh, K. (2020). Erosion of Fiscal Federalism in the Times of Covid-19: The Hindu Business Line. www.thehindubusinessline.com/opinion/erosion-of-fiscal-federalism-in-the-times-of-covid-19/article31670568.ece (accessed September 2020).

Government of Kerala (2020a) Corona guidelines, Department of Health and Family Welfare, Government of Kerala, 26 January 2020, http://dhs.kerala.gov.in/wp-content/uploads/2020/03/ncorona_26012020-1.pdf (accessed August 2020).

Government of Kerala (2020b). Kerala Epidemics Disease Covid-19 Regulations, Health & Family Welfare Department, Government of Kerala, 10 May 2020, http://dhs.kerala.gov.in/wp-content/uploads/2020/05/Daily-Bulletin-HFWD-English-May-10.pdf (accessed August 2020).

Heller, P. (2020). A Virus, Social Democracy, and Dividends for Kerala, *The Hindu*, 18 April.

Isaac, T.M.T. and P.K.M Tharakan (1995) Kerala – the Emerging Perspectives: Over (1–3), 4–36.

Isaac, T.M.T. and R. Sadanandan (2020). Covid-19, Public Health System and Local Governance in Kerala, *Economic and Political Weekly*, 55(23), 35–40.

Iyer, M. (2020) Migration in India and the Impact of the Lockdown on Migrants, *PRS India*, www.prsindia.org/theprsblog/migration-india-and-impact-lockdown-migrants (accessed September 2020).

Jenkins, R. (2007). Political Skills: Introducing Reforms by Stealth. In *India's Economic Transition: The Politics of Reforms*, ed. Rahul Mukherji, New Delhi: Oxford University Press, 170–201.

Lahoti, R., Bhasole, A., Abraham, R., Kesar, S. and Nath, P. (2020). Hunger Grows as India's Lockdown Kills Jobs: Results of a Survey from 12 States, *The India Forum*. www.theindiaforum.in/article/hunger-grows-india-s-lockdown-kills-jobs (accessed September 2020).

Madhavan, (2020). Dilution Without Adequate Deliberation: On Labour Laws. *PRS Online*, www.prsindia.org/media/articles-by-prs-team/dilution-without-adequate-deliberation-labour-laws (accessed August 2020).

Mudde, C. (2019). *The Far Right Today*. London: John Wiley & Sons.

Parayil, G. (1996). The Kerala Model of Development: Development and Sustainability in the Third World, *Third World Quarterly*, 17(5), 941–957.

Roy, C. (2020). What A Parliament Session Without Question Hour Would Mean. *Bloomberg Quint*, www.bloombergquint.com/opinion/what-a-parliament-session-without-question-hour-would-mean (accessed September 2020).

Schneider, A. and Ingram, H. (1993). Social Construction of Target Populations: Implications for Politics and Policy, *American Political Science Review*, 87(2), 334–347.

Scroll.in (2020a). PM CARES Fund received Rs 2,105 crore from government firms' CSR initiatives, reports Indian Express, https://scroll.in/latest/970764/pm-cares-fund-received-rs-2105-crore-from-government-firms-csr-initiatives-reports-indian-express (accessed September 2020).

Scroll.in (2020b). Parliament: Monsoon Session ends, Rajya Sabha passes 15 bills in last 2 days amid Opposition boycott. https://scroll.in/latest/973911/parliament-monsoon-session-ends-rajya-sabha-passes-15-bills-in-last-2-days-amid-opposition-boycott (accessed September 2020).

Sebastian, M. (2020). This Photo is Winning Kerala Government Praise for its Coronavirus Response, *Huffington Post*, www.huffingtonpost.in/entry/kerala-coronavirus-midday-meals-gokdirect_in_5e6b18fbc5b6dda30fc65c6d (accessed September 2020).

Skocpol, T. & Somers, M. (1980). The Uses of Comparative History in Macrosocial Inquiry. *Comparative Studies in Society and History*, *22*(2), 174–197.

Snyder, R. (2001). Scaling Down: The Subnational Comparative Method. *Studies in Comparative International Development*, *36*(1), 93–110.

Spinney, L. (2020). The coronavirus slayer! How Kerala's rock star health minister helped save it from Covid-19, *The Guardian*, May 14.

Thapar, K. (2020). Coronavirus Lockdown: 'Food Riots Are a Very Real Possibility,' Says Pronob Sen, *The Wire*, https://thewire.in/food/pronob-sen-karan-thapar-coronavirus-food-riots (accessed September 2020).

Vaishnav. A. (2020). Central Government's Response to the Covid-19 Pandemic (May 23–May 29, 2020), *PRS India*, www.prsindia.org/theprsblog/central-government's-response-covid-19-pandemic-may-23-may-29-2020 (accessed August 2020).

Vijayan, P. (2020). Challenges in the Midst of Covid-19 Pandemic', *Economic and Political Weekly*, 55(24), 13 June.

5

NEPAL AND COVID-19[1]

Ratna Mani Nepal

Developing countries are experiencing major shocks as the Covid-19 pandemic continues. The challenges for developing countries do not just stem from the increasing number of confirmed cases and deaths, but are also related to concerns about economic and political stability. In most countries public health has never been a substantial issue in electoral politics, but Covid-19 brings it to the fore of political discourse. This chapter presents an account of Nepal's experience in coping with Covid-19. This low-income developing country[2] represents a special case, in that it lies between China, where the virus appeared first, and India, which tops the list of developing countries in the number of cases. The case of Nepal is also noteworthy due to the government's response, which exacerbated the crisis.

Nepal's first case was detected in the third week of January in a migrant student from Wuhan, China. Widespread infection began only in late March when migrant workers from India started crossing the porous border, returning to their homes. In the face of a growing crisis, the government's initial responses were praiseworthy, and included border controls and lockdowns.[3] However, as migrant workers continued to arrive, from India especially, a constant increase of Covid-19 cases was not accompanied by a commensurate response. An inadequate number of holding centers, quarantine facilities, and testing equipment in hospitals further aggravated the crisis. Why could the government not continue the pace of its initial response? What led to its inadequate response in the later period? As the pandemic spread, government responses were mostly ill-informed short-term emergency measures that tended to lack perspective.

Nepal can be categorized as a state-led market economy (SME) (Nederveen Pieterse, 2018; Xing and Shaw, 2013). The county's largely agricultural economy was controlled by the King and his loyalists for about two and half centuries, and a small modern industrial sector also received the palace's patronage (International Commission of Jurists 1996; Pandey 2009). Protectionist policies adopted during the Panchayat period had supported the state's interests (Pyakuryal 2016). However, since 1990, free market ideology has guided the country's economic policies and long-established political-social institutions have gradually adjusted to increasingly powerful market forces. In this transition the country saw a gradual rise of powerful elites who exert influence over real estate, education, health, service and agriculture sectors (Adhikari 2008). Resource extractive groups have also gained influence in the economy. The impact of economic liberalization and privatization is today reflected in the low supply of services such as public transportation, accessible public healthcare and free higher education.

Different market economies have responded to the Covid-19 crisis disproportionately (Fukuyama 2020). This chapter narrates what the Covid-19 crisis reveals in Nepal's political and economic institutions. To what extent have they proven effective to contain the virus and its consequences? This chapter contextually analyzes preparedness, governance and leadership as well as societal perceptions of migrant workers. Next, the chapter analyzes the country's public health and economic capacities.

Covid-19 cases and preparedness

Nepal's preliminary response to the Covid-19 outbreak started in the final week of January. On January 22, *Gorkhapatra*, the official national daily newspaper reported about the n-SARs Cov 2 virus outbreak in Wuhan, China, and the Chinese agencies warning Nepal to be aware and alert of the possible outbreak. A day later, on January 23, the first Covid-19 case was detected in a student who had returned from Wuhan. After the first case appeared in Kathmandu, the capital city, the government took rapid action to prepare for an outbreak. By January 27 the Prime Minister organized cabinet-level discussions about the management of isolation wards in public hospitals in Kathmandu and had taken action to establish health checks at the international airport and border points.

Despite an initially low number of cases, the government maintained a substantial degree of preparedness. The Ministry of Health and Population organized training programs for transportation workers, nurses and ambulance drivers. Some local governments and police officers also organized Covid-19 awareness campaigns in different parts of the country (*Gorkhapatra* 2020a). In addition, 180 Nepalese students stranded in Wuhan were repatriated on February 17 (*Gorkhapatra* 2020b). The formation of a High-Level Coordination Committee (HLCC) at the beginning of March further demonstrated a high level of political commitment to contain the outbreak. This committee, comprised of cabinet ministers and top bureaucrats, was headed by the Deputy Prime Minister and was responsible for organizing Covid-19 responses at the central as well as local levels. This committee further extended its reach to provincial and district levels and delegated responsibilities to local bodies.

The HLCC approved considerable policy measures, including restrictions on all forms of gatherings, national and international flights, and visa issuances. Public hospitals across the country were designated as 'Covid-19 treatment special hospitals'. The committee also organized a series of conferences, inviting concerned stakeholders, including political parties in parliament, to forge a national consensus. There was very little political opposition concerning Covid-19 crisis management. Meanwhile, the federal government provided financial support to provincial and local governments, which they could spend on holding zones, quarantine centers and related activities. Nepal received assistance from China, India, Germany and international agencies such as the World Bank, World Health Organization (WHO) and United Nations (United Nations/Nepal 2020). In April, the WHO which had identified Nepal as a potential risk zone praised the government for its handling of the Covid-19 crisis.

In the third week of March, these processes were followed by the establishment of a fund worth NPR500m to fight Covid-19. On March 23, two months after the first case was identified, a second Covid-19 case was confirmed, and the next day, March 24, the government executed a nationwide lockdown order, a major response to cope with a potential outbreak. The lockdown lasted for four months and ended on 21 July. After three weeks, various districts issued an additional order to respond to surprising increases in detections. The government concurrently decided to involve private hospitals in Covid-19 treatment and to increase testing capacity in different provinces. (See Figure 5.1.)

The country's preparedness measures were first called into question at the beginning of April, which saw an exponential rise of cases. This trend continued, reaching 1,572 total cases by the end of May. Death rates continued to grow even during lockdown with 29 Covid deaths in June and 56 in July. By the end of December, Nepal had 238,861 total confirmed cases, 14, 255 active cases and 1,567 deaths.

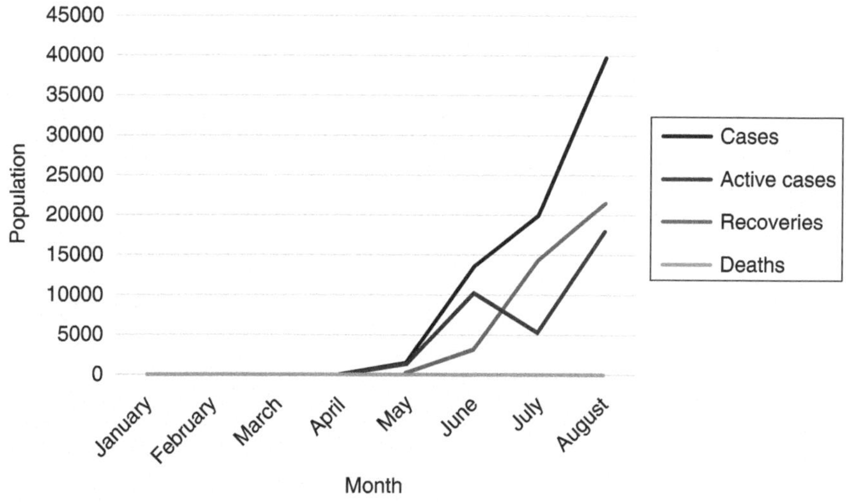

FIGURE 5.1 Covid-19 trends in Nepal

Source: Worldometer.info, 31 August 2020.

With cases surging, the majority government[4] seemed weak and faced growing public distrust. The spread of the virus called into question not only the effectiveness of the state but also the coping strategies implemented by state actors. Why did preparedness measures fall flat?

Governance and leadership: the crisis accelerator

The Covid-19 responses adopted by states are shaped by governance institutions and leadership (Duflo and Abhijit 2020, Fukuyama 2020, Weyl and Rajiv 2020). Nepali governance and leadership have often been defensive and lack legitimacy due to a stretched political transition that the country has endured since 1950. Conservative forces shut down attempts to adopt progressive institutional measures.[5] The first modern court was founded in 1952 and after the first general election was held in 1958, the country waited for more than three decades for the second. This long period was characterized by bureaucratic autocracy under the patronage of the King. The bureaucracy itself was developed by the King's cronies (Nepal 2013, Pandey 2009). This system continued to influence governance and leadership even with economic reforms in the 1990s. Since the first elected government took power, political coalitions have been weak and parties tend to practice clientelism (Gyawali 2018). Democratic leadership failed to escape entrenched bureaucratic conservatism.[6] Free market ideology introduced in this period further corrupted institutions and governance. Government actors often bypassed formal institutions and adopted short-sighted contingencies.[7] As a result the government distanced itself from the public. Lack of a developmental outlook, short-term political gain and corruption have damaged leaderships' image (Gyanwaly 2018). The handling of the Covid-19 crisis has profiled these features.

Government responses seemed more like 'contingency policy measures' than prospective and studied strategies. For example, the state decided to set up 'health desks' at airports and border points, despite planning more extensive health facilities. The health desk policy failed to detect Covid-19 cases entering from porous border points. The HLCC then directed local governments to manage holding centers and quarantine posts targeting migrant workers from India, without providing adequate equipment or resources. Further, the central government did not release financial support it had committed to local bodies until the four months of the lockdown were over.[8] With the rise of migrant workers entering the country, quarantine practices were overwhelmed. Local governments let people in quarantine simply walk to their homes, contributing towards community transmission of Covid-19.

This demonstrates a weak implementation of policy measures; frail governance marred the institutional response. For example, the lockdown could not control the movement of the public from one district to another, because the lockdown was ordered without early warning. Hence, thousands of migrants and non-local workers were stranded in cities when the lockdown was levied. Because of the continued lockdown and loss of jobs, they were compelled to simply walk back to their hometowns, often over large stretches of territory. Security personnel detained these migrants in some places while in other places, local governments guided them to their destinations. Both practices violated the lockdown law. Moreover, both central and local governments issued the 'entry pass policy' targeting those who needed to travel for emergency reasons. However, this privilege was monopolized by those who were close associates of the chair of local governments, parliamentarians and ministers in provincial and central governments.[9] Thousands traveled across the country even during the lockdown. This violated the principles of lockdown and exacerbated the Covid-19 situation.

Disobedience is punishable according to the law (The Infection Disease Act 1964, on the basis of which lockdown orders were issued), but implementation was so weak that security personal let violators go with brief warnings. If serious punishments were applied, they would often result in fierce opposition from political leadership. Indeed, public understanding of the disease seemed low. Many did not take lockdown seriously and did not abide by it. A study conducted by Nepal Health Research Council (NHRC) found that a quarter of public did not use masks in Kathmandu Valley, where population density is highest (population per square kilometer is 20,288).[10] Of those who wore masks, a quarter did not use them appropriately. Social distancing was also not followed as per the recommendation.

Downplaying the Covid-19 crisis and its use for political benefit have been present since the early response. Early in February, ministers confidently announced that they would not let the virus into the country. The secretary of the Ministry of Health claimed that Nepal was safe from the virus outbreak due to effective preparation. Later, the Prime Minister offered an inconsistent but conservative perception of the virus and its possible cure; he incorrectly predicted that Nepal's climate was unfavorable to Covid-19, Nepali's immunity power was high and indigenous herbal products such as turmeric and hot water could cure the sickness. He denied the number of deaths declared by the Ministry of Health and Population as caused by Covid-19, assuring that those deaths were caused by other critical diseases (TKP, Editorial 2020). The Prime Minister's response thus distracted from necessary actions to contain the virus.

Leadership not only distorted institutions but also played a nationalistic political game to conceal the weakness of preparedness measures, thereby further deepening the crisis. In the first week of May, India unofficially inaugurated a road passing through Nepal to Tibet, China's autonomous region. Then, fanning the flames of nationalism, the Prime Minister made a series of statements against India, demonstrating 'Machiavellian traits' (Wagle 2020). Turning towards political distractions rather than Covid-19 crisis management, the state published a new political map of the country that incorporated contested territories along the western border which both India and Nepal have long claimed as their own. By blaming India for increased Covid-19 cases due to an increasing number of migrant workers from India, Nepalese leadership weakened the country's international standing. The Prime Minister also blamed national mainstream media, social media users and civil society actors for not supporting the government's efforts to cope with the

Covid-19 crisis (Ghimire 2020). Indeed, a coordination failure among concerned stakeholders contributed towards governance failure.

Nepal's poor performance was exacerbated by acts of contingency institutions which complicated the usual role of state institutions. For example, the formation of the High-Level Coordination Committee (HLCC) by cabinet decision contradicted the functions of the National Emergency Coordination Committee (NECC) formed as per the Disaster Risk Reduction Act 2017. Ironically, the latter has provincial- and district-level committees responsible for coordinating actions related to both natural and non-natural disasters. A separate unit within the Ministry of Health called Health Emergency and Disaster Management Unit is actually chaired by the Minister for Health and is specifically designed to respond to a public health crisis. The new committee's policies contradicted and even obstructed the operations of the existing institutions. Why so many committees? In April the HLCC was itself a victim of contingency when another committee, the Covid-19 Control and Management Committee (CCMC), was formed, recruiting the chairman and other members from the HLCC.

Weak governance and weak institutions enable elite capture (Nederveen Pieterse 2018: 94). The committee approach led skeptics to believe that the government acted under the pressure of non-state actors that sought to control Covid-19 crisis management and procurement.[11] The committees broke the chain of command from the center to the local level, wasted resources and distorted the flow of information regarding the crisis. The decision to form new committees also turned a blind eye to constitutional decentralization that devolves power to local governments to apply necessary measures to maintain public health (GoN 2018). In sum, the contingency policies that prevailed over government institutions derailed the state's performance.

Migrant workers: a new low caste

In Nepal, caste has long been a major source of social stigma. The Covid-19 crisis led conservative society to encounter a *new low caste* – migrant workers. Amid the lockdown, the Indian government transported thousands of returnees to the Indian side of the Nepal-India border. Due to a lack of quarantine centers, Nepal hesitated to let them into the country. They were stranded along the border, foodless, shelterless, and without proper hygiene and safety measures. The Prime Minister advised them not to cross the border until the state could complete its preparations.[12] However, an increasing number of migrant workers entered the underprepared society, adding fear and furor. Some of the workers even risked their lives as they tried to swim across the border to their home country.

On May 18, Prime Minister KP Sharma Oli, who was already dissatisfied with India due to border issues, referred to the migrant workers as an *Indian virus*. He believed that coming from India, they were causing the Covid-19 outbreak in Nepal. According to Oli, the *Indian virus* was harder to contain than the comparatively mild Chinese and Italian viruses (Bill and Sapkota 2020). His statements promoted a sense of suspicion about incoming migrant workers. As Covid-19 cases increased with the entry of migrant workers, this suspicion was soon converted into hate. People did not let migrant workers eat and drink at restaurants and hotels. Villagers did not welcome migrants into their homes, and shopkeepers hesitated to take money from them when they sought to purchase food. In many cases, they were stopped from even entering villages. In quarantine centers and hospitals, many migrants were also mistreated (Adhikari 2020). Social stigma also extended to frontline health workers, Covid-19 infected and ambulance drivers. Some were even stopped from visiting their homes and apartments. In Kathmandu, people threw stones in a home where doctors were isolated.

The government treated migrant workers differently depending on class. Migrant workers from India were often suspected as virus carriers and were placed in quarantine (Puri 2020). The majority of these migrants work in unregistered informal sectors such as agriculture and hence send a relatively low volume of remittances. Workers from higher-wage countries received more attention. Earlier in February, for example, the government merrily chartered flights to bring back 180 students and workers from Wuhan.

Initially, Nepal showed apathy towards bringing people back from abroad, beyond India, as it lacked adequate quarantine facilities. When the number of workers wanting to come back to the country soared, the government issued a guideline, according to which most returnee workers had to pay for their own plane fare and 14 days of hotel quarantine costs.[13] According to the guidelines, only those migrant workers with valid labor permits and proof that their employers or host country were not paying for their airfare would be considered for free-of-charge repatriation. These guidelines violated the provision of the Foreign Employment Fund, which was supposed to be mobilized to bring workers back (Prasain and Mandal 2020). The government did not implement the Supreme Court's order that the fund be used for this purpose.

Unequal distribution of health services

Nepal's public health system clearly posed a challenge to government efforts to contain the pandemic. Underfunded, unequally distributed and limited health services constrained crisis coping strategies. Public investment in healthcare is low. At 1.8 percent of GDP in 2018/19, public health investment has only increased by 0.4 percent since 2014/15 (MoF 2019). This figure is far behind the universal standard of about 5 percent (Savedoff 2003). The health budget as a percentage of the national budget has been constant since 2014, at about 5 percent. Per capita health expenditures stand at US$5.8, a pointedly low figure. Doctors and nurses per 1,000 population are 0.67, which is significantly less than the WHO recommendation of 2.3 doctors, nurses and midwives per 1000 population (MoHP 2013: ii).

The government decided to develop hospitals as special Covid-19 treatment hospitals, but they quickly experienced equipment shortages. In addition, a lack of trained health workers complicated testing and response capacity (Poudel 2020a).

Low healthcare budgets mean low investment in health facilities and services, which further means a low number of RT-PCR tests. Until late August, total Covid-19 tests were 9, 4802, which means 30973 per million/population (Worldometers. info).

Private spending in the health sector has rapidly expanded, and today more than two-thirds of hospitals and nursing homes are privately owned, comprising more than 60 percent of the nation's doctors. Public use of private health centers is higher than of public health institutions and out-of-pocket healthcare expenses have been rising (Belay and Tondon 2015). The majority of the country's health system now operates in the private sector, in large part due to economic liberalization and privatization policies adopted in the 1990s.

Despite the possibility of fruitful engagement with the private health sector, private health services were not properly mobilized to cope with the Covid-19 pandemic. Private institutions too seemed reluctant, because Covid-19 cases could impact their 'health business' by spreading fear among the public, affecting revenues from regular services (Poudel 2020b). In mid-August, the government urged private hospitals to allocate 20 percent of beds for Covid-19 patients. However, the private sectors did not oblige, and the government had to issue a new order for the infected to be isolated at home.

It seems therefore that crisis management is more about facility arrangement than capacity. This is linked to the uneven distribution of health facilities across the regions. Related to Nepal's geographic diversity, only 61.8 percent of the population has access to health facilities within half an hour (CBS 2017), a number that varies greatly across the rural/urban divide. This means that many people need to travel far to visit health centers for a Covid-19 test. Lack of road connectivity and awareness in the rural regions has considerably affected government efforts of mass testing (Kathayat 2020). One of the coronavirus safety measures is frequent hand-washing with soap. Yet, only 47 percent of households use soap and water for hand-washing while 20 percent lack such facilities (CBS 2017). Province No. 2 where population density and average household size are the highest among the provinces (CBS 2019), has been hardest hit by the Covid-19 pandemic. This province contains just three RT-PCR testing laboratories and 13 public hospitals, which is low in comparison to the facilities in other provinces (Table 5.1).

Elite capture has also played a role in Nepal's plight. Early in March, the HLCC canceled due process procedures of health equipment procurement and made a fast-track decision to offer the procurement contract to 'Omni Group'. The private company, inexperienced in the health sector, is believed to be a supporter of the Prime Minister. The low-quality equipment that the company imported left health institutions facing shortages. The government has since decided to involve the Nepalese Army in procurement processes. This demonstrates a lack of effective decision-making and exposes rent-seeking behavior among authorities. On another occasion, despite the poor validity of the rapid diagnostic test (RDT) to confirm the Covid-19 virus, the government continued to purchase these comparatively low-quality tests. The cost of the more accurate RT-PCR

TABLE 5.1 Covid-19 and socioeconomic indicators by Provinces (31 August, 2020)

Provinces	*Deaths per cases (percentage)*	*Pop. density (people/km²)*	*HDI*	*Public hospital*	*No of RT-PCR testing labs*	*GDP per capita (US$)*
Province no 1	0.77	175	0.5	18	4	733
Province no 2	0.85	559	0.42	13	3	570
Bagmati	0.95	272	0.54	33	22	1094
Gandaki	0.56	112	0.51	15	2	760
Province no. 5	0.45	219	0.47	20	6	611
Karnali	0.16	41	0.43	12	4	475
Sudurpaschim	0.15	130	0.43	14	3	474

Source: MoHP 2020 (author's calculation).

Note: Deaths per cases = $\frac{total\ deaths}{total\ cases} \times 100\%$.

tests was higher, in part because of quality control measures for equipment and reagents, but critics believe that the government's decision was a result of pressure from the test's suppliers.[14] In any case, the diminishing capacity of the government to control the pandemic has been constrained by the increasing control of business elites in the health sector.

Economy: limitations and implications

In 2019, Nepal's GDP was US$29.813 billion (MoF 2019). One-third of this figure comes from remittances, the hardest hit sector by the Covid-19 pandemic, and the country is expected to lose remittances by 28.7 percent in 2020. Due to the cumulative effect of the crisis, the economy may shrink by 5.2 percent (UNDP 2020). Indeed, in the middle of the pandemic, revenue generation was only a third of total expenditures.[15] Hence, the economy will remain a challenge even during the post-Covid-19 period. But does only the economy matter? Was financial scarcity the only cause of ineffective response to the crisis and an increasing number of Covid-19 cases? Questions about economic behavior, procurement, expenditure, accountability, and transparency are interconnected.

An incommensurate return on a relatively expensive investment can be in part attributed to the 'committee approach' of the Covid-19 response. Not a single member of the committees, from the central level to the local level, rejected the 'meeting allowance' as well as reimbursement for transportation costs. Many ministers and high-level bureaucrats bought luxurious vehicles during the pandemic. Some provincial and local governments hiked their salaries. Reports of misuse of funds surfaced out from both central and local governments (Kantipur Daily 2020). Lack of transparency regarding the use of the Covid-19 crisis management fund (worth NPR 500 million) incited protests in the streets against the government. During the pandemic, transparency and accountability could have helped overcome resource scarcity by building broader coalitions and increasing trust in the government, but Nepal failed to forge these conditions.

At the end of March, the ministry of finance and the central bank announced relief packages. The packages did not contain household support of cash transfers or unemployment benefits, nor did they offer support to informal sector workers who were hit hardest by the pandemic. Rather, the packages seemed to primarily support the banking sector, big-debtors, and business elites.[16] For small entrepreneurs, the jobless and daily-wage people, the relief packages were meaningless. A study conducted amid the lockdown found that the policy had its greatest economic impact on street vendors, small shopkeepers and other small and micro-enterprises (UNDP 2020). Emerging shopping malls across the country were less affected and actually operated longer hours during the lockdown.

Covid-19 has disproportionately affected regions with low development performance (see Table 5.1). There has been a significant relation between per capita income and death per cases.[17] For example, Bagmati province had highest GDP per capita income and lowest death per cases. Conversely, the highest death per case was calculated in Karnali province, where GDP per capita is the lowest. Thus, poverty has been a major contributor to both virus spread and death. Perhaps the gravest impact of this crisis has been the stagnation of the country's underdeveloped economy.

Conclusion

Public health crises are hard to manage and are even more critical for developing countries that lack economic and political leverage. Underdevelopment is a major contributor to the Covid-19 crisis but was not the sole factor behind Nepal's diminishing performance. The deepening crisis exposed lapses in the system and was marred by contingency policies that worked to undermine established rules and protocols, limiting their effectiveness on the ground. Institutions and governance in Nepal are weak, the result of Nepal's complex political history, economic liberalization policies and a long history of feudal capture. As such, leadership is largely unresponsive to the masses, lacks accountability, and tends to prioritize the interests of elites. As a result, the state has difficulty mobilizing its institutions and enforcing its policies. Limited health and economic resources have not been the primary reason for Nepal's failed Covid-19 strategy, more so, it is the failure to effectively mobilize those resources and apply them effectively.

Notes

1 With thanks to Dr. Bhim Suwal, Associate Professor, Tribhuvan University.
2 According to United Nations, aggregate values of the three indices, namely gross national per capita (GNI per capita), the human assets index (HAI) and economic vulnerability index (EVI), determine the level of development of a country. Nepal is a least-developed

country with the values of the three indices US$ 1090, 71.2, and 28.4 respectively (UN 2018).

3 The responses began as early as the third week of January. The lockdown measure was issued on March 24.

4 The present ruling party bears a de facto-unification for the purpose of the election held in 2017. Before the formation of this majority government, the country observed 16 coalition governments in a period of two and half decades since 1990. Not a single government, elected or nominated by the kings, has held the office for full five years tenure since 1950.

5 The first democratically elected government formed by social democratic party Nepali Congress in 1959 was ousted by the king in 1960 and adopted a Panchayat political system for 30 years. The Nepali Congress' government had initiated some major reforms of social and economic modernization. See for detail Joshi and Rose 2007.

6 Mr. Ganesh Man Singh, the leader of the Unified Movement for Democracy in 1990, once said symbolically that the dog's tail is controlling its head, which referred to the bureaucracy that had prevailed over the political leadership in the country.

7 After the first constitutional assembly failed to draft the constitution, political parties could not forge consensus of who leads the government to hold second election in 2013. Finally, they agreed that the Chief Justice could be a neutral candidate. The Chief Justice became the prime minister and held the election but he did not quit his post at the Supreme Court.

8 One personnel at the Ministry of Health and Population said that until the end of July even the info graph prepared in early April was not disseminated to the local governments.

9 Top police personnel in a district confirmed that chairs of local governments and the political parties took 'pass policy' as a privilege to support their voters. They frequently put pressure on him to release those who were detained due to lockdown violation. They also forced him to let people cross the districts with a pass.

10 CBS 2019.

11 The HLCC took a fast-track decision to expedite health equipment procurement. It appointed Omni Group, a company less known in the field, for the purpose of procurement, canceling the due procedure initiated by the Department of Health. The decision pulled the HLCC in controversy.

12 On May 25, the PM KP Sharma Oli blamed them for flouting rules at the border and causing the Covid-19 spread in Nepal.

13 The Covid 19 returnee order, Ministry of Labor, Employment and Social Security. Available at https://drive.google.com/file/d/1ltgut4gpGkUZi-N5DYsejCG6W23y1Tl9/view?fbclid=IwAR2VViySYAUqdGRW8xzOVWD4gF9sjrxYTMeFGTAFIbEKzmkuCU5psEgFg_Y [Accessed 6/24/2020].

14 A public health expert working at the department of health said that pharmaceuticals and health equipment suppliers determine the cost of the treatment at the hospitals in the country. He argued that the government decision to continue the RDT test despite its tested ineffectiveness was taken because some suppliers in Kathmandu had tests kits in stock, which they wanted to sell during the pandemic.

15 The finance minister said in the third week of June that government current expenditure was three times higher than revenue.

16 See for detail of the both relief packages, Reanda Biz Serve 2020 Potential impact of Covid-19 on Nepalese economy: 61–62. The report is available at www.reanda-ternational.com/News_Photo/pdf/P_i_C_N_E.pdf [Accessed 7/12/2020].

17 The data of Table 5.1 were calculated to find if there is a correlation between Covid-19 cases and provincial development indicators. The correlation between death per case and HDI was 0.57, between death per case and GDP per capita income was 0.75 and between death per case and distribution of RT-PCT testing labs was 0.51. The results show that the relationship between death per Covid-19 case and GDP per capita was significant.

References

Adhikari, Deepak 2020 Coronavirus in Nepal: Laborers returning home allege bias in hospitals, April 9. Available at www.aa.com.tr/en/asia-pacific/coronavirus-in-nepal-laborers-returning-home-allege-bias-in-hospitals-/1798135 [Accessed 8/9/2020].

Adhikari, Jagnnath 2008 *Land reform in Nepal: Problems and Prospects*. Kathmandu: Actionaid.

Belay, Tekabe and Ajay Tondon 2015 *Assessing Fiscal Space for Health for Nepal*. Washington DC, World Bank.

Bill, Peter and Janak Raj Sapkota 2020 Covid-19: Nepal in crisis, *The Diplomat* 29 June.

Central Bureau of Statistics (CBS) 2017 *Nepal Demographic Health Survey, 2016*. Kathmandu, Ministry of Health, New Era and ICF.

Central Bureau of Statistics (CBS) 2019 *Nepal in Figures*. Kathmandu: CBS.

Duflo, Esther and Abhijit Banerjee 2020 Coronavirus is a crisis for the developing world, but here's why it needn't be a catastrophe, *The Guardian*, 6 May.

Fukuyama, Francis 2020 The pandemic and political order: It takes a state, *Foreign Affairs*, July/August.

Ghimire, Binod 2020 Oli seizes May Day address to take the media to task for 'promoting instability', *The Kathmandu Post*, 1 May.

Government of Nepal (GoN) 2018 *The Public Health Service Act, 2018*. Kathmandu: Nepal Law Commission.

Gorkhapatra Daily, 2020a, 2 February 2020, *P. 1*.

Gorkhapatra Daily, 2020b, 17 February 2020, *P. 1*.

Gyanwaly, Ram Prasad 2018 Introductory note: In quest of self-reliant, balanced, and inter-dependent economy. In idem, ed. *Political economy of Nepal*, 1–7. Kathmandu: Central Department of Economics, TU and FES.

International Commission of Jurists (ICJ) 1996 *Human Rights and Agrarian Relations in Nepal: A Study of Relations*. Kathmandu: International Commission of Jurists.

Joshi, B. L. and Rose, L. E. 2007 *Democratic Innovations in Nepal: A Case Study of Political Acculturation*. Kathmandu: Mandala Publications.

Kantipur National Daily, *Editorial*, 3 June 2020.

Kathayat, Chandani 2020 Covid-19 tests proving difficult in remote regions of Karnali province, *The Kathmandu Post*, 25 August.

Ministry of Finance (MoF) 2019 *The Economic Survey Report 2018/19*. Kathmandu: MoF.

Ministry of Health and Population (MoHP) 2013 *Health Resource for Health: Nepal Country Profile*. Kathmandu: MoHP.

Nederveen Pieterse, Jan 2018 *Multipolar Globalization: Emerging Economies and Development*. London, Routledge.

Nepal Health Research Council (NHRC) 2020 Assessment of compliance with SMS measures against Covid-19 in Kathmandu Valley. Kathmandu Available at http://nhrc.gov.np/wp-content/uploads/2020/08/SMS_Report-1.pdf [Accessed 8/11/2020].

Nepal, Khemraj 2013 *Samaj sanskar ra shasan*. Kathmandu: InLogos.

Pandey, Devendra Raj 2009 *Nepal's Failed Development: Reflections on the Mission and the Maladies* (Revised ed.). Kathmandu: Nepal South Asia Centre.

Poudel, Arjun 2020a Contact tracing is key, but a lack of human resource is making it ineffective, *The Kathmandu Post*, August 14.

Poudel, Arjun 2020b Private hospitals not taking fever patients, forcing patients to seek treatment at state-run health facilities. *The Kathmandu Post*, March 30.

Prasain, Sangam and Chandan Kumar Mandal 2020 Supreme Court orders government to use welfare fund to repatriate Nepali workers stranded abroad, *The Kathmandu Post*, June 17.

Puri, Shiva 2020 Poor management continues to afflict people quarantined in Tarai districts. *The Kathmandu Post*, June 29.

Pyakuryal, Biswambhar 2016 *Nepal's Development Tragedy: Threats and Possibilities*. Kathmandu: Fine Print.

Rodrik, D., A. Subramanian and F. Trebbi 2004 Institutions rule: The primacy of institutions over geography and integration in economic development, *Journal of Economic Growth* 9(2): 131–165.

Savedoff, William 2003 *How Much Should Countries Spend on Health?* Discussion paper 2. Geneva: WHO.

TKP, Editorial 2020 Stop peddling, pseudoscience. *The Kathmandu Post*, 19 June.

United Nations/Nepal 2020 *Covid-19 and Nepal: Preparedness and Response Plan* (NPRP). Kathmandu.

UNDP 2020 *Rapid Assessment of Socio-economic Impact of Covid-19 in Nepal*. Kathmandu: United Nations Development Program/Nepal.

Wagle, Achyut 2020 How KP Oli failed the nation? *The Kathmandu Post*, July 6.

Weyl, Glen and Rajiv Sethi 2020 *Mobilizing Political Economy Resources for Covid-19*. Edmond J. Safra Centre for Ethics Covid-19 White Paper 3.

WHO 2020 Novel Coronavirus (2019 n-COV) Situation report 12, 1 February 2020. Available at www.who.int/docs/default-source/coronaviruse/situation-reports/20200201-sitrep-12-ncov.pdf?sfvrsn=273c5d35_2 [Accessed 7/29/2020].

Xing, Li and Shaw, Timothy M. 2013 The political economy of Chinese state capitalism, *JCIR* 1(1):88–113. http://kropfpolisci.com/chinese.state.capitalism.pdf [Accessed 6/20/2020].

6

INDONESIA AND COVID-19

Decentralization and social conflict

Rebecca Meckelburg and Charanpal S. Bal

Seven months after the first Covid-19 case was officially confirmed, it is clear that Indonesia has failed to control the pandemic. By the end of October 2020, the country has recorded 353,461 cases and 12,347 deaths. Testing rates, at 14,000 tests per million of population, are amongst the lowest in the world, and positivity rates, at between 14–20 percent of those tested, are amongst the highest. The Indonesian central government's pandemic response has been characterized by hesitancy in enforcing lockdowns, extremely limited testing capacity, inability to secure personal protective equipment (PPE) for frontline workers and an overall apathy towards the responsive capacity of public health services. At the same time, local governments at provincial, district and municipal levels responded to address some of these limitations with varying levels of success. Alongside this, the earliest frontline responses to the social, economic and health crises caused by the pandemic came from independent community initiatives. They attempted to fill key gaps in public health and social service provision through the self-coordination of social safety nets, implementing health protocols and even local lockdowns. These observations reveal tensions and rivalries at different levels of governance that mainstream pandemic analyses do not examine.

We adopt a scalar politics approach to explaining pandemic governance outcomes in Indonesia to date. In keeping with the volume's emphasis on institutions, we focus on how competing social forces have harnessed or mobilized different institutions, at different scales of governance, in order to forward or defend their respective agendas and interests. This involves understanding Covid-19 responses in Indonesia as a result of ongoing contestations between social groups within the process of political decentralization. Our analysis reveals that pandemic responses at different scales of governance – national, local, and community – are products of different configurations of social forces and political coalitions. Accordingly, we argue that pandemic responses have been fractured and fractious to the point that it is highly problematic to speak of an 'Indonesian response'. While local-level responses reflect ongoing tensions between crony-capitalist and reformist forces, the national government response reflects a far narrower oligarchic consensus over prioritizing economic growth over public health. Predictably, this has led to considerable tensions between governance actors at different scales and presents significant impediments to a coordinated whole-of-government response. These findings imply that pandemic responses are best understood as distributional conflicts over political and economic power rather than as a global collective action problem.

Decentralization and democratization in Indonesia

In January and February 2020, with infection numbers swelling in Southeast Asia, key figures in the Indonesian central government sought to deny the existence of the virus. On March 2, President Joko Widodo reported the first known case. The central government then vacillated on enforcing lockdowns amid miserably low testing capacities and concerns that the impact of lockdowns on the economy would lead to social unrest. Despite inaction at the top, some local governments at the provincial, district and municipal levels responded reasonably swiftly, implementing local pandemic policies and coordinating social safety nets. These responses were further buttressed by grassroots mobilizations at the neighborhood and village levels that implemented health protocols, assisted in the delivery of welfare services and instituted village and neighborhood lockdowns. Yet, these efforts were let down by the lack of material support and effective coordination from the top. Limited testing facilities, problems with provisioning PPEs and the central government's refusal to implement any form of nationwide lockdown became key sources of friction between different governance actors. It was only in early May that the central government announced a limited movement restrictions order for one month in the wake of large movements of people from urban centers to rural areas just prior to the *Idul Fitri* holidays. By July 2020, the central government had all but opened the country back up for business while testing and tracing rates continue to remain amongst the lowest in the world. By mid-October 2020, Indonesia had not hit the peak of the first wave, with numbers still rising at record levels.

Invariably, explanations for pandemic responses have largely focused on state capacities. Emerging studies have focused on the nature and quality of institutions in determining the efficacy and implications of state responses (Capano et al. 2020). Political explanations for institutional forms, particularly in cases where efficacy is lacking, have been varied. The 'democratic backsliding' argument holds that a retreat from forms of democratic accountability and liberal norms will not only undermine pandemic responses, but also suffer from further democratic erosion because of the pandemic (Croissant 2020). In the Indonesian context, Mietzner (2020) argues that the rise of anti-scientific religious populism, increasing religious conservatism, worsening political corruption and clientelism prevented an objective assessment of risks while damaging the capacity of state institutions to respond appropriately. While acknowledging the real limitations of institutional responses in the country, the democratic decline argument does not account for the proliferation of independent community organizing that provided many of the frontline responses to the social, economic and health crises that followed the pandemic.

The neoliberal state transformation argument demonstrates that state capacities since the 1970s have increasingly been restructured to protect capital and markets while capacities to provide public goods have been increasingly retrenched (Hameiri 2020). The varieties of capitalism model, largely adopted in this volume, seeks to taxonomize different forms of market economies. It reveals that state-market models that are more responsive to public interests tend to produce better governance outcomes. Both these perspectives have important implications for the Indonesian case – the neoliberalization of the state in post-New Order Indonesia has increasingly pushed healthcare provisions towards the market while a crony-dominated free market model means that institutional capacities are geared towards the agendas of elite networks. However, as initial pandemic responses indicate, such arrangements are neither absolute nor uncontested. Lane (2020) and Wijaya (2020), for instance, point to political rivalries and conflicting agendas as drivers of poor pandemic responses.

Variations and tensions between national, sub-national, and informal grassroots pandemic responses have been evident in other cases such as the United States, India and Thailand (see this volume). The state is clearly not a unitary actor. In Indonesia, these variations and tensions point towards deeper pre-existing tensions over the political project of decentralization. Following the fall of the New Order regime in 1998, the country embarked on a program of decentralization that would give regions considerable autonomy and control over budgets and policymaking. While decentralization was largely a neoliberal project that was articulated together with a slew of market-building policies, it was also a key democratic demand from the *Reformasi* movement of the late 1990s. The impacts of decentralization, however, have been uneven. In large part, decentralization has led to the proliferation of crony networks, largely consigned to Jakarta during the New Order, to a 'bewildering range of individuals and organizations' all over the archipelago (Hadiz and Robinson 2013, 36). Yet, oligarchic capture of local government institutions is by no means complete or uncontested. While elite interests from the New Order era continue to dominate, the actual dynamics of political struggle in different regions at different times present a picture of ongoing uncertainty and conflict rather than consolidated hegemonic power. In particular, the implementation of sub-national and village autonomy, coupled with the emergence of mid-level provincial capitalist classes, has presented unusual spaces for temporary alliances and opportunities for elite and non-elite actors to test out different strategic and tactical approaches.

In order to capture how these dynamics shape overall pandemic responses, we adopt a scalar politics[1] approach that highlights how different actors have mobilized or latched on to different institutions at different scales of governance to forward often conflicting agendas. Institutions are important in explaining pandemic governance outcomes. Their form and capacity, however, are results of struggles and conflicts between social groups over the control and exercise of power and access to and control over resources through these institutions (Kannankulam and Georgi 2014; Poulantzas 2000). We therefore understand institutions and their capacity for responses as outcomes produced by conflicts and tensions over political decentralization and state-building in the post-New Order era.

Empirical material for this chapter was primarily drawn from media, government and civil society reports. These were supplemented with interviews with five civil society activist and rural community leaders in Jakarta and Central Java, conducted by Meckelburg between June 16 and August 29, 2020. Respondents interviewed included an activist with the Urban Poor People's Network in Jakarta, a human rights and women's activist in Yogyakarta, as well as three rural community farmer activists in Semarang, Temanggung and Magelang districts of Central Java. Meckelburg, based in Central Java, was also able to directly observe local government and community initiatives in the municipality of Salatiga and surrounding rural districts. As data was largely drawn from the islands of Java and Bali, and specific nuances from outer Indonesia may not be sufficiently captured, we hope our analysis of the scalar politics of pandemic responses would lend itself well to other contexts. Analyses of scalar politics are not new and have been useful in revealing the types of interests and conflicts that underscore the governance of a myriad of issues such as the avian influenza pandemic, transboundary haze, and migrant worker rights in Southeast Asia (Hameiri and Jones 2013; 2015; Bal and Gerard 2018).

Our analysis reveals that different sets of social forces and material conditions underpin responses at district/municipal, grassroots, provincial and national levels. Lower levels of social differentiation and the ascendency of reformist social and political forces at the local level tend to produce relatively better outcomes that are responsive to community needs. However, any positive developments in the early months of the pandemic, including those at the provincial levels, were severely undercut by the national government's apathy towards public health. The latter response is driven by a national oligarchic consensus over GDP growth and infrastructural developments which have, in turn, truncated district and provincial lockdowns and states-of-emergencies, while driving public health provisions towards the market. At the base is the continued inability of both provincial and national governments to manage informality at the grassroots level. It is precisely this contrast in drivers that explains conflicts between actors at different scales of pandemic governance. Underlying these conflicts is a collective distribution problem – the distribution of power and access to resources that could be mobilized to protect different groups of people from both the pandemic and its adverse economic impacts. It is the dynamics of these struggles over power and resources at different scales that determine the responsiveness, or otherwise, of institutions.

Local government responses

As political decentralization in Indonesia has rescaled the governance of key public services into the hands of district and municipal governments, local governments have, understandably, become the critical focal point of pandemic crisis management. District and municipal governments have primary control and responsibility for staff management and budgets for regional and city schools, hospitals and community health centers, social welfare programs and crisis response protocols and enforcement. District and municipal governments made the key pandemic policies, including declarations of local state of emergencies; infectious disease management and control; provision of PPEs for medical staff; restrictions of medical services to hospitals to limit community transmission; as well as school and university closures. In addition, these governments swiftly announced and enacted social safety net provisions. Many regional governments acted not only out of a desire to demonstrate their political credentials to their constituents but for social and economic reasons, including the limitations of health systems if the virus was left unchecked.

The relative success of some district and municipal governments in mobilizing resources for pandemic response appears to be contingent on the extent of social differentiation and the balance of social forces within respective regions. In districts and municipalities with histories of popular social and political mobilization, as well as electoral campaigns for district heads and mayors driven by local organizations, local officials demonstrated more rapid responses in providing social assistance. These district governments were able to swiftly secure PPE for health workers in hospitals and local health centers (Puskesmas) and did not experience high levels of infection amongst health workers.

Access to land in the global south plays a significant part in the dynamics of capitalist social relations at the level of local political economies. The structure of landholdings and local power relations, particularly within the island of Java, is shown to have some impact on local government responses (Meckelburg 2019). This provides spaces and opportunities – material, institutional and ideological – for contestation by multiple contending social actors and groups over access to and control of land. The decentralization of state authority in Indonesia has had the effect of intensifying contestation as local powerbrokers at district and village levels sit between investors offering considerable economic perks and the local electorate that powerbrokers rely on for votes.

In several districts in inland Central Java, for instance, smallholder agriculture dominates local political economies. These districts tend to demonstrate more limited social or class differentiation across the district population and hold strong traditions of mutual assistance and support for vulnerable members of their communities. These regions have been places of refuge for many returned internal and overseas migrant workers as families and kin groups still have access to land. It is precisely in these districts that village communities were able to deliver effective public health messages as well as mobilize resources to quarantine and isolate large numbers of people who arrived from the epicenter of the crisis in Jakarta and West Java. In the early months of the pandemic, these measures were successful in limiting the spread of the virus in many rural areas reasonably successfully.

Conversely, in northern coastal districts of Java where industry, agribusiness and forestry are more dominant, political-economic dynamics in these regions have long been favorable for the interests of industrial capital and agribusiness. Here, district governments have been generally less responsive both in the preparation of district health services as well as in the distribution of social assistance. Further, with limited access to land, local populations in these regions are more dependent on employment in industries with little concern for health and safety protocols and the informal sector which often involves travel between regions with high levels of Covid-19 transmission. It is, therefore, of little coincidence that it is several of such districts that have experienced more widespread transmission in the general population and higher levels of infections amongst health workers in the initial months of the pandemic.

While political decentralization in Indonesia has been a neoliberal project, the actual development of local political structures reflects the extent of elite capture or conversely, the adoption of reformist programs that are more responsive to community interests. Despite the ascendency of crony-capitalist forces, many aspects of governance and distribution of regional resources remain unresolved. The past decade has seen a rise of reformist district heads, city mayors and provincial governors riding on broad-based popular support that stands in contrast with more regular practices of riding solely on money politics or patronage networks. While these nascent reformists are not entirely separate from crony networks, they draw considerable popular support outside these networks and represent more diverse elements within society as opposed to just elite networks. In this sense, the social actors actively making competing claims on local-level institutions significantly influences the efficacy of responses. The pandemic has provided opportunities for reform-minded district leaders to strengthen popular support by being more responsive to the needs of local communities. This contrasts with crony-capitalist elites whose relationship with voters is generally limited to one-off gifts or payments in return for votes.

At the provincial level, responses have been similarly uneven. Provincial governments elected on relatively broad-based popular support, such as those in West and Central Java, were able to produce or secure medical supplies, coordinate regional lockdowns and tracing regimes and provide social assistance budgets. Yet, in provinces such as South Sulawesi, provincial and district governments actively misused social assistance funds to strengthen party cartels and attract voters before upcoming regional elections. However, the more proactive responses were in large part stymied as the national government failed to secure global supplies of testing equipment and actively pushed back against provincial lockdowns. At the same time, public communications by provincial governments, particularly in Jakarta, were largely addressed to middle-class electorates with little attention paid to the challenges faced by workers in the informal sector (Achmadi 2020). Indeed, across provincial levels of governmentality, there are limited initiatives to develop effective public health responses for more than 60 percent of the population who work in this sector.

Grassroots mobilizations

Initial public health responses in Indonesia were strongly tied to community mobilizations and forms of social solidarity that included village and neighborhood-based lockdowns, including support for health workers and vulnerable members of the community The phenomenon of community initiated public health measures and social welfare support enacted by urban neighborhood groups and rural villages prior to national or district initiatives was widespread across the archipelago (Bennett 2020; Krismantari 2020). These occurred largely independently of, but sometimes in tandem with, district and municipal government responses. Local leadership, both formal and informal, backed by mobilized communities has been critical in securing resources for Covid responses and in delivering social assistance.

In the cramped and densely populated urban poor neighborhoods of Jakarta, neighborhoods that have historically been marginalized, ignored or threatened with eviction were able to draw on informal organizing capacities forged in long histories of self-advocacy (Varagur 2020). In North Jakarta, the Urban Poor People's Network (Jaringan Rakyat Miskin Kota) were able to mobilize networks and resources in communities that already had histories of facilitated social organizing (Interview with MS 24 August 2020).Volunteers organized the distribution of food and supplies through home delivery to whole neighborhoods, significantly reducing the movements of many residents. Communities organized crowdfunding efforts and pooled savings to meet everyday needs during the first few months of lockdown. We note that these networks are not universally existent across densely populated areas in large metropolises such as Jakarta and there have been many cases of 'every person for themselves'. However, where these networks with strong reserves of social capital exist, they have histories of grassroots campaigns organized through independent local initiatives or community programs supported by activist-based NGOs.

In smaller urban centers such as Yogyakarta and Salatiga in Central Java, community kitchens (Syambudi 2020) or locally organized meal packages were rapidly established to provide support for vulnerable informal sector workers from online transport sector workers, small traditional market traders and *becak* drivers to sex-workers (Bennett 2020). Other initiatives have coordinated collection and distribution of food goods, clothes and cash for surrounding urban and rural areas (Interview with BS 16 August 2020). Some of these initiatives sprang from local working-class communities, while other initiatives came from urban-dwelling social activists who have links to networks and groups from different social sectors.

In urban regions, high levels of informality in social and economic life have demonstrated a strong capacity for adaptability. The pandemic has had the effect of semi-formalizing social relations between workers in the informal sector and economically secure middle classes who have come to rely more on their relations with people in precarious work. Here informality has been a source of resilience and an ability to adapt rapidly to challenging circumstances. Achmiadi (2020) notes the empathy that is generated between social classes where relationships are built initially on informality. At the same time, the state has been strikingly absent in these developments. Indeed, historically there is significant tension between governmentality and informality – whether formal governance actors are prepared to acknowledge the role of urban informality or not, it has contributed significantly to mitigating the scale of the crisis.

In rural villages, local mitigation measures have had a different character. In the early months of the pandemic crisis, tens of thousands of people living precariously in informal work or who had lost industry jobs left urban cities to return to rural homes. At the village level, communities responded quickly, establishing quarantine facilities and other logistics to support return migrants (Interview with SA June 16, 2020). Many 'shut down' their villages, only allowing residents to enter while ensuring that returned residents completed quarantine protocols. Practical initiatives including the initiation of basic health protocols were largely organized by local groups at village level. In the face of widespread economic hardship, many self-initiated local farmers' groups set up mechanisms to distribute produce to urban and rural communities worst affected economically (Interview with BT, August 22, 2020). Regions dominated by smallholder farmers continue to demonstrate strong capacities to mitigate the spread of the virus through limited interactions outside of local villages as well as the capacity to provide basic social security guarantees including adequate food supplies for village residents.

What is striking in observations of the pandemic responses is that it is these local grassroots initiatives that have been critical in mitigating the potential for large-scale social or economic crises for large sections of the population in the early period of the pandemic, despite significant losses in income for these same populations. Community support at the grassroots level, together with some (very uneven) delivery of financial assistance from various levels of government, have significantly cushioned these negative impacts. Here the pandemic has highlighted the limited function of governmentality in responding to social, economic and health needs of large sections of both rural and urban society. The self-initiated organizing capacity of sections of society across rural and urban spaces in a time of crisis demonstrates the significant spaces that operate beyond state governance structures or are neglected by the state.

While the initial impact of the Covid-19 virus was felt mostly by middle-class or wealthier citizens, as the pandemic has taken hold it is increasingly a disease more likely to impact the marginal and more vulnerable (majority) members of society. The profile of patients is increasingly dominated by factory workers, market vendors, healthcare workers, transport workers and workers in sales and distribution that involve high levels of mobility between regions or are working on healthcare frontlines. For these sections of society, it is likely that where grassroots organizations have mobilized in the early months of the pandemic, they will continue to play a crucial role in mitigating the threats facing these more vulnerable groups.

Narrow elite consensus: the national government response

The central factor in Indonesia's failure to control the pandemic lies with the decision-making of the Widodo government at national level. The Covid-19 pandemic in Indonesia produced a national government response that was framed by oligarchic consensus over the Widodo administration's national infrastructure drive and the prioritization of GDP growth. Correspondingly, the pandemic agenda at the national scale revolved around mitigating risks and threats posed by the pandemic to these broad economic objectives rather than public health per se.

Widodo's second term since reelection in 2019 has involved the building of a 'grand coalition' of oligarchic interests tied to various national infrastructure projects. Widodo's grand coalition includes all but two national political parties, all of whom have obtained strategic ministries, including Prabowo Subianto, his prime presidential opponent in the 2019 election who now heads the Ministry of Defense. This grand coalition undermines potential for an electoral opposition at the national level of politics. The centerpiece of this coalition is the distribution of project benefits to supporters and former political adversaries in return for elite political support. This includes infrastructure projects in places where coalition figures currently hold land concessions and commercial stakes in industrial installations. It is projected that the spoils of this national infrastructure drive will be shared around, thus healing rifts caused by intra-elite conflicts that characterized the 2017 Jakarta and 2019 general elections. At the same time, popular legitimacy for the 'grand coalition', particularly from middle-class constituencies, is to be secured by delivering on GDP growth. Meanwhile, securitization of the pandemic provides cover for increasing repression of any opposition from the majority poor.

The key prongs of the national government response focused on ameliorating economic contraction and economic hardship that might cause potential social unrest in order to avoid major disruptions to national infrastructure and economic growth policies. This approach, in the early months of the crisis, put the national government at odds with many provincial and more local responses. Provincial and local governments needed action at a national level to restrict citizen movements, provide testing infrastructure and protective equipment for medical personnel. Meanwhile the central government provided only a single point of testing, based in Jakarta, whilst encouraging international and domestic tourism in the early months of 2020.

Consequently, open disputes arose between national and local governments in the early months of the pandemic included resources for mass testing capacities; the provision of protective equipment for medical staff that triggered a massive fallout between the Ministry of Health and the Indonesian Medical Association (IDI); and the national government's refusal to impose movement restrictions. Notably, medical experts such as the IDI, who played key roles in local responses, were sidelined in the national response by narrow oligarchic interests. By August 2020, district governments fell in line behind the national imperative to protect the economy while testing and contract-tracing levels remained extremely low. Six months into the crisis, ongoing shortages in adequately trained staff demonstrates the lack of any substantive commitment by national government to provide this as a matter of urgency. Procurement of PPE remains a problem across many regions (DTC 2020) and the central government through its failure to act decisively has effectively dismissed any responsibility for this. Regulations imposed in the name of controlling movement of citizens between regions were mere formalities as citizens were encouraged to take short holidays in order to support the kick-start of local economies dependent on the service sector and tourism.

Initial economic stimulus measures budgeted by central government that included social assistance for the poor and financial incentives for medical staff, failed to be managed and delivered effectively through their respective state ministries and departments (Detikcom 2020). Poor coordination between national ministries and incompetence in the case of health and social ministries exacerbated the crisis (Akhlas 2020). No executive measures have been taken to ensure more effective action at these levels. Rather the Covid-19 mitigation response was repurposed as the Covid-19 Response and Economic Recovery team headed by Erick Thohir, the state-owned enterprises minister, with the army chief-of-staff appointed as his deputy director. Thohir has said that the military would work to discipline the public as the key to public safety (Akhlas 2020).

With the reopening of the economy in early July 2020, case numbers rose significantly and the demographic of patient cases reported showed a significant shift to middle- and lower-class people working in factories, offices, local markets, transport and hospitals (Herlambang 2020). While urban and rural poor activist communities and organizations in some regions have managed to advocate for more responsive local government action, these groups remain localized and not coordinated enough to influence policymaking on a national scale.

By early September 2020, some national elites argued publicly that not solving the health crisis would only deepen the economic crisis facing Indonesia. However, attempts by the Jakarta provincial governor to re-implement large-scale movement restrictions due to an escalating crisis in the Jakarta public health system were actively sabotaged by national ministers. This most recent conflict highlights how sub-national government responses can often be driven by a more diverse range of social interests, while the national government's response is driven by the narrow interests of oligarchic elites. It is this ongoing contestation that creates major problems in coordination and sometimes points of open conflict.

The national government's continued apathy has further pushed healthcare provisions towards the market where state-owned pharmaceuticals and private healthcare providers stand to gain. Unlike other countries in Southeast Asia, voluntary testing of people with symptoms is user-pays. Further, in July and August 2020, data indicates that hospitals across many regions of Indonesia, in particular in Jakarta and West, Central and East Java, are close to or have reached full capacity, in some cases turning away Covid patients (*The Jakarta Post* 2020). While the government promised that all Covid treatments would be covered by government budgets, there are reports of hospitals charging self-isolating positive patients for treatment and medication (Interview with SD August 18, 2020). All of these factors indicate the increasing adoption of a user-pays system for Covid detection and treatment which further undermines any potential for pursuing an effective trace, track and treat public health approach.

Conclusion: unresolved contention amid escalating crisis

Economic contraction has been unavoidable during the pandemic and in the second quarter of 2020 Indonesia suffered its sharpest economic downturn since the 1998 economic crisis (Akhlas 2020). While the overall contraction has not been as significant as other countries, in October 2020, the first wave of the pandemic has not yet peaked. Financial reports show that the largest contractions in GDP have been in household spending and investment. With no strategy or even intent to effectively control the pandemic, these sectors are unlikely to show any significant recovery and indeed may worsen as new daily cases continue to rise.

Some provincial governments continue to attempt to improve public health facilities in particular testing capacity and isolation beds. However, the failure of central government to act decisively in supporting the procurement of approved standard equipment and raw materials, instead leaving this to the market, has stymied many of these attempts when provinces receive faulty sub-standard equipment or chemical reagents that do not work. The efforts of many district governments now appear to have been pared back to providing some forms of public health education about wearing masks, washing hands and physical distancing, alongside punitive local enforcement of health protocols. This apparent compliance with the national political agenda of 'economy first' places a question mark over the capacity and willingness of district governments to engage in open conflict with provincial and national governments over resourcing public health infrastructures to improve testing, tracing and treatment capacities. At the same time some local governments face rising community protest if they have no demonstrated plan of action in the face of rising case numbers and Covid deaths.

The appointment of the army chief-of-staff as vice-chairperson of the national government's Covid and economic recovery response team indicates that it is anticipated that stability may require management by force or at least punitive methods of control. At the same time, the scale of population and scale of mobilities between regions tends to outpace any ability to effectively regulate or police this. Restoring international diplomatic and business confidence in Indonesia however may require more overt securing of public space in Jakarta specifically to ensure that the management and delivery of infrastructure and other economic growth targets can proceed relatively normally.

As the disease spreads more widely to poor workers in factories and the informal sector and to rural regions, the capacity for grassroots mobilizations to effectively mitigate the health and economic consequences is not yet known. We cannot yet measure the resilience of these networks in the face of longer term economic and social hardship, in particular if domestic demand for basic goods remains depressed. We can say that risks in the 'new normal' will disproportionately affect workers in industries where support for health protocols is harder to guarantee or with limited ability to demand safe working conditions. Furthermore, those in the informal sector, people dependent on mass transport and regions where community organizations find it hard to mobilize adequate social resources will also be disproportionately affected. The other group being sacrificed as a result of economic priorities is frontline health workers which invariably weakens the capacity of the health system to respond. Virus transmission risk will continue to rise across Indonesia while testing rates remain some of the lowest in the world. Coupled with a health system showing signs of reaching existing capacity and essential mitigation measures such as testing being available largely on a user-pays basis, this will mean that growing numbers of people infected will not be identified nor will they be able to access medical services if their condition becomes acute.

Note

1 A scalar politics approach emphasizes the importance of different tiers of governance within and across states. Scales of governance are never neutral with each scale presenting a different set of actors, resources and political opportunities that privilege certain social interests over others. Scalar politics are, therefore, ensuing struggles between social groups over how power and resources are distributed across and controlled at various tiers of governance (Hameiri and Jones 2013).

References

Achmadi, Armanda. 2020. 'Talking Indonesia: Covid-19 and the City.' Indonesia at Melbourne. July 30, 2020. http://indonesiaatmelbourne.unimelb.edu.au/talking-indonesia-covid-19-and-the-city/. Accessed September 1, 2020.

Akhlas, Adrian. 2020. 'Indonesia Looking at Near-Zero Growth as Govt Struggles to Spend Budget, Sri Mulyani Says.' *The Jakarta Post*, August 21, 2020, sec. Business. /www.thejakartapost.com/news/2020/08/19/indonesia-looking-at-near-zero-growth-as-govt-struggles-to-spend-budget-sri-mulyani-says.html. Accessed September 1, 2020.

Bal, Charanpal S. and Kelly Gerard. 2018. 'ASEAN's Governance of Migrant Worker Rights.' *Third World Quarterly*, 39 (4): 799–819. https://doi.org/10.1080/01436597.2017.1387478.

Bennett, Linda. 2020. 'Too Much Reporting on Covid-19 in Indonesia Is Missing Context.' *Indonesia at Melbourne*. May 5, 2020. https://indonesiaatmelbourne.unimelb.edu.au/too-much-reporting-on-covid-19-in-indonesia-is-missing-context/.

Capano, Giliberto, Michael Howlett, Darryl S.L. Jarvis, M. Ramesh and Nihit Goyal. 2020. 'Mobilizing Policy (In)Capacity to Fight Covid-19: Understanding Variations in State Responses.' *Policy and Society*, 39 (3): 285–308. https://doi.org/10.1080/14494035.2020.1787628.

Croissant, Aurel. 2020. 'Democracies with Pre-existing Conditions and the Coronavirus in the Indo-Pacific | The Asan Forum.' *The ASAN Forum* (blog). June 6, 2020. www.theasanforum.org/democracies-with-preexisting-conditions-and-the-coronavirus-in-the-indo-pacific/.

Detikcom. 2020. 'Jokowi's Five Harsh Reprimands to Ministers During the Pandemic' (in Indonesian). *Detikfinance.com*, July 9, 2020. https://finance.detik.com/berita-ekonomi-bisnis/d-5086697/5-teguran-keras-jokowi-ke-menteri-di-tengah-pandemi. Accessed August 30, 2020.

DTC. 2020. 'Urgent, Health Ministry and Covid-19 Taskforce Prepare Quality PPE' (in Indonesian). *SuaraMerdeka.com*, September 1, 2020, sec. Nasional. www.suaramerdeka.com/news/nasional/239369-mendesak-kementrian-kesehatan-dan-satgas-covid-19-siapkan-apd-berkualitas. Accessed August 26, 2020.

Farisa, Fitria. 2020. 'SMRC Survey: 49 percent of Citizens believe that Covid-19 Social Assistance Does Not Reach its Targets' (in Indonesian). *KOMPAS.com*, May 12, 2020, sec. Nasional. https://nasional.kompas.com/read/2020/05/12/15082801/survei-smrc-49-persen-warga-menilai-bansos-covid-19-tak-capai-sasaran. Accessed August 30, 2020.

Hadiz, Vedi R. and Richard Robinson. 2013. 'The Political Economy of Oligarchy and the Reorganization of Power in Indonesia.' *Indonesia*, no. 96: 35. https://doi.org/10.5728/indonesia.96.0033.

Hameiri, Shahar. 2020. 'Covid-19: Time to Bring Back the State.' *Progress in Political Economy (PPE)* (blog). March 19, 2020. www.ppesydney.net/covid-19-time-to-bring-back-the-state/. Accessed August 20, 2020.

Hameiri, Shahar and Lee Jones. 2013. 'The Politics and Governance of Non-Traditional Security.' *International Studies Quarterly*, 57 (3): 462–473. https://doi.org/10.1111/isqu.12014.

———. 2015. 'Governing Transboundary Pollution: Southeast Asia's Haze.' In *Governing Borderless Threats: Non-Traditional Security and the Politics of State Transformation*. Cambridge, United Kingdom: Cambridge University Press.

Herlambang, Adib. 2020. 'East Java Has 141 Covid-19 Clusters, This Is the List of Locations' (in Indonesian). *AyoSemarang.com*, July 16, 2020, sec. Nasional. www.ayosemarang.com/read/2020/07/16/60395/jatim-miliki-141-klaster-penyebaran-covid-19-ini-daftar-lokasinya. Accessed August 20, 2020.

Jakarta Post. 2020. 'Time to Hit the Brakes.' *The Jakarta Post*, September 2, 2020. www.thejakartapost.com/academia/2020/09/02/time-to-hit-the-brakes.html. Accessed September 3, 2020.

Kannankulam, John and Fabian Georgi. 2014. 'Varieties of Capitalism or Varieties of Relationships of Forces? Outlines of a Historical Materialist Policy Analysis.' *Capital & Class* 38 (1): 59–71. https://doi.org/10.1177/0309816813513088.

Krismantari, Ika. 2020. 'Expert: People's Initiatives in the Covid-19 Pandemic were Born Because of the Slow Government Response' (in Indonesian). *The Conversation*. https://theconversation.com/ahli-inisiatif-masyarakat-saat-pandemi-covid-19-lahir-karena-lambannya-gerak-pemerintah-136708. Accessed September 2, 2020.

Lane, Max. 2020. 'The Politics of National and Local Responses to the Covid-19 Pandemic in Indonesia.' Working Paper 46. Perspective. Singapore: ISEAS –Yusof Ishak Institute. www.iseas.edu.sg/wp-content/uploads/2020/03/ISEAS_Perspective_2020_46.pdf. Accessed July 20, 2020.

Meckelburg, Rebecca. 2019. 'Subaltern Agency and the Political Economy of Rural Social Change.' Doctoral Thesis, Perth: Murdoch University. https://researchrepository.murdoch.edu.au/id/eprint/57177/1/Meckelburg2019.pdf. Accessed July 10, 2020.

Mietzner, Marcus. 2020. 'Populist Anti-Scientism, Religious Polarisation, and Institutionalised Corruption: How Indonesia's Democratic Decline Shaped Its Covid-19 Response.' *Journal of Current Southeast Asian Affairs* 0 (0): 186810342093556. https://doi.org/10.1177/1868103420935561. Accessed July 10, 2020.

Poulantzas, Nicos. 2000. *State, Power, Socialism*. London:Verso Books, new edition.
Syambudi, Irwan. 2020. 'Corona Pandemic Solidarity Actions: Community Kitchen Donates 50 Million Rupiah' (in Indonesian). *Tirto.id*, April 1, 2020. https://tirto.id/aksi-solidaritas-pandemi-corona-dapur-umum-hingga-donasi-rp50-juta-eJVL. Accessed August 30, 2020.
Varagur, Krithika. 2020. 'Indonesia's Government Was Slow to Lock Down, so Its People Took Charge.' *History & Culture*. May 13, 2020. www.nationalgeographic.com/history/2020/05/indonesia-government-slow-lock-down-people-took-charge/. Accessed July 10, 2020.
Wijaya, Trissia. 2020. 'Covid-19: The Politics of Local Responses in Indonesia.' *Melbourne Asia Review* (blog). August 17, 2020. https://melbourneasiareview.edu.au/covid-19-the-politics-of-local-responses-in-indonesia/. Accessed August 30, 2020.

7

THAILAND AND COVID-19

Institutions and social dynamics from below

Chantana Wun'Gaeo and Surichai Wun'Gaeo

The Coronavirus pandemic reached Thailand when a Chinese woman tourist tested positive on January 8, 2020. Later, on January 31, the first Thai, a taxi driver who had picked up that tourist, triggered the pandemic from within the country. On February 4, the number of infections rose to 25, and Thailand was ranked second for Covid-19 infection risk after China (Matichon Online 2020a). By May 13 however, Thailand's Center for Covid-19 Situation Administration (CCSA) reported zero new cases for the first time (Thairat Online 2020). As of October 28, the Global Covid-19 Index (GCI) ranks Thailand as 4th out of 184 countries for Covid-19 recovery, with zero identified cases internally, except those under quarantine after entering the country. Against this achievement, Thailand faces an economic contraction of 7–8 percent in the second half of 2020 (NESDB 2020). The complexity of the pandemic crisis is reflected in the high cost of disease control measures, which have created an unprecedented crisis of social and economic disruptions.

The pandemic has been managed under an atmosphere of political tension. As the consequence of a coup d'état in 2014, this upper income country of 67 million has been under military rule for six years. The new 2017 constitution made it possible for the coup leader to return as Prime Minister in the 2019 general election, and crisis administration has relied on a special law giving the Prime Minister an authority that goes even beyond disease control. Under these circumstances, it is easy to jump to the conclusion that successful crisis management requires command and control. Thus, in addition to its review of state measures and mechanisms against Covid-19, this chapter will also explore the dynamics of society at play through the crisis.

Thailand's Center for Covid-19 Situation Administration (CCSA) was set up on March 12, 2020, in response to a series of risks from super spreader clusters, including 35 people infected at a boxing match in Bangkok, the return of an

Islamic Dawa group from Indonesia, and a group of undocumented Thai workers returning from South Korea. The CCSA is primarily composed of key medical doctors with the Prime Minister at its head. As the outbreak peaked, the numbers of infected reached nearly 1,000 cases, and a lockdown was imposed, affecting specific enterprises mostly in the service sector. Following the first specific lockdown came the Emergency Decree on March 26, recommended by the key medical group. This included a tighter national lockdown, closing of borders and airports, provincial lockdowns, and the establishment of a curfew between 10 pm–5 am.

Though the epidemic was not yet contained, within a month, the lockdown and curfew started affecting people of low-income and daily wage earners. To calm public outcry, cash distributions were allocated for Covid-19 affected people, providing 5000 Baht (US$166) per month for three consecutive months. Subsequently, several cash distribution packages have been launched to boost consumption and tourism, for instance, เที่ยวด้วยกัน (*let's tour*), เที่ยวปันสุข (*sharing happiness tour*), คนละครึ่ง (*each pay 50 percent*). Substantial concerns accompanied the government's passage of three decrees to secure a 1.9 trillion Thai baht loan for Covid-19 relief and reconstruction measures.

Curving the pandemic: institution mechanisms

While the most notable mechanisms for the epidemic control are the CCSA and the Emergency Decree, the true drivers of Thailand's Covid response have been the teams of medical doctors (especially from university hospitals) and health volunteers operating under the auspices of the county's long-established primary health system. In addition, the crisis has also revealed the underlining social capital seen by the work of community members in reaching out and lending a hand during the new normal practices. The private sector played an important role as well, providing much-needed medical supplies and PPE to support the new normal.

Responding to the disease

The CCSA, set up by the Cabinet Resolution on March 12, is the central locus for Thailand's multi-dimensional pandemic control and mitigation strategy, and is headed by the singular command of the Prime Minister. From March 28 to April 21, 13 different functional centers were set up as the county's response become more comprehensive, covering a range of issue areas, including information, medical appliances, transportation, telecommunication, research and innovation and national security. The CCSA held daily committee meetings and updated the situation on public television and Facebook Live especially during the first 3–4 months. The daily report has been a very important means of risk communication and Covid-19 literacy to keep the nation alert and calm at the same time.

The Emergency Decree, with no participation of parliament, was used instead of the Communication Disease Act which already announced Covid-19 as a dangerous contagious disease prior to the decree. The Decree controls lockdown,

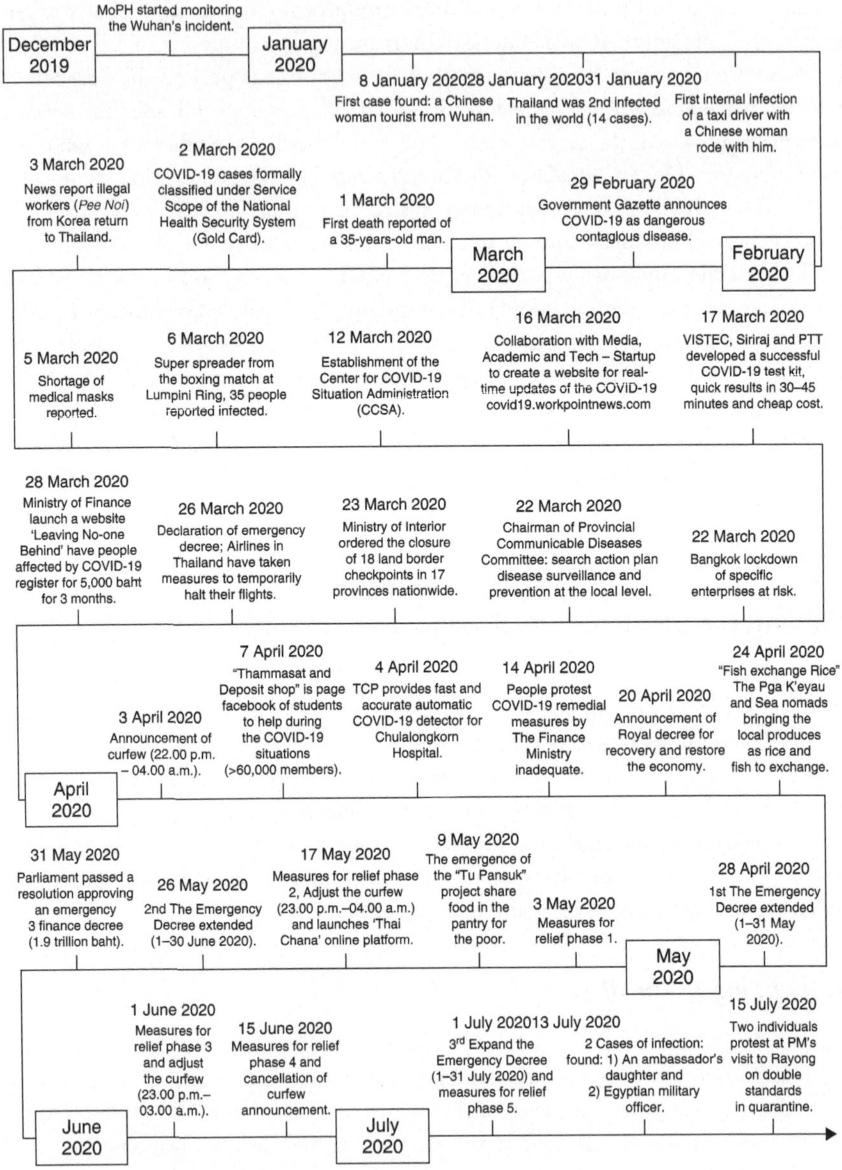

FIGURE 7.1 Covid-19 trends in Thailand

curfews, people's mobility, public gatherings, distorted or false communication as well as the mobilization of resources and personnel to respond to the Covid-19 situation. The justification for the decree, not without criticism, was that CCSA required a higher authority than existing laws, and was needed to integrate different government departments (Thansettakij 2020). Many arrests were made for breaking curfew, traveling outside lockdown provinces (The Standard Team 2020) and the ban of political gathering (see Human Rights Watch 2020). The Decree, as much as it was needed by the CCSA, faced much skepticism as it was used for arbitrary arrest and unclear charges (iLaw 2020). The corporate sector also found the Emergency Degree harmful for business so it should be used only for a short period. In October 2020, the Decree still remains but no longer applies to political gatherings to avoid further skepticism.

The village health volunteer (VHV) also plays a critical role in curbing the pandemic. The VHV has existed since the 1970s as a part of Thailand's primary health care system. There are 1,095,572 village health volunteers throughout the country (Primary Health Care Division 2020). The VHV operates using a bottom-up approach, which is very efficient in terms of handling the pandemic crisis. Volunteers are able to keep officials informed with surveys of endemic infections, and are also able to distribute necessities. In the context of a crisis, the operations of VHVs have been very helpful to control the disease using technology to track and trace people in areas so as to prevent the infection from spreading (Kertesz et al. 2020).

Responding to people's vulnerabilities

The first few months of the lockdown were devastating for daily wage earners and small enterprises; these groups quickly lacked cash for food, rent, utilities and children's education, not to mention masks and alcohol for virus prevention. To address this, cash distribution programs covered five groups of people, including: freelancers and the self-employed, students who were also working part-time, employees in the social security system, small enterprise entrepreneurs (SME) and farmers. Although a large number were excluded and mismatched due to the problem of the digital divide and a cumbersome registration procedure, over 15 million registrants were approved for cash distributions (Bangkok Insight Editorial Team 2020). Other measures were also imposed such as debt postponement, soft loan arrangement, exemption of utility bills for small users and free public transportation. Migrant workers, however, were excluded from these programs, and were not included in relief provided by the state in spite of being in the Thai social security system; it fell to non-profit organizations to provide daily necessities to migrants on a limited scale (Prachatai 2020).

Troubles with the new normal

Thai people were informed of 'new normal' practices, including social distancing, wearing masks, washing hands and checking-in to places with the tracking application called 'Thai Chana' (Thai winning). Once the lockdown was released, a protocol for business operation was imposed. For example, hotels could only accept guests by following SHA (Safety and Health Administration) standards. An SHA certificate would be provided to a hotel that managed to pass the standard.

Living with Covid-19 is accepted now as the new reality. In the context of mask wearing, Thai people had already gotten used to wearing a mask as a result of PM2.5 effects in the past few years. However, compliance also depends on the availability of such protective gear and accessibility or ability to comply. Many incidents have indicated problems with living in the new normal. First, in the beginning of the crisis, there was a lack of personal protective equipment and the market did not work in distributing the needed merchandise. This affected medical doctors a great deal. Government intervention during critical times when markets do not work is crucial (Bangkokbiznews 2020). The Thai government did not handle this well in the beginning. Second, social distancing is not possible for a big family in a small house. Congested communities, especially in those in Bangkok or other urban areas, face a shortage of space, lack of hygiene and perhaps clean water. Social distancing by means of physical space is often not possible for low-income households. Third, some small enterprises like homestays or street food stalls require additional effort to comply. Last but not least, 'work from home' measures, when applied to schooling, created a disruption in education due to problematic online learning measures. Only 57 percent of poor students in marginal communities are able to access the internet, for reasons like being in remote areas or being unable to afford online study. Those limitations are not the only hurdles for studying through online media, but they reveal the inequities of education and the digital divide (Workpoint News 2020). Workers in the service industry were also tremendously affected, and lay-offs were prevalent. In short, compliance with the new normal measures has revealed wide social inequalities.

It is already evident what Covid-19 has done to the economy globally and domestically. The severity of the crisis perhaps does not come primarily from the disease but from the way our economy and development are structured. The disease's direct impact is reported daily in the numbers of deaths and infected. Indirect impacts are the consequence of disease control measures. The Ministry of Public Health reports that during Covid-19, suicide rates have increased by 22 percent (Thai PBS News 2020). However, a survey found that levels of anxiety increased over time, with those reporting *low anxiety* rising from 5.6 percent in the first week to 72.4 percent in the 21st week (Department of Mental Health 2020a).

Based on the analysis of the Health Footprint of Covid-19, the Department of Mental Health has divided the pandemic into four waves: the first is characterized by the immediate mortality and morbidity of Covid-19; the second wave reflects the impact of resource restrictions on non-urgent Covid-19 conditions; the third wave is the interrupted care of chronic conditions; and the fourth wave includes psychic trauma, mental illness, economic injury and burnout shown in four indications including depression, stress, burnout and suicide. The Department of Mental Health relies on a multi-disciplinary mechanism called MCATT (Mental Health Crisis Assessment and Treatment) which was established in 2012 to take action extending from medical centers to the community level, with the mobilization of village health volunteers (Department of Mental Health, Ministry of Public Health 2020b).

Amidst intense efforts to handle the epidemic, concerns were raised as to whose priorities count. One dramatic story, among others, concerns 100,000 Thai migrant workers in Malaysia who were trapped and could not return home. They simply could not afford to cover the cost of the new normal reentry protocol. Although the situation was gradually resolved with the help of local civil society, this created a bitter feeling among Malayu Muslims in the southern border provinces. Along the same line, a couple of protesters in Rayong province expressed their anger over discrepancies of how the new normal measures were enforced when a group of military diplomats were not quarantined despite the fact that one among them was infected. This resulted in almost 100 percent hotel cancellation in Rayong for fear of the spread. These may not be a big issues individually, but gaps in the handling of Covid-19 have added up, contributing to simmering political frustration over the issue of inequality.

Local and community initiatives: social capital and resilience

What emerges from the pandemic crisis is the rediscovery of sharing society, even after a long decade of political polarization. The recent political crisis has divided people in to rival camps, red and yellow shirts, creating the atmosphere of deep social distrust. The unprecedented impact of Covid-19 especially on the vulnerable groups changed the political biases. People volunteered and supported those in need of protection without concerning the color of the factions like before. One common factor among countries that have managed to curve the pandemic is that people comply with protection measures (Sawasdee 2020). As discussed before, Thai people comply, but they must first have the ability to do so. It is no exaggeration to say there are numerous individuals, groups and organizations that have contributed to the resilience of society under the crisis. Civil society and individuals function in diverse aspects of crisis management, for example, information platforms, knowledge sharing, fund raising, food sharing, village health volunteers, producing protective gear and sanitizers. In parallel, the corporate and provincial governors have also made a difference.

The first Covid-19 tracking platform and application was not done by the government but by volunteer professionals. These programs tracked the spread of the disease and helped inform decision-making processes. Other innovative ideas were also implemented such as Tu Pan Suk (Happiness Sharing Food Cabinet). Once a lot of people were laid off or could not carry out their business due to the lockdown, sharing food was the least people could do. The Tu Pan Suk spread throughout communities, helping those in need without having to travel too far.

Fundraising is common in civil society. However, during the Covid-19 lockdown, social network crowdfunding was widely experimented with. One incident raised 8 million Baht in just a couple of days to help a taxi driver. Social trust was surprisingly high during the crisis. People were often one step ahead of the government in distributing protective gear and sanitizers. When hospitals faced shortages of protective gear for medical professionals, people managed to raise funds, importing what was needed to donate to those hospitals. The project *Covid Relief Bangkok*, established by organizations in the civil society sector, collected a targeted THB 900,000 for the most vulnerable (BKK Kids 2020).

With regard to the role of the private sector, social enterprises collaborated on ad hoc projects to mobilize funds for protective gear for public health workers, teaching courses for making hand sanitizer and face masks with the support of village health volunteers across the country. For example, the *Socialgiver Group* that runs its business online donated revenues for Covid-19 assistance (www.socialgiver.com/en/give/covid-relief-bangkok). Perhaps the most astonishing experience was when farmers from the north and northeast communities collected rice and vegetables in their stock and sent it to fishing communities in the south in exchange for dried fish. This type of exchange can only be done with the support of existing networks of community development.

Conclusion: transformative possibilities?

The power and legitimacy of health and medical professionals as a trusted authority has been central to Thailand's success. The spread of Coronavirus galvanized many local communities and self-organization has played an important role outside of the central government's assistance. The central role of village health volunteers working with local government organizations during the lockdown has been evident. Local mechanisms filled in gaps where more centralized forms of crisis management did not work. Here is evidence of decentralization at work as a crucial tool for actualizing local governance.

Inequality matters both in the context of policy implementation by the centralized state and in correcting administrative gaps and policy biases. In response to suffering, Thailand has witnessed many spontaneous social responses across different social and cultural regions. A 'whole-society' perspective gives a more comprehensive picture of interactions between state and society at different levels. The pandemic has helped to articulate the roles of the state and civil society, though not without tensions.

Every crisis is a window of opportunity. It takes Covid-19 to realize that the country has been under threat of environmental hazards for a long time. The lockdown for a week suddenly turned PM 2.5 haze into the clearest sky for the first time in the past several years. People reported seeing whales and sea animals coming closer to the shoreline when the beaches were empty of the usual crowd of tourists. This changes people's perspective about our development and human security. If this moment was picked up, a policy change toward sustainability could have been anticipated.

Some people are satisfied with the ability to curve the epidemic, and some are struggling to survive the lockdown and fear for an unknown future. The Covid-19 crisis is actually seen from different perspectives. There is a saying that 'we are all in the same storm but we are not all in the same boat' (Tett 2020). Whether Covid-19 has made Thailand more capable of dealing with a crisis in the future and if the opportunity for change is being seized should receive timely attention. How does the crisis defined today determine a transformative future? Positive Covid-19 statistics is one side of the story; the other side is the high cost of the crumbling economy. The country faces entangled double crises. The new normal of disease prevention paradoxically jeopardizes the economy and democratic governance. Thus, a new norm should also apply to our business as usual in the economy, politics and governance. The short episode of Thailand's responses to Covid-19 raises awareness of major concerns for transformative agendas. First, as uncertainty becomes certain, a long debate over the investment in primary health care and health security coverage needs to be pursued further. Second, social resilience in time of crisis is not exclusively based on command and control but on social cohesion and networking. This is an outcome of long-term social capital development of local and civil society organizations. Third, local communities that are able to retain their autonomy over resources and sustainable livelihoods have a better chance of cope with uncertainty. This points to the significance of a transition to a sustainable society. The pandemic crisis has opened an opportunity to rethink, among other things, existing international supply chains and the viability of mass tourism as a backbone of the economy, meaningful local self-government, investment in social protection, the indifference in inequalities, and specifically for Thailand, the addiction to command-and-control methods such as the Emergency Decree.

The second wave of the pandemic broke out again in January 2021 as anticipated. The super spreader this time was from the Samut Sakhon Central Shrimp Market where thousands of migrants working in the market were found to be infected. The government wasted the opportunity during the control period to create conditions for social resilience by neglecting migrant workers. The incident reveals a chronic problem of governance over the issue of migrant workers that in the end affects the management of the pandemic. Judging from the conservative Thai political atmosphere today, the opportunity for a transformative agenda emerging from the crisis is not seized.

References

Bangkokbiznews. 2020. 'ไทม์ไลน์บริหารจัดการหน้ากากอนามัย เรามาถึงจุดนี้ได้อย่างไร,' *(Face Mask Management Timeline: How are we facing to this problem?)* [https://www.bangkokbiznews.com/news/detail/870637, accessed September 27, 2020].

The Bangkok Insight Editorial Team. 2020. 'โค้งสุดท้าย เราไม่ทิ้งกันส่งไม้ต่อสู่ คนละครึ่ง แจกเงินเยียวยาประชาชน.' *(The final stretch of the project No One Left Behind is being forwarded to the other one to distribute assistance to people)* [https://www.thebangkokinsight.com/437912/, accessed September 27, 2020].

Bello, Walden. 2020. 'How Thailand contained Covid-19: Why a public health system with popular support matters,' *Focus on the Global South* [https://focusweb.org/how-thailand-contained-Covid-19-why-a-public-health-system-with-popular-support-matters, accessed September 8, 2020].

BKK Kids. 2020. 'Who are Covid Relief Bangkok' [www.bkkkids.com/blog/who-are-Covid-relief-bangkok/, accessed August 21, 2020].

CARE. 2020. *Raks Thai Rapid Gender Analysis Gendered Impact of the Covid-19 Pandemic on Migrants in Thailand.* [https://reliefweb.int/report/thailand/rapid-gender-analysis-Covid-19-gendered-impact-Covid-19-pandemic-migrants-thailand, accessed September 8, 2020].

Court of Justice. 2020. 'เลขาธิการสำนักงานศาลยุติธรรม เผยสถิติฝ่าฝืน พรก.ฉุกเฉิน 1-15 พค.' *(The Secretary General of the Court of Justice Office reveals a number of breaking the Emergency Decree cases during 1–15 May 2020)* [www.coj.go.th/th/content/page/index/id/193207, accessed September 8, 2020].

Department of Disease Control, Ministry of Public Health. https://ddc.moph.go.th/viralpneumonia/eng/index.php.

Global Covid-19 Index (GCI) [https://covid19.pemandu.org/Thailand.html, accessed October 28, 2020].

Human Rights Watch. 2020. 'Thailand: State of Emergency Extension Unjustified,' [www.hrw.org/news/2020/05/27/thailand-state-emergency-extension-unjustified, accessed September 27, 2020].

iLaw. 2020. 'ศาลสั่งจำคุกแรงงานพม่า 3 เดือน 15 วัน นั่งเล่นโดมิโน 4 คน ฝ่าฝืน พรก.ฉุกเฉิน.' *(4 Burmese labors sentenced to 3 months and 15 days for breaking the Emergency Decree by playing domino game)* [https://ilaw.or.th/node/5704, accessed September 8, 2020].

Jala, Idris and Michael Barber 2020 *Global Lessons in Tackling Covid-19: The Global Pathfinder Initiative August 2020.* Permandu Associates and Delivery Associates. [https://covid19.pemandu.org/download/GPF%20Full%20Report.pdf, accessed October 29, 2020].

Kertesz, Daniel, Richard Brown, and Sushera Bunluesin. 2020. 'Thailand's 1 Million village health volunteers- unsung heroes- are helping guard communities nationwide from Covid-19.' [www.who.int/thailand/news/feature-stories/detail/thailands-1-million-village-health-volunteers-unsung-heroes-are-helping-guard-communities-nationwide-from-covid-19, accessed September 2020].

Mental Health, Department. 2020a. 'รายงานผลการคัดกรองความกังวลต่อไวรัสโควิดข19.' *(The report of anxiety screening to the Covid-19 virus)* [www.dmh.go.th/covid19/, accessed September 8, 2020].

Mental Health, Department. 2020b. แนวทางการฟื้นฟูจิตใจในสถานการณ์การระบาดของโรคติดเชื้อไวรัสโคโรนา 2019 Covid-19. (The mental rehabilitation measures in a pandemic situation of infectious Corona virus 2019: Combat the fourth wave of Covid-19: C4) [www.dmh.go.th/covid19/pnews/view.asp?id=23, accessed September 8, 2020].

Matichon Online. 2020a. 'ยอดตายไวรัสอู่ฮั่นพุ่ง 492 ติดเชื้อ 23,892 คนไทยรั้งที่ 2 ติดเชื้อ 25 แซงญี่ปุ่น' *(Wuhan Death toll reaches 492 with 23,892 infected people; Thai ranks 2nd with 25 infected people, overtaking Japan)*, 5 February 2019 [www.matichon.co.th/foreign/news_1945952, accessed October 29, 2020].

Money Buffalo. 2020. 'ผีน้อยคืออะไร? ผีน้อยพา Covid-19 กลับไทย?' *(What is Pee Noi? Does Pee Noi bring Covid-19 to Thailand?)* [www.moneybuffalo.in.th/ธุรกิจและเศรษฐกิจ/ผีน้อย-พาCovid-19-กลับไทย, accessed August 21, 2020].

National of Infectious Disease Commission. 2020. 'ข้อแนะนำป้องกันโควิด-19 ช่วงเดือนรอมฎอน.' *(Suggestions for preventing Covid-19 in a Ramadan month)* [http://healthydee.moph.go.th/view_article.php?id=752, accessed August 21, 2020].

NESDB Economic Report. 2020. [www.nesdc.go.th/ewt_dl_link.php?nid=10519&filename=QGDP_report, accessed October 28, 2020].

Ong-arj Decha. 2020. 'วิถีปกาเกอะญอเกราะหยี ปิดหมู่บ้านต้านโควิดการให้และแบ่งปันในยามวิกฤติโควิด-19.' *(Pga K'nyau way, Kro-yhi, village lockdown and sharing in the midst of Covid-19 pandemic)* วารสารผู้ไถ่ *(Journal of Savior)* 41: 113, 60–67.

Parichat Chk. 2020. 'ไวรัสโคโรนาระบาด: ยิ่งมีคนติดเชื้อเพิ่มขึ้นกระแสเหยียดจีน เกลียดกลัวคนจีนยิ่งรุนแรง' *(Corona Virus Outbreak: The more increase of infectious people, the more severely discriminate Chinese people)* [https://brandinside.asia/coronavirus-outbreak-xenophobia-raising/, accessed August 22, 2020].

Phukhao Post. 2020. 'โครงการปันสุขปลูกผัก สานพลังรัก บ้านวัด ราชการ (บวร) สร้างแหล่งอาหารในชุมชน.' *(Sharing Happiness project, planting for strengthening love among home, temple and officials to build food sources in a community)* [http://phukhaopost.com/news/28-0-10487-โครงการ-ปันสุข-ปลูกผัก-สานพลังรัก-บ้าน-วัด-ราชการ-(บวร)-สร้างแหล่งอาหารใน%EF%BF%BD, accessed August 22, 2020].

PPTV Online. 2020. 'ผลสำรวจเผยคนจนกว่าครึ่งเข้าไม่ถึงมาตรการเยียวยาโควิด-19.' *(A survey reveals that over a half of poor is not able to get into the official measure for relief from Covid-19 impact)* [www.pptvhd36.com/news/ประเด็นร้อน/126670, accessed September 27, 2020].

Prachatai. 2020. 'แรงงานข้ามชาติในวันที่มาตรการเยียวยาโควิด-19 ยังไปไม่ถึงพวกเขา.' *(Migrant workers with lack of relief measures for Covid-19)* [https://prachatai.com/journal/2020/05/87542, accessed September 27, 2020].

Primary Health Care Division. 2020. 'รายงาน อสม. ระดับประเทศ.' *(Report on National Village Health Volunteers)* [www.thaiphc.net/phc/phcadmin/administrator/Report/osm/province.php, accessed September 27, 2020].

Standard Team. 2020. 'เปิดสถิติ 5 เดือน กับการดำเนินคดีชุมนุมทางการเมืองภายใต้ พรก.ฉุกเฉิน คุมโควิด-19' *(A number of litigations to political gatherings under the enforcement of the Emergency Decree)* [https://thestandard.co/5-month-statistics-on-the-prosecution-of-political-rallies/, accessed September 8, 2020].

Tett, Gillian. 2020. Covid: We're in the same storm but not in the same boat, *Financial Times*, 30 September.

Thai PBS News. 2020. 'สธ เปิดสถิติฆ่าตัวตายเพิ่ม 22% จ่อตั้งทีมป้องกันเชิงรุกบนโซเชียล' *(Ministry of Public Health reports suicide rate increase by 22 %)*, 10 September 2020 [https://news.thaipbs.or.th/content/296311, accessed September 2020].

Thaiger. 2020. 'Thailand seals its 2,000 kilometer border with Myanmar' [https://thethaiger.com/news/national/thailand-seals-its-2000-kilometre-border-with-myanmar, accessed September 27, 2020].

Thaipost. 2020. 'ทบ.แจงกักตัวทหารสหรัฐยึดกฎ ศบค. ไม่มีข้อยกเว้นชี้จำเป็นฝึกต่อเนื่อง-แลกเปลี่ยนผู้เชี่ยวชาญ' *(The Army explains the quarantine of U.S. service men abiding by the Center of Covid-19 rules without exceptions, continuing military practice and experience exchange are necessary)* [www.thaipost.net/main/detail/73310, accessed September 2, 2020].

Thairat Online. 2020. 'สรุปไทม์ไลน์ .โควิด-19 ในไทย จากวันที่พบผู้ป่วยรายแรกสู่วันไร้ผู้ติดเชื้อ' *(Covid-19 Timeline in Thailand from the first infection found to the day with no infection)* posted 17 May [www.thairath.co.th/news/society/1843259, accessed October 28, 2020].

Thansettakij. 2020 'พรก ฉุกเฉิน ทำไมยังไม่ยกเลิก ฟังเหตะผลจาก ศบค' *(Why continue with the Emergency Decree – Listen to CCSA's justification)*. 20 July 2020 [www.thansettakij.com/content/politics/442887, accessed October 7, 2020].

Worapoj Singha. 2020. 'โรคโควิด-19 แรงงานข้ามชาติถูกละเมิดโดยความจำยอม เสียงจากคนทำงานด้านแรงงานข้ามชาติคุณอดิศร เกิดมงคล.' *(Migrant workers' right are breaking with undeniability, opinions of Adisorn Kerdmongkol, a person who works with migrant workers)* วารสารผู้ไถ่ *(Journal of Savior)* 41: 113, 60–67.

Workpoint News. 2020. 'เด็กพื้นที่ห่างไกลไม่พร้อมเรียนออนไลน์ช่วง Covid-19 เหตุไร้ไฟฟ้าสัญญาณอินเตอร์เน็ต.' *(Children in remote areas are not ready for online study during the Covid-19 outbreak because of lack of electricity and internet)* [https://workpointtoday.com/covid-19-education/, accessed September 27, 2020].

World Health Organization. 2020. 'Covid-19 Explorer.' [https://worldhealthorg.shinyapps.io/covid/, accessed September 26, 2020].

Middle East

8

IRAN AND COVID-19

Institutional configurations

Ali Asghar Mosleh and Abbas Jong

Due to its extensive ties with China, Iran was one of the first countries to face the Covid-19 crisis. Although the first case of the disease was officially confirmed by the government on February 19, there was evidence of its outbreak and spread in some parts of the country weeks before. Iran, which at that time was involved in various domestic, regional and international crises, was not prepared to face this one. With the 2018 withdrawal of the Trump administration from the Joint Comprehensive Plan of Action agreement and the imposition of unilateral sanctions, Iran has faced the intensification of various economic, political and cultural crises, impacting an economy in which the government plays a pivotal role, with oil revenues and foreign relations as central factors. These sanctions coincided with the escalation of Iran's involvement in regional and international conflicts, which further intensified the pressure on Iranian society, leading to widespread protests in November 2019 and the subsequent assassination of Iranian General Qassem Soleimani by the United States. Crises, political problems and a decline in its governing capacity characterized the Iranian state as it was forced to further confront the global pandemic.

On May 18 the Iranian Minister of Health, while presenting a report on Iran's performance to the World Health Organization, described the Iranian experience in two phases: readiness and treatment (defense) followed by extensive screening (attack). On the same day Iranian President Hassan Rouhani stated that the crisis has been brought under control, despite additional difficulties stemming from US sanctions.[1] In an earlier cabinet meeting, while criticizing the Chinese quarantine model as well as the collective security model of European countries, Rouhani emphasized the 'Iranian model' of dealing with the coronavirus pandemic as a successful model; a model which, in his opinion, could set a balance for the equation of economy and health.[2] How can we make sense of Iran's confrontation with the

Covid-19 crisis at the governmental level? How did Iranian governance strategies succeed after early failures? What institutional configurations were involved?

The current research examines Iran's Covid strategy, focusing on official administrative and government-directed institutions. It draws on official reports and accounts of the coronavirus crisis from January to April. Daily news items and reports were coded and contextually analyzed, identifying institutions, organizations and actors as well as institutional functions. Sources include official organizations, research centers and official news agencies, especially Iranian Students' News Agency (ISNA)[3] and Mehr News Agency.[4] Our analysis examines institutions based on seven functional categories.

Theoretical and empirical remarks

Francis Fukuyama (2020) has claimed that effectiveness in dealing with the Covid-19 crisis is based 'not the type of regime, but the state's capacity and, above all, trust in government.' Meanwhile, the efficiency of governments to concentrate power in their executive and bureaucratic branches in times of crisis is also of great importance. State capacity along with the independence of bureaucracy are two key aspects that can indicate quality of governance. Government capacity is highly dependent on access to resources and expenditure processes as well as levels of expertise at the executive level (Fukuyama, 2013, 2016). Governance and its components can be understood as interconnected and complex networks of different social elements and variables (Nederveen Pieterse, 2018; World Bank, 2007), what Guy Peters, following the idea of 'implementation structure' in public administration, calls 'governance structure' (Peters, 2014, 2016). In general, governance can be considered as 'the ability of government to make and enforce rules, and to deliver services' (Fukuyama, 2013) inwardly and through 'the interactive processes through which society and the economy are steered towards collectively negotiated objectives' (Ansell and Torfing, 2016: 4). These processes are embedded in and contingent on given institutional (implementation) structures (Peters, 2014, 2016). The key point in this definition is that although government itself (in terms of different political regimes) can have different relations to these processes, abilities and functions are limited and conditioned at an institutional level.

Accordingly, the study of different countries' reactions to the Covid-19 crisis in terms of different systems of governance can reveal institutional structures and their specific characteristics. For a country such as Iran with an indeterminate and uneven institutional structure that emerges from a complex and indeterminate regime of interests and power, any policy or governance intervention is accompanied by heterogeneous reactions at the institutional level. These institutional features make it difficult to simply locate Iran in macro-theoretical categories. These reactions should thus be considered as institutional configurations, following Boike Rehbein's (2015, 2018) notion of 'heterogeneous configuration.' Beyond any prior categorization and any kind of teleology, the quiddity of institutions and their relations will be meaningful only concerning a precisely defined experimental field and its historical and structural implications. Perceptions of relations (internal, external and between institutions) have a significant role in understanding objective reality. Since each configuration is regarded at a point between the universal and the singular, in an epistemological sense, it can also represent specific institutional conditions. These configurations are articulated when encountering specific problems at a definite time and place. Different issues and contexts allow us to identify institutions, configurations and their various relations.

Through modernization processes in Iran, the state imposes authority over institutional structures, which, in the Islamic Republic, are blended with a kind of political Islam. Due to embodied regimes of interests and powers, the Iranian state possesses a high level of indeterminacy and complexity (Katouzian, 1981, 1997; Skocpol, 1982; Abrahamian, 2008). Figure 8.1 represents the official political structure in Iran, which reveals multiplicity and hybridity of existing institutions. However, in practice, conflicts and incursions between different parts of the government are waged over political and economic interests. Due to an indeterminate institutional structure as well as the multifaceted nature of certain functions, many institutions do not remain within their boundaries. The judiciary in contemporary Iran, for instance, has been widely involved in many functional territories of the state and the economy. In addition to its sacred functions, religious institutions play a significant role in the construction of governance as well as the economy of Iran, in many cases conflicting with executive functions. Iran's system of government is thus best considered as a complex configuration of forces, actors, institutions and dominant organizations, which interact in a variety of indeterminate, fluid and uneven relations articulated through various regulatory forces.

The current study, beyond any conceptual essentialization of Iran's political structures, attempts to illustrate how the relative success of the Iranian government in controlling the first wave of the coronavirus was as the result of a kind of governmental configuration. It's important to note that this configuration is not the regular and ordinary governmental configuration. Rather, the efficient activation of regulatory forces represents an exceptional situation in which interfering, competing and distorted institutions fulfilled functions in a well-organized and effective configuration. The active participation of the Iranian people and society within this configuration played an important role in the effectiveness of the state's strategy.

Outbreak timeline

The city of Qom (the center of Shiite authority in Iran with extensive transnational relations) and then the city of Rasht in northern Iran (a popular recreational city; many from Tehran travel there for leisure) were the first two centers of the spread of this disease. The ensuing spread of the disease throughout Iran was facilitated by a lack of preparedness of medical institutions, a lack of foresight by relevant authorities and a lack of access to required equipment. Figure 8.2 shows the number of daily confirmed Covid-19 cases and deaths announced by the Ministry of Health of Iran.

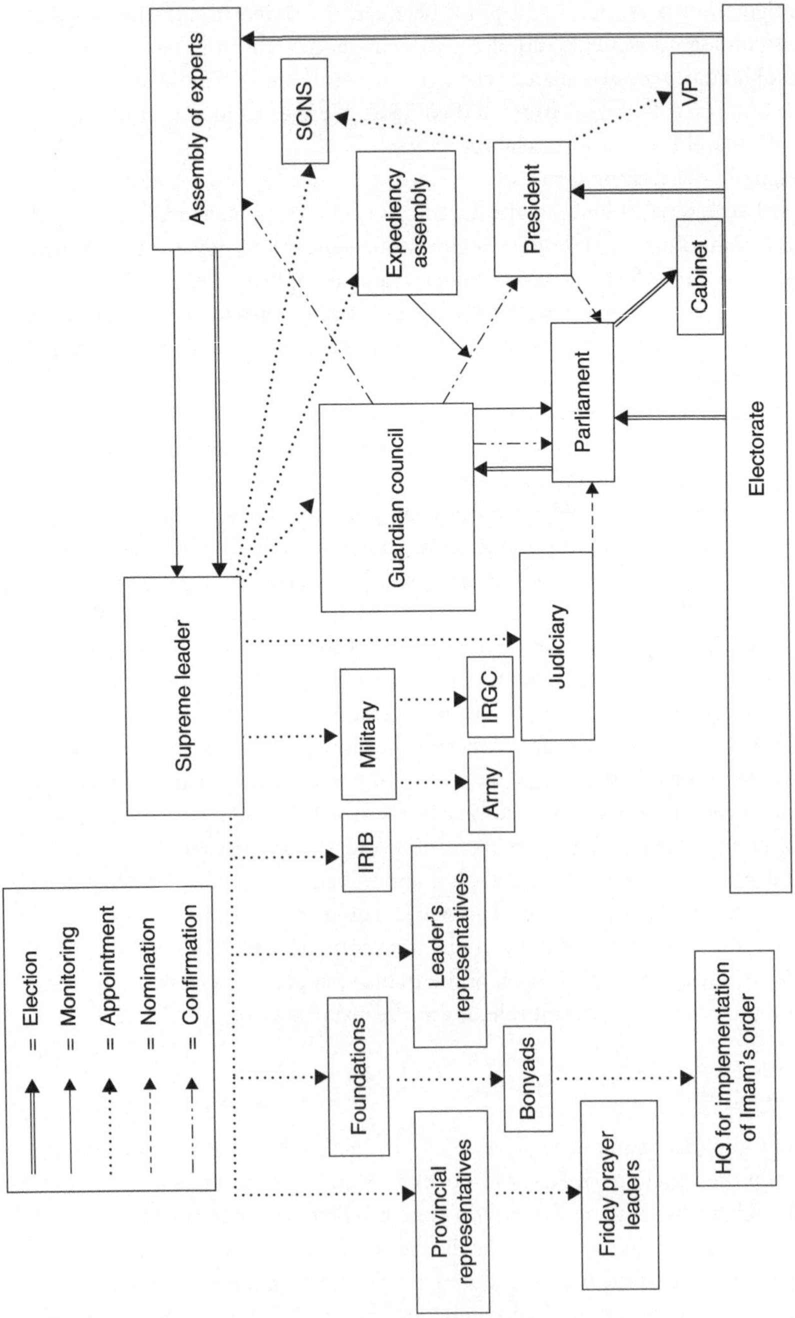

FIGURE 8.1 Political structure of power in contemporary Iran

Source: Retrieved from Boroujerdi and Rahimkhani (2018: 37).

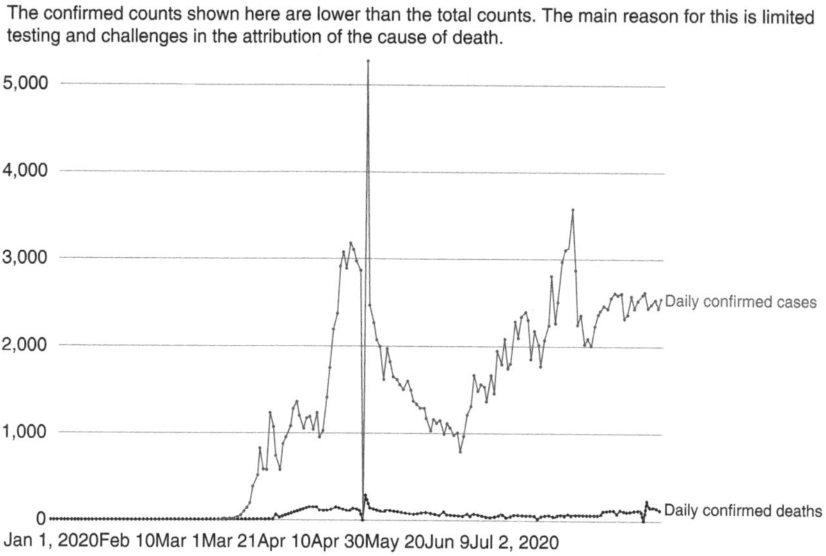

FIGURE 8.2 Daily confirmed Covid-19 cases and deaths, Iran

As in many countries, Iran's encounter with the disease began with rumors, denial, conspiracy delusion, ambiguity in the number of cases and deaths, and initial confusion and lack of efficient plans, which eventually led to the formation of a special headquarters to manage the various aspects of the pandemic. After several days of confusion and disorientation within the state, on February 23 with the order of the President and with the authorization of the Supreme National Security Council and the approval of the Supreme Leader of Iran, the Minister of Health was tasked to establish the National Anti-Corona Headquarters. The members of this headquarters include the Minister of Interior, Minister of Roads and Urban Development, Minister of Education, Minister of Science, Minister of Cultural Heritage and Tourism, Minister of Culture, Chief of General Staff of the Armed Forces, Attorney General, Head of Program and Budget Organization, Head of Radio and Television, Head of the Hajj and Pilgrimage Organization, the government spokesman, the commander of the police force and a member of the Guardian Council. All decisions and affairs related to the crisis, including public notices and policies became centralized. This concentration of power in the executive branches played a key role in efficiently managing this crisis in Iranian society by flattening existing institutional interferences and rivalries. Even religious institutions were subject to the decisions of this powerful medical institution.

The establishment of this headquarters was followed by a series of executive policies, which closed and restricted public places and events, including universities, schools, public meetings, religious, political and cultural ceremonies, sports competitions, cinemas, and so on. Additional measures included restrictions on domestic and foreign travel, the implementation of prevention and treatment protocols, social distancing, disinfection of some public spaces, removal of certain legal restrictions in the economic field, and provisioning of medical facilities.[5] Due to the intense pressure of US sanctions against Iran the provision of many medical items proved difficult. However, due to existing medical and productive infrastructure in Iran, the state was able to manage; the Chinese government also played a pivotal role in supplying many items. By creating and expanding local production capacity for testing kits, extending free sampling centers, and preparing detailed statistics for each region, as well as increasing the number of medical centers dedicated to the disease and classifying patients, Iran was able to successfully overcome the first wave of Covid-19 in late April.

Apart from a small amount of global aid and imports of required items and technologies from China, Iran claimed to have been able to produce three models of coronavirus detection kits, relying on local technology by knowledge-based companies and to mass-produce them with government and military assistance to greatly increase the speed of test and detection. During this period, many of the required hygienic items began to be produced domestically (Islamic Parliament Research Center of the Islamic Republic of Iran, IPRC, 2020b). The government's financial constraints, as well as the structure of Iran's economy, culture and society, prevented the implementation of many successful strategies and techniques adopted and exercised by other countries in the face of coronavirus such as severe lockdowns and interpersonal tracking. Given available resources, Iran concentrated on the expansion of testing and detecting capacities, as well as special hospitals and health centers for the treatment of Covid-19 patients. The government's strategy was assisted by good practices of self-regulation by Iranians in the absence of a system of widespread supervision and discipline. The strategy, as the President put it, was accompanied by the cooperation of more than 80 percent of the population, helping Iran to overcome the first wave of the disease by the end of April.

Governance in phase I

As mentioned above, the advancement of these policies simultaneously required coordination and cohesion among governmental and administrative institutions along with support of social institutions. Based on our review, the institutions involved in Iran's response to the Covid crisis can be placed within seven functional categories: macro-policymaking (strategies and priorities); specific policymaking; policy implementation and enforcement; regulatory adaptation; medical and hygienic activities; provision and facilities; and surveillance and disciplinary activities. Each category needs to be examined in detail to identify its elements, institutions and relations. Some of the institutions that have shaped Iran's Covid response include government and administrative institutions, religious and market institutions, economic cartels, military and security organizations, nongovernmental social institutions, such as families, NGOs, charities, cultural institutions, media, scientific and academic institutions. While some institutions may be confined to a single category, others span multiple categories. The Ministry of Health and police force, for example, performed several institutional functions. The alignment of interests within a complex regime of power is an exceptional situation. The crisis has revealed the ambiguity of the boundaries between state, religious and economic institutions which have different and even contradictory functions. Institutional relations in this crisis have been mostly complementary due to common interests, with the exception being market institutions.

Macro-level policymaking has been carried out by the National Anti-Corona Headquarters, chaired by the President and led by the Ministry of Health, which became legal and operational through the support and approval of Iran's Supreme Leader, obliging other apparatus, organizations and institutions to follow and obey its decisions. In recent years, a lack of intervention by the Supreme Leader has been associated with political crises and functional problems for executive bodies that have been mired in power conflicts. However, with the permission of the Supreme Leader, the state was able to withdraw one million euros from the National Development Fund, and at the time of the parliament's closure, the Supreme Leader agreed to delegate the approval of the 1399 budget (2020–2021) to the Parliamentary Integration Commission so as not to disrupt government performance. These functions should be performed by the parliament, however, due to its deteriorating influence and the expansion of supranational governing institutions, parliament has fallen into dysfunction, exacerbated by a crisis of active domestic participation.

In the context of regulatory adaptation, institutions increasingly turned to cyberspace. Education, with the support of the Ministry of Communications, introduced the 'Shad' virtual network, which was able to meet the educational needs of schools to some extent. Universities also continued their activities virtually. Holding social events was banned and with the support of religious institutions, many religious centers and religious occasions and rituals were closed or transferred to cyberspace, all of which are innovations. Closures, reduction of working hours, expansion of telecommuting, leave for prisoners, conscription postponements, and so on, were also part of regulatory adaptation. Together, the Ministry of Communications, Islamic Republic of Iran Broadcasting and police force were able to achieve a substantial information monopoly during the Covid-19 pandemic. Various media campaigns with the widespread support of religious and cultural institutions have been among the most important measures taken by the government in this regard.

In the field of medical and hygienic care, the Ministry of Health played an important role by implementing the strategy of follow-up, diagnosis, containment and treatment, as well as the intelligent distribution and provision of health facilities and medical items. The Red Crescent and military forces also played an important role in meeting immediate medical and hygienic needs. The Ministry of Health compiled health protocols for medical centers, patients and other social groups, including protocols for collective ceremonies, social distancing, different guild activities, virtual health counseling and supporting indigenous treatment methods. When it comes to surveillance and discipline, the role of the judiciary, police force, the Ministry of the Interior, municipalities and Ministry of Communications has been significant. Their role has been to oversee the implementation of policies formulated by the National Anti-Corona Headquarters. These tasks included dealing with groups that disregard health protocols, countering hoarding and overselling hygienic and medical items, controlling the activities of manufacturers and trade guilds, supervising trips and entries and exits to and from cities, surveillance of cyberspace violations, controlling published news and dealing with fake publishers, combating the damage caused by this pandemic, and so on.

In the field of provision and facilities, various institutions have played important roles providing medical and hygienic items as well as economic support for the vulnerable classes, including governmental institutions such as the Imam Khomeini Relief Foundation and the Foundation for the Oppressed. With the support of state financial institutions, the Ministry of Industry, Mining and Trade implemented policies and permits for the import of health items, essential goods and services from foreign markets. Allocations to fight Covid-19 are estimated at over 100 thousand billion Iranian Tomans,[6] including 12.6 thousand billion Tomans for the Ministry of Health, 2,300 billion Tomans for health insurance. Other allocations have been made for unemployment insurance as well as four subsequent support packages to three million Iranian households under economic pressure. In additionone million loans have been granted to 23 million households with the support of subsidies. Based on its budget revenue management, the government withdrew €1 billion from the National Development Fund to fight the Covid-19 pandemic, making up the deficit by selling shares of state-owned companies. The Ministry of Foreign Affairs also tried to free up resources blocked under sanctions, which achieved some successes.

Despite the success of government's strategy in getting the pandemic under control by the end of April, Iranian society has faced additional pressures with a second wave of the coronavirus pandemic, which began in early July. This second wave has been accompanied by intense market reactions, increasing economic pressure, and the lack of a dynamic strategy for the post-crisis situation. Since late June, the value of the national currency appears to have reached its lowest level in contemporary Iranian history as a result of the state's budget deficit, exacerbated by the Covid-19 crisis, a sharp decline in state revenues and poor economic performance. Negative economic growth in 2018 and 2019 has reduced the formation of fixed capital as a result of a reduction of potential production capacity and lowering the level of public welfare. This situation, in light of US sanctions, along with inflation above 40 percent and instability in the foreign exchange market, has led to the closure of many economic enterprises and put Iran's economy in a state of recession and uncertainty. As a result of the Covid-19 crisis, demand for Iranian products in world markets has decreased and domestic demand also declined due to lessening household incomes as well as diminishing goods and services (transportation, restaurants, tourism, etc.). The economy has also faced supply shocks due to disruptions in the raw material supply network. The Parliament Research Center estimates that between 5.7 and 11 percent of the economy's supply has fallen as a result of the coronavirus outbreak and between 2.9 and 6.4 million current employees will lose their jobs due to the virus (IPRC, 2020b). Another report of the Ministry of Welfare estimates that 3.7 million jobs were affected by the Covid-19 crisis, with low-income earners disproportionately affected (Deputy Minister of Economic Affairs and Planning of the Ministry of Cooperatives, 2020).

Conclusion

Iran faced the Covid-19 crisis at a time of tough US sanctions and deep crises, but was able to get through the first wave of the crisis with a strategy that mobilized institutions under a centralized authority. This configuration and its relative success reveal an important aspect of the institutional structure and the capacities of contemporary Iran. Iranian society has demonstrated a high degree of resilience in the face of the coronavirus outbreak. This can be at least partially attributed to the country's tumultuous history, including the Eight-Year War between Iran and Iraq, various sanctions, and political and economic pressures. These experiences have provided Iran with an important advantage in dealing with crises.

The Covid-19 crisis has exacerbated current crises in Iran and has imposed unprecedented pressure on the market and society. This crisis has changed some of Iran's domestic and international relations and behaviors. Despite the relative success of the Iranian state and government in controlling the first wave of the crisis, severe economic and social pressures have caused subsequent Covid-19 waves and the state has been unable to reemploy its previous strategy. The government's executive capacity has drastically declined, which has paved the way for the emergence of rival and non-elected government institutions alongside destructive political and economic forces. The entanglement of issues and crises in contemporary Iran, in which the Covid-19 crisis is just one of several serious crises, has left the future of the post-Covid-19 situation in an ambiguous state. The Iranian people are left in a critical situation as a result of a widening governance cap, brutal pressure from the US government and the Covid-19 crisis. Taken together, the situation seems to put Iranian society at the brink of economic and social collapse, providing a unique opportunity for Special Forces and currents to consolidate and expand their power.

Notes

1 ISNA. Rouhani: If it was not for the support of the Supreme Leader, we certainly could not have achieved the current success in the fight against Corona: www.isna.ir/news/99022921224/روحانی-حمایت-مقام-معظم-رهبری-نبود-قطعا-نمی-توانستیم-در-مبارزه
2 ISNA. Supporting businesses in trouble/social distancing plan has been helpful: www.isna.ir/news/99011306435/کمک-به-کسب-و-کارهایی-که-دچار-مشکل-شدند-طرح-فاصله-گذاری-اجتماعی
3 www.isna.ir
4 www.mehrnews.com
5 http://president.ir/fa/114345
6 The Iranian toman is a superunit of the official currency of Iran, the rial. One toman is equivalent to ten rials. The rial is the official currency, Iranians use the toman in everyday life.

References

Abrahamian, E. (2008). *A History of Modern Iran*. Cambridge: Cambridge University Press. Retrieved from https://doi.org/10.1017/CBO9780511984402 (accessed July 1, 2020).

Amable, B. (2003). *The Diversity of Modern Capitalism*. Oxford: Oxford University Press.

Ansell, C. and Torfing, J. (2016). *Handbook on Theories of Governance*. Northampton: Edward Elgar.

Boroujerdi, M. and Rahimkhani, K. (2018). *Postrevolutionary Iran*. Syracuse: Syracuse University Press. Retrieved from https://doi.org/10.2307/j.ctt20p56tf.

Deputy Minister of Economic Affairs and Planning of the Ministry of Cooperatives, L. and S.W. (2020). *Effects of Coronavirus Outbreak on Business and Household Welfare, Protectionist Policies in Iran and the World*. Retrieved from www.mcls.gov.ir/fa/article/1558/ (accessed July 1, 2020) آثار-شیوع-ویروس-کرونا-بر-کسب-وکار-و-رفاه-خانوارها-سیاست-های-حمایتی-در-ایران-و-جهان

Fukuyama, F. (2013). What Is Governance? *Governance, 26* (3), 347–368. Retrieved from https://doi.org/10.1111/gove.12035.

——— (2016). Governance: What Do We Know, and How Do We Know It? *Annual Review of Political Science, 19* (1), 89–105. Retrieved from https://doi.org/10.1146/annurev-polisci-042214-044240.

——— (2020). The Thing That Determines a Country's Resistance to the Coronavirus. Retrieved from www.theatlantic.com/ideas/archive/2020/03/thing-determines-how-well-countries-respond-coronavirus/609025/ (accessed July 1, 2020).

Islamic Parliament Research Center of the Islamic Republic of Iran (IPRC). (2020a). *On Coping with Corona Outbreaks (16) Assessing the Roadmap and Leadership Requirements (Second Edition)* (21016962 No. 16). Retrieved from https://rc.majlis.ir/fa/report/show/1490085 (accessed July 1, 2020).

——— (2020b). *On Coping with Corona Outbreaks (40) Assessing the Macroeconomic Dimensions of the Coronavirus Outbreak (First Edition)* (17011 No. 40). Retrieved from https://rc.majlis.ir/fa/report/show/1510373 (accessed July 1, 2020).

——— (2020c). *On Coping with Corona Outbreaks (46) Capacities and Challenges in Knowledge-Based Activities and Technology Businesses* (27017058 No. 46). Retrieved from https://rc.majlis.ir/fa/report/show/1531396 (accessed July 1, 2020).

——— (2020d). *On Coping with the Corona Outbreak (28) The Challenges of the Iranian Family in the Face of Corona* (27016976 No. 28). Retrieved from https://rc.majlis.ir/fa/report/show/1502819 (accessed July 1, 2020).

Katouzian, H. (1981). *The Political Economy of Modern Iran*. London: Palgrave Macmillan UK. Retrieved from https://doi.org/10.1007/978-1-349-04778-9.

——— (1997). Arbitrary Rule: A Comparative Theory of State, Politics and Society in Iran. *British Journal of Middle Eastern Studies, 24* (1), 49–73. Retrieved from https://doi.org/10.1080/13530199708705638.

Momeni, F. (2017). *Social Justice, Freedom and Development in Contemporary Iran*. Tehran: Naghs o Nashr.

Nederveen Pieterse, J. (2018). *Multipolar Globalization*. London: Routledge.

North, D. (1990). *Institutions, Institutional Change and Economic Performance*. Cambridge: Cambridge University Press.

Peters, B. G. (2014). Implementation Structures as Institutions. *Public Policy and Administration, 29* (2), 131–144. Retrieved from https://doi.org/10.1177/0952076713517733.

——— (2016). Institutional Theory. In C. Ansell and J. Torfing (Eds.), *Handbook on Theories of Governance* (pp. 308–321). Northampton: Edward Elgar.

Rehbein, B. (2015). *Critical Theory After the Rise of the Global South Kaleidoscopic Dialectic*. New York: Routledge.

——— (2018). Critical Theory After the Rise of the Global South. In *Social Theory and Asian Dialogues* (pp. 49–67). Singapore: Springer. Retrieved from https://doi.org/10.1007/978-981-10-7095-2_4.

Skocpol, T. (1982). Rentier State and Shi'a Islam in the Iranian Revolution. *Theory and Society*, *11*(3). Retrieved from https://doi.org/10.1007/BF00211656.

Wimmer, A. (2002). *Nationalist Exclusion and Ethnic Conflict: Shadows of Modernity*. Cambridge: Cambridge University Press.

World Bank. (2007). *A Decade for Measuring the Quality of Governance*. Washington, DC.

9

SAUDI ARABIA AND COVID-19

Religious institutions

Frank Fanselow

Covid-19 poses a crisis of legitimacy for governments in many societies. Daily league tables of the number of new infections, tests, ICU cases, recoveries, deaths and reproduction rates published in the media have turned into an international competition for showcasing the effectiveness of their policies and serve domestically as an opportunity for governments to parade their efficiency in bringing the public health crisis under control, and for opposition forces an opportunity to challenge governments over their ineffectiveness and negligence in handling it.

But when the curves started to flatten and the initial shock subsided, attention turned to the economic fall-out, and further down the line to the political and security consequences of the global economic downturn. Apart from public health statistics, now financial and economic performance indicators, governments are navigating the seemingly incompatible demands of the health of their population and the health of their economies. GDP rates, unemployment figures, trade deficits, housing evictions, as well as public health budget increases, sizes of stimulus packages, job support packages, and tax relief compete with the number of new infections and recoveries for public attention.

The Arab Gulf countries

While most governments had to quickly develop emergency programs for their citizens, who were becoming sick, un(der)employed and homeless, to soften the economic crisis and pre-empt potential political instability, the Arab Gulf states were in some ways much better prepared than most others. Their governments were already providing extensive social security for citizens long before Covid-19 struck. These states are in a position to afford the highest public sector employment rates in the world: In Saudi Arabia about 72 percent of the citizen workforce are employed in the public sector, in Kuwait about 72 percent, in Qatar about 86 percent. Following the Arab Spring uprisings, the UAE even increased its public sector employment of citizens to about 90 percent for political reasons (Asaad and Barsoum 2019). Public sector jobs provide not only a salary but also security: not just job security but other social benefits, such as access to interest-free or cheap housing loans, residential land grants, free health care, and free education to university level.

On the other hand, the private sector in these Gulf Cooperation Council (GCC) countries is overwhelmingly staffed by foreign employees: over 90 percent of private sector employees are foreigners in Qatar and the UAE, and over 80 percent in Saudi Arabia (Karasapan 2020). Although the private sector is hard hit by the economic fall-out of the crisis, without access to permanent residence or citizenship its overwhelmingly foreign workforce is politically irrelevant. For the relatively small number of their citizens working in the private sector, some GCC countries have implemented relief measures. In Saudi Arabia the government introduced a furlough system, promising to pay 60 percent of salaries over three months (al-Monitor April 2020). Job losses are concentrated among the non-national workforce with many migrant workers forced to return to their home countries whose governments' economic policies had relied to a significant extent on exporting their unemployed and generating foreign currency inflows from migrant laborers. As a result, in countries like Pakistan, Bangladesh, and the Philippines, substantial numbers of returning migrant workers add to the already growing unemployed numbers, and the fall in remittances widens budget deficits at a time when governments have sharply increased financial commitments. In this reverse migration the unemployed, originally exported by their countries of origin, are now being re-imported with all the potential for economic and political instability that this has for their home countries (Slater and McQue 2020).

The capacity to sustain a huge public sector that enables the state to employ almost the entire economically active citizenry, depends on the continued flow of oil and gas revenues and income from accumulated investments. In such rentier political economies, the main source of state revenue is not derived from taxation of economic productivity of its population, but from external rents derived from accidents of geology or geography, such as the sale of raw materials, in this case oil and gas. Instead of the state redistributing social wealth collected in the form of taxes from the rich to the poor, in the political economies put the state in the unique position to distribute wealth without having to tax its citizens. The social contract of such 'Shellfare' states is therefore very different from other types of states: the state is expected to provide social security and economic rewards to its citizens – or the king to his subjects – who in return are expected to remain loyal despite the absence of formal political representation and institutionalized democratic participation.

Rentier state theory has in recent years come under criticisms, for example for overlooking the effects of economic diversification and of informal, non-conventional forms of political participation by a supposedly depoliticized population (Hvidt 2011, Zicchieri 2016). While it is true that Gulf economies have begun to diversify and no longer depend solely on oil exports, their success still largely depends indirectly on oil, maybe not their own but that of their neighbors. Dubai stands out in transforming itself into a real estate economy, but much of the money that flows into real estate is generated by in the oil industry in its neighborhood, including not just in Abu Dhabi but also in Saudi Arabia and other GCC states. The 'Dubai Model' could hardy succeed in a poorer neighborhood, as the case of Brunei shows which has the least diversified economy of all oil-producing rentier states. Although in need of revision, rentier state theory remains a powerful explanatory tool in the case of political economies that, despite the lack political representation and democratic participation, maintain a high level of legitimacy as a result of the dominant role of the distributive state over the society (Yamada 2020).

The great Covid-19 gamble

While oil rentierism gives the state a uniquely dominant position over society, it also makes it deeply dependent on external, global market forces and vulnerable to global economic crises. In the post-1973 period during which the Kingdom of Saudi Arabia emerged as the world's largest oil exporter, the country could use its monopolistic powers – in coordination with other OPEC producers – to exercise significant influence over global oil prices through supply-side measures.

But in the last decades its ability to control oil prices has sharply declined. The emergence of post-Soviet Russia as a major oil and gas exporter outside OPEC, the rise of the US shale oil industry which has made the US the largest producer in the world, as well as the development of new low-energy and alternative energy technologies has meant that the kingdom's global market share has declined to a level where it can no longer rule the markets.

Recognizing its problematic dependence on global energy markets, the Saudi government has in recent years adopted policies intended to turn the country into a developmental state ('Vision 2030') – similar to the UAE or Singapore – in which economic diversification and capitalist expansion take place in the context of strong state intervention and regulation of the economy, including heavy infrastructural investment to attract foreign investment. The reasoning is that by jump-starting the private sector and delivering rapid economic development, the state would be able to reduce, and eventually relinquish, its costly responsibilities of employing and paying almost its entire population.

In pursuit of this '2030 Vision', but faced with declining oil revenues, and no longer in a position to exert monopolistic powers in the global energy market, the Saudi government has in recent years turned to high-risk gambling to play the oil markets. In the first oil price war that started in 2014, Saudi Arabia sought to bankrupt US shale oil producers by undercutting global prices. By increasing output and pushing prices down, the kingdom hoped to push shale oil producers out of the market, but these turned out to be more resilient than anticipated and managed to cut production cost to a level that allowed them to stay in the market below the break-even price of the Saudi state budget and were therefore too costly for the kingdom to sustain in the longer term. The price war ended in 2016 with an agreement between OPEC and Russia (OPEC+) to cut production in order to maintain prices at sustainable levels.

But when the Covid-19 crisis began to unfold in March 2020, Saudi Arabia took another gamble on the global oil market. At first, when the Covid-19 outbreak brought about a sharp drop in oil prices, the government sought to get OPEC+ again to cut production to keep prices high, but Russia refused to follow suit. By mid-March the Saudis reversed gear to punish US shale producers – as well as the Russians – by further undercutting the already low oil prices to increase their market share and push their competitors out of the market. The gamble turned out to be disastrous as – amidst falling demand – oil prices spun out of control and remained well below the break-even price of all major players, in some cases even pushing prices into negative territory due to high storage costs for future oil deliveries.

Domestic implications: shaking the foundations of rentier state social contract

In the face of the dual challenge of the Covid-19 crisis and the oil price war, the Saudi government had little option but to adopt unprecedented austerity measures, such as a tripling ofVAT and cuts in salary allowances for the public sector that had been introduced during the first oil price war to offset the effect of increased petrol prices. Such austerity measures were the opposite of policies adopted in many other countries intended to help alleviating the consequences of the economic crisis, such as tax cuts and income supplements.

That is one of the paradoxes of the rentier state economics: when global prices fall, in non-rentier states domestic prices fall as well, but for governments of rentier states falling oil prices mean declining revenues and they face the difficult choice of cutting subsidies and implementing tax increases to offset the loss of revenue from external sources. From the perspective of citizens of these countries, responding to falling oil prices by raising domestic prices is counter-intuitive and this becomes politically difficult to sell domestically. Such austerity measures shake the very foundations of the social contract on which the rentier state is based. Decades of distributive state policies have nurtured a culture of entitlement and dependence which is difficult to counter, except at considerable political costs. As the ability of the state institutions to fulfil their side of the bargain declines, the specter of political dissatisfaction arises.

Religion and political legitimacy

In Saudi Arabia, this comes at a time when the government's pursuit of the 'modernizing' developmental state has already alienated many 'traditional' tribal and religious leaders. In recent years the balance of power in the Saud-Wahabi alliance has shifted towards one particular faction of the royal family, leaving other factions of the family as well as the conservative religious establishment out in the cold.

For Muslim nations in general, and Saudi Arabia in particular, the Coronavirus could not have come at a worse time, hitting them right at the beginning of a season of intensified religious activities. Ramadan family gatherings for breaking the fast (*iftar*), followed by prolonged community prayers (*tarawikh*), the minor pilgrimage (*umrah*) season during the month of Ramadan, followed at the end of July by the annual *haj* pilgrimage to Makkah, one of the world's largest religious gatherings attracting 2.5 million pilgrims from all over the world – all these constitute ideal conditions for the spread of a virus both through local communities and global networks as pilgrims carry it back home all over the world.

There have been private hostility and public protests to restrictions imposed on religious activities in other religions, including Jewish (e.g. Holmes 2020, Kershner 2020) and Christian communities in different countries (Duin 2020, Song, Buseong and Edward White 2020). But in the context of secular states, the state's alleged interference in religion does not have the same implications it has in a state like Saudi Arabia, where Islam has historically been the pillar of legitimacy of the state and where such measures are therefore particularly sensitive.

Historically the Saudi dynasty has used its custodianship of the two holiest places of Islam as a source of religious legitimacy domestically as well as internationally. Already long before the Saudi conquest of the Hijaz, the western part of the country where Makkah and Medina are located, the Saudi dynasty had entered into a symbiotic alliance with the Wahhabi religious movement to gaining religious legitimacy in return for economic support for Wahhabi *ulama* and their institutions. Following the Battle of Makkah in 1924, in which the Sauds defeated the Hashemite dynasty of the Hijaz, the Saudi dynasty began ruling the holy cities in Islam and claiming the role of 'protectors of religion', and in the 1980s the Saudi kings officially assumed the ancient title 'Custodian of the Two Holy Mosques' formalizing that claim.

Since its conquest of the Makkah almost a hundred years ago, the Saudi state has regarded the organization of the annual *haj* pilgrimage – widely seen as one of the largest and most complex collective events globally – as their most important religious function as well as a measure of the administrative competence and efficiency of their state. Apart from its religious and political importance, the pilgrimage also has huge financial value to the country's economy. Before the discovery of oil, it was the state's most important source of income, and in the '2030 Vision' it plays a major role in a diversified post-oil economy.

In the last decades, enormous resources have been spent on the organization of the pilgrimage, both in terms of its physical infrastructure and the huge bureaucratic apparatus tasked with regulating all aspects of the pilgrimage, including public health. In some ways Saudi Arabia was therefore better prepared for an epidemic than most other countries. Since a meningitis outbreak during the 1987 pilgrimage, and the Middle East Respiratory Syndrome (MERS) in 2013, the public health authorities had been concerned about the threat of new epidemics and imposed drastic public health regimes to prevent outbreaks of communicable diseases among pilgrims.

As the news of the Coronavirus spread at the beginning of the year, Saudi authorities, therefore, were quick to react. They closed the country's borders to foreign pilgrims on February 27, 2020 at a time when according to official figures no cases had yet been found in the country (*The Guardian*, 27/2/2020). Three days later on March 2 the first case was identified: a Saudi citizen who had returned from a trip to Iran, which by that time had already been heavily affected (Arab News, 2/3/2020). The Saudi government does not officially allow its citizens to travel to Iran, but many Shi'ites in the eastern provinces of the country visit Iran via Bahrain, and Iranian immigration officials do not stamp their passports, which made it difficult to identify potential carriers (Abdo and Jacobs 2020, Hanna 2020).

The virus immediately became ethnicized and politicized in the local and social media where some referred to it as the 'Iranian virus'. Shi'ite citizens were accused of importing and spreading it, and the government put the restive, predominantly Shi'ite eastern Qatif province under curfew on March 12. Apart from anti-Shi'ite sentiment, social media also stoked racist sentiments against foreign migrant workers who stood accused of bringing the virus into the country and spreading it through their careless hygienic habits. As in other countries, the virus thus stoked nationalist sentiments by casting it as a threat to the Saudi body politic emanating from foreign bodies.

Following the closure of its external borders, the government issued orders for the closure of all mosques, including those at Makkah and Madinah, on March 17 (Al Arabiya 17/3/2020). After an extended period of uncertainty and speculation about the *haj* pilgrimage, on June 23 the government announced that international pilgrims were banned from the *haj* this year and, while it would not be entirely canceled, the *haj* would only be conducted on a minimalist and symbolic scale with a tiny number of pilgrims who already live in the country representing different Muslim countries (Al Arabiya, 23/6/2020).

The orders to close mosques and cancel the normal *haj* came from the Ministry of Health, not from the religious authorities. But these orders were strongly supported by the entire official religious establishment, including the Ministry of Islamic Affairs, the Council of Senior Scholars, the State Mufti, and other state-linked religious organizations. Public reactions criticizing the move remained muted and did not coalesce into any collective expressions of criticism domestically. The state's control over the religious establishment seems to have remained intact (Wehrey et al. 2020). Most Saudi citizens appear to have accepted the medical need for restricting the performance of religious duties. Outside the kingdom, however, the Saudi government's measures attracted criticism from Islamist voices that took the opportunity to challenge Saudi authority over the holy sites and its leadership role in the Muslim world.

The wider context: reactions in other Muslim nations

Saudi Arabia's religious response to Covid-19 must also be considered in the context of its special role in the wider Muslim world. In the global Muslim community (*ummah*), Saudi Arabia is not just one Muslim nation among others, but for historical reasons and by virtue of its custodianship of the holy cities of Makkah and Madinah occupies a pivotal position in the Muslim world. It is not just the geographical center for the performance of prayer and pilgrimage rituals, but also a theological point of orientation through the voices of its religious establishment (*ulama*). Saudi religious policies therefore have repercussions around the Muslim world, either providing a model for others to follow or a front to attack the kingdom.

The first country to introduce Covid-19 restrictions was Kuwait when on March 13 its Ministry of Religious Endowment ordered the closure of mosques for the five daily prayers as well as Friday prayers (Reuters, 13/3/20). Widely reported internationally was the change of wording of the call to prayer (*adhan*) from 'come to prayer' to 'pray at home'. Two days later the UAE National Crisis and Emergency Management Authority and the General Authority for Islamic Affairs and Endowments jointly announced the closure of mosques (The National, 16/3/20), and as soon as Saudi Arabia did the same on March 17, governments of most other Muslim countries in the region and beyond introduced similar restrictions.

While these measures provoked little public opposition in Saudi Arabia and other Arab countries, they were met by criticism and open resistance in some of the largest Muslim countries with a more developed civil society, greater political participation, and more independent religious authorities. In Indonesia, the world's largest Muslim nation, the government avoided issuing orders for the blanket closure of mosques and called on Friday prayers to be suspended for two weeks from 20 March, but this was not enforced and many mosques defied the request (Siregar 2020). The weakness of the state revealed itself in continuing resistance to mosque closure by Islamist preachers and some religious organizations (Syafiq 2020). The government set the tone when it was also hesitant to cancel a large regional meeting in Sulawesi by the Tabligh Jamaat in Sulawesi, an international movement that seeks to educate Muslims to perform their religious duties more strictly. After an initial letter asking the organizers to cancel the meeting was ignored, the government only forced a cancelation under widespread pressure at the last minute on March 19 when thousands of the participants had already arrived at the venue (Muhtada 2020).

In Malaysia the federal government left it up to religious authorities to impose the closure of mosques. According to the constitution, religious matters are left to the authority of sultans of the different federal states, who in turn refer it to their respective state mufti. As a result, there was no uniform date for the closure of mosques. The government also allowed a three-day Tabligh Jamaat meeting near Kuala Lumpur to go ahead on February 27 to March 1. The number of participants was reported to be 16,000 from all over Southeast Asia as well as South Asia, and became a major source of infection in Malaysia, Singapore, Indonesia, and Brunei (Aljazeera, 18/3/20).

The Pakistani government found itself unable to enforce a ban on religious gatherings in the face of opposition from Islamist political parties and movements

(Khan 2020). A request by the government to cancel a Tabligh Jamaat meeting in Lahore attended by up to 100,000 people was rejected because of the 'stubbornness of the clergy' as the Minister for Science and Technology put it (Naeem 2020). In some instances where police tried to enforce a ban on Friday prayers, clashes with worshippers ensued. On March 26 a council of prominent religious scholars (*ulama*) met and decided to keep mosques open with only one dissenting voice from a Shi'a cleric (Kugelman 2020). While some scholars agreed with government directives to limit the number of congregants to five, others rejected such restrictions.

Criticisms of these restrictions were not limited to the governments of these countries, but also reflected back on the precedent that Saudi Arabia had set and hence culminated in challenging the Saudi authority over the holy sites. The controversial Kuwaiti Salafi scholar Hakim al-Mutairi, for example, tweeted that it was contrary to religious scriptures to ban worshippers from mosques, criticizing his own country's government and implicitly also the Saudi government (Saudi24news, 14/3/20). The Moroccan Salafi preacher Abu Naim was arrested for similar comments made in a video (North Africa Journal, 17/3/20). Pakistani mullahs argued that the virus should be fought through prayer inside mosques, rather than outside of them. While these were individual voices, the 'International Commission to Monitor Saudi Administration of the Two Holy Mosques' also known as 'Al Haramain Watch', demanded that the two holy mosques be administered by an international body rather than the government of Saudi Arabia (Saudileaks 103/20). This organization was founded in 2018 by non-Arab, mainly Malaysian and South Asian, religious scholars opposed to Saudi control of the two holy sites (Middle east Monitor, 28/5/20). Of course, there is no prospect of the Saudi government handing over control of the holy sites and such demands are really intended to challenge the legitimacy, and thereby authority, of the Saudi government, including its religious establishment, not just to control the administration of the two mosques but also the religious and intellectual space that the kingdom had commanded in the past as the epicenter of Salafi and Wahhabi ideas but that it has recently vacated.

Conclusion

Covid-19 hit Saudi Arabia in the middle of a period of transition making an already uncertain situation even more uncertain. Its economy had already been badly affected by the sharp decline in global oil prices, which made it difficult for the state to keep its side of the rentier state social contract. In its pursuit of the post-oil 2030 Vision, the regime was already attempting to shed some of its neo-traditional and theocratic ideological legitimacy in favor of ideological elements more in line with the model of a modernizing developmental state that seems to value rational decision-making and scientific evidence. So far, the state has largely been able to remain on course, but Covid-19 has put more obstacles in the way and the longer-term repercussions for the political economy and ideological legitimacy of the current regime remain uncertain.

References

Abdo, Geneive and Anna L. Jacobs. (2020). 'Are Covid-19 Restrictions Inflaming Religious Tensions?' Brookings Blog (April 13). www.brookings.edu/blog/order-from-chaos/2020/04/13/are-covid-19-restrictions-inflaming-religious-tensions/ [accessed 18/02/2021].

Al Arabiya. (17 March 2020). 'Saudi Arabia Suspends Prayers at Mosques to Stop Spread of Coronavirus'.

Aljazeera. (18/3/20). 'Made in Malaysia: How Mosque Event Spread Virus to SE Asia'.

Al-Monitor. (2020). 'Saudi Arabia to Pay Some Private Sector Salaries Amid Coronavirus Fallout' (April 3) www.al-monitor.com/pulse/originals/2020/04/saudi-arabia-pay-private-sector-coronavirus-fallout.html [accessed 18/02/2021].

Arab News. (2 March 2020). 'Saudi Arabia Announces First Case of Coronavirus'.

Assaad, Ragui and Barsoum, Ghada. (2019). 'Public Employment in the Middle East and North Africa', *IZA World of Labor*. https://wol.iza.org/articles/public-employment-in-the-middle-east-and-north-africa/long [accessed 18/02/2021].

Chulov, Martin. (2020). 'Saudi Arabia Closes Two Holiest Shrines to Foreigners as Coronavirus Fears Grow', *The Guardian* (February 27).

Duin, Julia. (2020). '"This Is All about Jesus": A Christian Rocker's Covid Protest Movement', *Politico* (October 10). www.politico.com/news/magazine/2020/10/25/sean-feucht-christian-rocker-covid-protest-movement-431734 [accessed 18/02/2021].

Hanna, Andrew. (2020). 'What Islamists Are Doing and Saying on Covid-19 Crisis', The Wilson Center: Insights and Analysis, 14 May.

Holmes, Oliver. (2020). 'Israeli Politicians Argue Over Covid Curbs on Protests and Prayers', *The Guardian* (September 28).

Hvidt, Martin. (2011). 'Economic and Institutional Reforms in the Arab Gulf Countries', *Middle East Journal*, Vol. 65, No. 1: 85–102.

Karasapan, Michael. (2020). 'Pandemic Highlights the Vulnerability of Migrant Workers in the Middle East'. Brookings Blog (September 17). www.brookings.edu/blog/future-development/2020/09/17/pandemic-highlights-the-vulnerability-of-migrant-workers-in-the-middle-east/ [accessed 18/02/2021].

Kershner, Isabel. (2020). 'Israel's Coronavirus Lockdown Fuels Protests, Violence and Confusion', *New York Times* (October 5).

Khan, Arsalan. (2020). 'Why Pakistan Isn't Closing Mosques Despite the Coronavirus threat'. *TRT World* (27 March). www.trtworld.com/opinion/why-pakistan-isn-t-closing-mosques-despite-the-coronavirus-threat-34913 [accessed 18/02/2021].

Kugelman, Michael. (2020) 'Pakistan's Government Is Caught between a Mosque and a Hard Place'. *Foreign Policy* (April 24).

Middle East Monitor. (28/5/20). 'Islamic Scholars, NGOs Call for Makkah, Madinah to be Placed Under International Control'.

Muhtada, Dani. (2020). 'Religion and the Covid-19 Mitigation', *The Jakarta Post*, March 26.

Naeem Mubarak. (2020). 'Corona and Clergy – The Missing Link for Effective Social Distancing in Pakistan: Time for Some Unpopular Decisions', *International Journal for Infectious Diseases*, Vol. 95 (June 2020).

North Africa Journal. (17/3/20). 'Salafist Preacher for Publicly Opposing Anti-Coronavirus Measures'.

Reuters (13/3/20). 'Gulf States Cancel Events, Kuwait Shuts Mosques Over Coronavirus'.

Saudi24News. (14/3/20). 'Professor at Tafsir and Hadith at Kuwait University: Closing Mosques and Banning Worshipers is Forbidden by the Text'.

Siregar, Kiki (2020). 'Covid-19: Mass Prayers Still Held in Parts of Indonesia Despite Guidance Issued by Central Government'. *Channelnewsasia* (April 30). www.channelnewsasia.com/news/asia/indonesia-covid-19-mass-prayers-mosques-aceh-sumatra-12690702 [accessed 18/02/2021].

Slater, Joanna and Katie McQue. (2020). 'Migration, in Reverse', *The Washington Post* (October 1).

Song Jung-a, Kang Buseong and Edward White. (2020). 'South Korea's Megachurches Take on Government in Coronavirus Battle', *Financial Times* (September 19).

Syafiq Hasyim. (2020). 'Covid-19, Islamic Civil Society and State Capacity in Indonesia', *ISEAS Perspectives*, No. 39 (May 5).

The National (16/3/20). 'Coronavirus: UAE Cancels Public Prayers at Mosques and Churches'.

Wehrey, Frederic, Nathan J. Brown, Bader Al-Saif, Intissar Fakir, Anouar Boukhars and Maysaa Shuja Al-Deen (2020). 'Islamic Authority and Arab States in a Time of Pandemic', *Carnegie Endowment for International Peace* (April 16). https://carnegieendowment.org/2020/04/16/islamic-authority-and-arab-states-in-time-of-pandemic-pub-81563 [accessed 18/02/2021].

Yamada, Makio, (2020). 'Can a Rentier State Evolve to a Production State? An "Institutional Upgrading" Approach', *British Journal of Middle Eastern Studies*, Vol. 47, No. 1, 24–41.

Zicchieri, Alessandro. (2016). 'Is Rentier State Theory Sufficient to Explain the Politics of the UAE?' *e-International Relations* (4 February) www.e-ir.info/2016/02/04/is-rentier-state-theory-sufficient-to-explain-the-politics-of-the-uae/ [accessed 18/02/2021].

Europe

10

THE UK AND COVID-19

Colin Tyler

This chapter explores the institutional and ideological tensions that shape the United Kingdom government's responses to the Covid-19 pandemic. Political responses to Covid-19 within the UK are formulated and implemented by the relevant devolved administrations in its constituent nations (for England the UK or Westminster Parliament, the Scottish Parliament, the Welsh Assembly and Northern Ireland Executive), with some powers being further devolved to local councils and other public bodies. While there are numerous practical differences between the nomenclatures, approaches and timetables adopted in the four countries, broad similarities do exist in all four areas. What follows concentrates on the responses of the Westminster government (which has competence on English health matters), as the devolved administrations have mostly framed their respective responses in light of those of the Westminster government. Adopting usual practice, where the terms 'UK government' and 'government' are used in this chapter, they refer to the Westminster government alone, rather than also to the devolved administrations.

The chapter is structured as follows. The first part presents the UK government's response to the pandemic from January to September 2020. The second part sketches the movement, post-1979, of the UK state from being a social democratic institution towards a competition state. The third part explores the attitudinal context of the current government's response, by focusing on a powerful non-interventionist trend within contemporary centrist and right-wing UK political parties. The chapter concludes by highlighting the key lesson to be drawn from the government's actions during the pandemic: namely, that institutions can reassert themselves against and even within a formerly populist government.

Pandemic dynamics and the government's responses

Prior to Covid-19 cases being identified in the UK on 31 January 2020, various public bodies had gradually been raising their threat levels and planning various response scenarios (Oxford University, continuing). Initially, the government resisted calls to impose significant restrictions on the freedoms of its citizens and those entering the UK from abroad. Restrictions were introduced gradually. From 7 February, the government advised new arrivals from Wuhan, China to self-isolate for 14 days, with quarantine measures being tightened three days later, when limited testing was also introduced in England. On 1 March, as infection and death rates continued to rise, the government moved the UK response from the delay phase to the contain phase. Basic statutory sick pay was introduced for those required to self-isolate, with the scheme being made more generous over the coming days. Business rates were suspended for various sectors of the economy. Gradually, support for the wider population was introduced, including more generous welfare benefits for the unemployed and those in rented housing. On 11 March, the Chancellor of the Exchequer Rishi Sunak announced a £5 billion (bn) relief fund for the National Health Service (NHS) and related public sector organizations. Six days later he announced a £330 bn business stimulus package. Simultaneously, the government advised against all non-essential international travel. On 17 March, an Ipsos MORI poll revealed 51 per cent of UK citizens in favour of completely closing the national borders. Despite being a slight majority, the proportion was the lowest of 12 other countries polled: Vietnam (79 per cent) Italy (76 per cent) to France (53 per cent) and Germany (57 per cent) (Beaver, 2020a). (The UK figure rose to 74 per cent in a poll published on 24 March, the day after lockdown was imposed in England (Beaver, 2020b).) On 20 March, the government closed all schools and introduced a furlough scheme covering 80 per cent of the pay of anyone temporarily laid-off from work (Sunak, 2020a). Leisure and entertainment businesses were closed, as were all non-essential shops. The UK entered its first lockdown on Monday 23 March 2020. English employees who could were required to work from home, and social distancing measures were introduced in every establishment that remained open. English citizens were instructed to shop for food only when necessary and to avoid unnecessary journeys. During March and April, government ministers mooted adopting a 'herd immunity' policy, where Covid-19 would be allowed to spread in order to build up viral resistance within a significant proportion of the UK population. However, the approach was widely criticized by the press, wider UK population, domestic political parties and authoritative international bodies, not least the World Health Organization (Forrest, 2020).

The delay in imposing lockdown was reflected in the UK's poor performance in containing the virus' spread. According to Worldometer data (which combine figures for England, Scotland, Northern Ireland and Wales), the UK's first wave peaked in April, reaching 1,170 daily deaths on 21 April, approximately a month after the imposition of lockdown. By 16 June, the UK had recorded 298,136 cases of the disease, with 41,969 associated deaths. By 11 August, the UK recorded 312,789 cases (1.52 per cent of the global total), with a total of 46,628 deaths. Hence, by 11 August, the UK had recorded the fourth highest number of deaths among 215 countries included in Worldometer data, while having the twelfth largest total of cases (312,789 cases) and twenty-first largest population (67.9 million). The UK had the third highest number of deaths at 6,868 per million of the population, behind only San Marino (1,238) and Belgium (852), despite coming only fiftieth in the number of total cases per million (4,605). This trend continued in the following months, meaning that the UK has one of the world's highest per capita coronavirus death rates.

UK death rates vary significantly by gender, age, wealth and ethnicity, with men and many minority ethnic groups faring much worse than women and members of the white majority. Hence, the Office for National Statistics (ONS) reported (10 April) that in March 2020, the death rate increased significantly with age and that males had twice the death rate of females (Campbell and Caul, 2020a). June data showed that, when discounted for age, the rates were '65.1 deaths per 100,000 males compared with 43.3 deaths per 100,000 females' (Campbell and Caul, 2020b). The ONS reported (7 May) that in England and Wales from 2 March to 10 April, discounting for age, the rate was 420 per cent times higher for black males and 430 per cent for black females, than for their white counterparts (White and Natfilyan, 2020). (Here, 'Black' refers to 'Black Caribbean; Black African; Black Other', 'White' to 'White British; Irish; Gypsy or Irish Traveller; Other White'.) Discounting for 'age and other socio-demographic characteristics and measures of self-reported health and disability at the 2011 Census', the death rate among the black community was 190 per cent times higher than among the white community (White and Natfilyan, 2020). The ONS concluded that some but not all of the differences in the mortality rates between ethnic groups could be traced to greater poverty and greater self-reported pre-existing health problems among members of ethnic minority communities, as noted below.

Early in the English lockdown, the population recognized the threats to business (Ipsos MORI, 2020). The pandemic has had a devastating effect on the UK economy and globally. According to ONS figures, the UK economy shrank by 2.2 per cent in the first quarter of 2020 (January to March), but by an unprecedented 20.4 per cent in the second quarter (April to June) (Scruton, 2020). Together, these falls constituted the UK's worst recession on record. Using the first six months of 2020, the ONS noted that the UK's fall was 0.6 per cent less than Spain's contraction (22.7 per cent) but a little over twice the US contraction (10.6 per cent). The UK's economic recovery was slower than the government and some experts predicted (at 2.1 per cent in August), before being hit again by the second wave of infections from the end of September 2020 (Sardana, 2020). The ONS attributed the economic differences to the diverse durations and stringency of lockdown measures in the respective countries. These measures were multifaceted and highly dynamic, with the government introducing and extending various measures throughout the period, at the same time as relaxing other restrictions. For example, the furlough scheme was made less generous on 1 July, English bars, restaurants and hairdressers re-opened on 4 July, and on 10 July England relaxed some of the overseas travel restrictions that it had imposed nearly two months earlier, only to re-impose and redesign other travel restrictions at other times subsequently. The government introduced a confusing multidimensional response with significant regional variation when the second wave hit in October, provoking significant opposition (Johnson, 2020c).

The government's approach contrasted significantly with earlier lockdowns and lower death rates across much of Europe and globally. The UK's later lockdown dates can be partly attributed to the timing and rate of the disease spreading across the world. It can also be partly attributed to different medical advice. The pattern in the four countries of the UK was that initially all parties supported the introduction of restrictive measures, in both domestic and border policies, becoming increasingly critical as shortfalls occurred in the provision of Personal Protective Equipment (PPE), safety in the health care sector, especially nursing and care homes, 'track and trace', and so on. Moreover, opposition parties, media commentators across the political spectrum, voluntary and third sector organizations and members of the general public, as well as members of the scientific community, have highlighted the UK's rapidly growing death rate, particularly relative to other rich countries, often focusing on the high death rate among vulnerable groups such as the elderly, those with underlying health conditions, the poor and ethnic minority citizens, as well as the mounting economic costs (Anderson et al., 2020). Criticisms have been extended to the government's decisions to moderate lockdown conditions after the first wave grew more quickly than overseas. Why has the government's response been so problematic?

From social democracy towards the competition state

The first reason for government's sluggishness in imposing and maintaining lockdown is the increasingly neoliberal character of the UK's public institutions and policies. For 40 years, successive governments have undermined and dismantled the social democratic structures that constituted the UK state for the majority of the twentieth century. This process began with the first Thatcher administration in 1979 and reflected its intense skepticism regarding the state's ability to manage the economy efficiently. The state's role has been gradually reduced throughout the economy and society ever since, being undermined by a faith in private enterprise. Where previously workers had been protected by relatively robust legal rights, these rights were eroded, empowering employers. Underpinning this gradual destruction of social democratic institutions was a shift to a morality that emphasized virtues of self-reliance and personal responsibility. This worldview attacked what Thatcherites portrayed as the poor exploiting the aspirant and industrious rich. In line with their individualist morality, they saw the primary role of the state as being to create opportunities for citizens to earn and spend money as they saw fit. It was a deeply controversial position, of course. Thatcher's infamous 1979 claim that 'there is no such thing as society' is still viewed by many as a crude denial of community (Thatcher, 1987: 28–29, 29–30). At the time, Thatcher's publicity team responded by emphasizing her anti-paternalism and traditional Tory belief that the 'living tapestry' of social institutions could be sustained only through the daily actions of Burke's 'little platoon[s]' of self-directed, socially responsible individuals (Thatcher,

1987: 30; Burke, 1909–14: 75; Saunders, 2020). Viewed thus, extensive state action undermined social institutions and moral character.

Despite these protestations, Thatcher's exhortation of personal responsibility sounded hollow and insulting to the millions of UK citizens whose communities she appeared to willfully abandon (or to actively punish) during her premiership (1979–90). This attitude drove the diminution of the state's competences for many years. Hence, its roles were further reduced by subsequent governments, as with David Cameron's (UK Prime Minister (PM) 2010–16) 'Big Society' policies. Critics respond that there was no necessary link between personal responsibility and the weakening of the UK institutional infrastructure. Hence, the New Labour governments of Tony Blair and Gordon Brown (PMs in 1997–2007 and 2007–10, respectively) invoked ideals of rights and responsibilities (Blair, 2002). Yet, they saw the solutions to poverty as being institutionally driven. The key actor was an interventionist state, even if often Labour relied on the management-delivery arrangements of Public-Private Partnerships. Yet, even the centre-left plans of New Labour struggled within capitalist structures. Hence, Brown's efforts to create a New Marshall Plan to address global poverty crumbled due to opposition from foreign liberal markets, neoliberal governments and large corporations (Tyler, 2017: 268–76).

The UK liberal marketization project was renewed by the Conservative and Liberal Democrat Coalition government of 2010–15, and has been pushed further by subsequent Conservative governments. At the macro-level, the process pushed the state away from moulding capitalism to serve the common good, to that of serving capitalist interests. In practical terms, this transformation has entailed the gradual weakening and then removal of the social welfare supports, especially the undermining of the UK's system of socialized health care (free at the point of delivery for all citizens), the NHS and other support systems for families, the unemployed and elderly. Hence, public spending accounted for only 35 per cent of GDP in 2018–19, having accounted for 42 per cent in 2009–10, with public spending being reduced in deprived areas of the UK by double the amount it was reduced in affluent areas (32 per cent and 16 per cent, respectively) (Marmot, 2020). The UK has witnessed a significant reduction in funding increases to the NHS (to 1 per cent in 2019) and real term cuts to the budgets of other crucial institutions, including Public Health England (PHE) and adult social care, especially in deprived areas (Marmot, 2020). These and other austerity policies have made it far harder for UK institutions and the general population – and particularly the poor – to weather the Covid-19 pandemic.

Since 1979, the UK has shifted decisively towards being the competition state. This has made it difficult for the Johnson government to respond effectively to the pandemic. A competition state is an analytic category (or 'ideal type') against which actual states can be measured (Genschel and Seelkopf, 2015, 239–40.) It focuses on the supply-side of the economy, shunning the macro-economic interventions that characterize Keynesian welfare states. It sets itself a minimal remit, shifting what were previously state functions to private agents and institutions, especially corporations and the market. A competition state strongly favours the reduction in public welfare schemes, placing much greater emphasis on individual self-reliance and agency against the pressures of capitalist economic and social structures. By thus reducing its capacities and desire to act in favour of a neoliberal agenda, a competition state diminishes the voters' capacity to exert meaningful democratic control over their collective life.

In the present context, to the extent that the UK state fulfils these characteristics of a competition state, it lacks the institutional infrastructure to develop and execute effective anti-Covid strategies and tactics. These deficiencies are reflected in the intensification of underlying institutional fragilities within the UK state and their associated effects within the UK polity. A key area is the state's inability to prevent worsening income inequalities. Indeed, Covid-19 has highlighted once again profound inequalities riven throughout the UK population, and, as noted above, death rates have been much higher among the poor than the rich, and for members of ethnic minorities (especially black people) than for white people (Marmot, 2015; Wilkinson and Pickett, 2018). Moreover, Covid-19 highlights significant problems that just-in-time supply chains create for the poor, particularly during the hoarding that characterized the initial stages of the first lockdown (Power et al., 2020).

Certainly the government has pursued some policies that run counter to the minimalist ethos associated with competition states. Hence, as noted above, the UK government promised to pump money into the NHS and similar organizations (£5 bn announced in March), to inject £330 bn into businesses, and inaugurated a furlough scheme for workers, in a manner that initially at least seemed to recall post-Second World War reflationary Keynesian governments. It has lived up to these promises to some degree. Yet, concerns persist regarding the government's commitment to such measures (Anandaciva, 2020; Parker and Strauss, 2020).

Other concerns exist. For example, on 16 August the government's Health Secretary Matt Hancock announced the government's decision to replace PHE with the National Institute for Health Protection (NIHP), to focus on the control of infectious diseases. The new arrangements will combine PHE with parts of the Joint Biosecurity Centre and the NHS Track and Trace agency. The decision attracted much criticism across the political spectrum. It was felt to be ill-timed. Moreover, the decision to appoint Baroness Harding as the interim head was deeply controversial, given that the Conservative peer has no health background and appears to have had little success in similar leadership roles previously. More fundamentally, commentators criticize the way in which the present government and its immediate predecessors have instituted not merely this change, but a series of 'chaotic institutional overhaul[s]' (Dixon, 2020).

Critics see the hurried replacement of PHE as yet another attempt to avoid responsibility for government failures to respond adequately to the pandemic. Many allege that the government blames its scientists for what are ultimately political decisions, even where the government is subsequently shown to have disregarded the advice of official health advisory bodies including the Scientific Advisory Group for Emergencies (SAGE) (Gallagher, 2020). A particularly high-profile instance of the government shifting blame for its pandemic mistakes occurred in the aftermath of the release of deeply controversial school Advanced-Level results, which led to the apparently forced resignations of Jonathan Slater, a high-level civil servant at the Department of Education, and Sally Collier, the head of the school examinations board Ofqual. These evasions echoed other perceived missteps. The most prominent included a reversal over the government's 'track and trace' scheme, its delay in imposing lockdown and travel restrictions, problems with the procurement of PPE and self-serving amendments to its data collection regime. Events such as these have repeatedly harmed public trust in the government over the course of the pandemic (Reuters Institute/University of Oxford, n.d.).

Yet, other institutions have proved resilient in the face of these uncertainties and evasions. All sections of media scrutinize and criticize the government, often vigorously. Initially, some attacks from the right-wing media have been levelled not at the Conservative government, but at the civil service which allegedly hinders the Johnson government (Nuki, 2020). However, now most right-wing papers, including the usually loyal *Daily Mail*, have attacked the Johnson government directly. Within the state itself, parliamentarians continue to hold the government to account in many areas. For example, the government's lack of economic planning was criticized in July 2020 by the Commons Public Accounts Committee (Bridge-Wilkinson, 2020). An August 2020 Home Affairs Committee report criticized the government's sluggishness in imposing border restrictions and the abrupt changes made to restrictions thereafter (Home Affairs Committee, 2020). In the same month, parliamentarians from many parties launched legal action through the Good Law Project (a not-for-profit campaigning organization) to pursue their concerns regarding the government's probity when awarding over £5 bn of PPE contracts (Savage, 2020). Throughout, Parliament has continued its research and advice functions with, for example, the Lords Economic Affairs Committee launching an inquiry into the government's post-pandemic employment policy (Parliamentary Committees and Public Enquiries, 2020). The likely effectiveness of parliamentary scrutiny is open to debate however, given that the Johnson government was elected with a very significant majority in the House of Commons (80 seats in August 2020) and has won every subsequent parliamentary vote. Nevertheless, such examples of institutional resilience have led scholars, who had been outspoken pessimists regarding the strength of the UK polity prior to the crisis, to see life under the pandemic as a unifying experience. Hence, in May 2020 Crouch wrote: 'Not only are vast numbers of citizens deeply interested in the struggle against the coronavirus, but bonds of community and neighbourhood have been strengthened by our solidarity during the lockdown. Civil society has rarely been stronger' (Crouch, 2020b; for earlier pessimism, Crouch, 2020a). Again, caution is needed here, as every lockdown brings protests, resistance and blatant disregard for the rules by some citizens and even some councils.

The culture and structure of the British state places important constraints on the government, constraints that have been only partially overcome during the pandemic. Yet, the government has deliberately sought not to act for reasons that are explored below.

The ideological roots of the UK government's response

There is much evidence that the inherent limitations on the acceptable role and power of the UK state are not as great a source of regret for Johnson's government as they have been for many others. Beyond the fact that the UK has moved significantly closer to being a competition state, the second reason for the government's reluctance to impose and maintain lockdown is Johnson's self-professed instinctive resistance to state action, a resistance that is shared by many members of his party. Three days before the start of the UK's lockdown, Guto Harri, Johnson's former spokesman, claimed that Johnson 'has a more benign view of human nature than the assumption that everyone needs to be treated like a child and be told by daddy what to do' (Smith, 2020). This recalls Thatcher's exhortation of the 'living tapestry' of individuals taking responsibility for themselves and those nearest to them, noted above (Thatcher, 1987, p. 30). Interestingly, however, Johnson explicitly rejected Thatcher's associated claim that 'there is no such thing as society' in a Twitter video posted on 29 March (Johnson, 2020a). Similarly, on 30 June, he characterized his government's promised additional public expenditure as an instantiation of that great American Keynesian policy – the New Deal. Yet, as with the proponents of all former Anglo-American New Deals, he stressed that its goal was to help the masses by reviving capitalism (Johnson, 2020b). Chancellor Rishi Sunak reiterated this position in October 2020, promising that those who wish to develop themselves will find 'that the overwhelming might of the British state will be placed at your service' (Sunak, 2020b).

The government's resistance to state action has been tested by the pandemic. Even staunch right-libertarians within his own party supported Johnson's time-limited lockdown measures (Baker, 2020). On 29 June, following his own treatment for Covid-19, Johnson announced a break with his previous self-described 'very libertarian stance to obesity' due to the increased vulnerability to the disease that obesity brings (Honeycombe-Foster, 2020). Yet, Johnson's fundamental anti-statism remains largely intact. Hence, he remains reluctant to impose and maintain restrictions of the type that many scientists see as necessary to counter the spread of the disease. While often personally and professionally unprincipled, he strongly supports unfettered markets (Sylvester, 2020; Johnson, 2020b). He describes Britain as a 'land of liberty', where the state rarely imposes extensive restrictions on its citizens (O'Donoghue, 2020). He characterizes himself as a One-Nation Tory, someone who sees the elite as being duty-bound to help the disadvantaged, but to retain existing social structures (Brogan, 2020).

Another reason for the government's relative reluctance to impose and maintain restrictions is the new Conservative administration's apparent unwillingness to learn from abroad, especially the European Union (EU) and Germany, something that is heavily influenced by Johnson's obsession with the Second World War PM,

Winston Churchill. This obsession is possibly most evident in Johnson's book, *The Churchill Factor* (Johnson, 2014). Commentators have seen Johnson's Churchillian posturing as delusional, with too much of the imperial knight about it, as well as resting on a poor understanding of the historical Churchill (Klos, 2016; Wood, 2019; Wheatcroft, 2020). Yet, it is a self-image that plays extremely well with many Conservatives and other British people. A 2019 YouGov survey revealed that 95 per cent of Conservative Party members admired Churchill, 2 per cent more than admired Thatcher (Smith, 2019). Many on the right revel in Johnson's attempt to present himself as a heroic latter-day Churchill, pursuing British interests in the face of foreign opposition (Roberts, 2019; McKinstry, 2020). Johnson's faux Churchillianism seems to have encouraged him to respond to the coronavirus pandemic in any way that clearly differs from that of other nations, especially France, Germany and Italy, which many reactionaries see as Britain's historical enemies. This cause dovetails with another factor (Ross, 2016).

The final reason for the UK's deeply flawed responses to the coronavirus pandemic is the legacy of the Brexit Leave campaign, which Johnson fronted under the guidance of his chief political adviser Dominic Cummings. He ascended to the parliamentary throne as PM in no small part because of his repeated claim that the UK would thrive outside of the EU (Tyler, 2020). It is now politically unthinkable for him to respond to the coronavirus outbreak in what his supporters would see as a fundamentally 'European' way, and especially not with the help of their former EU exploiters. Politically, Johnson has to ensure that there at least seems to be clear blue water between the UK and continental Europe. Hence, the government's recent political victory seems to have made the current Conservative leadership highly resistant to learning from the experiences of EU member states and to participating in EU responses to the pandemic, for example through collective procurement rounds for PPE and ventilators (Hopkins, 2020). Critics have argued that Johnson initially adopted the 'herd immunity' policy to indicate his government's rejection of the EU's more rapid and interventionist alternative (Mason, 2020). The long-term effects of the Johnson government's political need and predilection to ensure that it is not viewed as relying on the EU seem stark. For example, the Brexit Health Alliance has warned that the UK can only maintain its institutional resilience if it is part of EU data-sharing and early-warning mechanisms, agrees common trade standards in relations to medical supplies, negotiates appropriate joint research and development programs with the EU and ensures that EU citizens feel their jobs are secure when working in the UK health sector (Draper, 2020). However, instituting these arrangements would be politically disastrous for the Johnson government. The feeling against the EU remains too strong, especially among its electoral base, even during the pandemic (What UK Thinks, 2020).

Conclusion: populism rejected, institutions reasserted

Of the many lessons to learn from the UK's government's response to the Covid-19 pandemic, possibly the most striking is the transitory nature of UK populism and the resilience of institutionally based politics. Johnson became PM of a minority government on 24 July 2019, after Theresa May was forced from office. To gain an overall parliamentary majority, he called a general election, which he won on 12 December, with a huge majority of 80 seats. The first UK cases of Covid-19 were detected on 31 January 2020. Immediately, the government shifted from the crude populist stance that had characterized Johnson's politics since he assumed the leadership of the official Brexit Leave campaign referendum in February 2016 (Tyler, 2020). Johnson's Brexit campaign had been based squarely on such populist tropes of fake anti-elitism (the Johnson campaign was run by some of the most privileged people in the world), an attack on established institutions such as the judiciary and the press and a strident rejection of expertise. (In the words of Gove's deputy in the official Leave campaign, 'People in this country have had enough of experts' (Mance, 2016).) The government's pandemic response represented a radical rejection of this earlier populism.

Certainly, populist elements remained. For many weeks, members of the general public would stand outside their houses at 8 pm every Thursday evening to clap their gratitude for health care workers. This ritual was promoted by the government, with NHS workers being habitually referred to as 'heroes', a label usually reserved for military personnel, on the US post-9/11 model. Yet, notice that even this organized mass emotional outburst was aimed at supporting an institution which many British people see as core to the national identity: the NHS. Many citizens saw the government's promotion of this ritual as deeply hypocritical, given years of sustained failure by many Conservative governments to fund the NHS adequately, and the Johnson government's failure to provide adequate PPE and its refusal to improve the immigration status of the many foreign health professionals on whom the NHS relies. There were other, less mixed rejections of the populist logic, as when the government immediately put experts and expertise at the centre of its pandemic campaign. From 16 March, every Monday to Friday the government hosted a press briefing led by ministers and government scientists, which broadcast live in the early evening. Speaking for SAGE, the UK Chief Medical Adviser Professor Chris Whitty, the Chief Scientific Adviser Sir Patrick Vallance and other experts presented relatively detailed technical data on infections, deaths and the economy, as well as explaining and justifying the government's disease control measures. These broadcasts had such an impact that Vallance, and particularly Whitty, became minor celebrities in the UK for a time.

The briefings were discontinued on 23 June. Partly, this reflected the government's decision to ease lockdown. Partly, however, it was becoming harder for the government to silence dissenting voices among its scientific advisers. A recurring point of conflict was the government's refusal to discipline Johnson's key political adviser and architect of his Brexit Leave campaign, Dominic Cummings, for violating lockdown rules. Key experts such as England's Chief Nursing Officer Ruth May were dropped from the daily briefings over their refusal to defend Cummings. The publication of expert advice has exposed times when the government has not followed the guidance of SAGE, the official health body (Demianyk, 2020).

Even usually loyal newspapers such as *The Telegraph* criticized the government for such moves (Donnelly and Mikhailova, 2020). The government's stance came on the back of a decline in trust in the government's honesty and its handling of the pandemic, a decline that was not reflected in any decline in trust in other, more resilient institutions, including the press (Reuters Institute/University of Oxford, continuing). Institutional forces did much to counter the Johnson's earliest populist tactics. The lesson is clear, then: one should not underestimate the resilience of the UK's institutions as a counter to government power.

References

Anandaciva, S. (2020), 'What does the 2020 spring Budget mean for health and care', *King's Fund*, 13 March www.kingsfund.org.uk/blog/2020/03/spring-budget-mean-health-and-care. Accessed: 16 October 2020.

Anderson, R.M., T.D. Hollingsworth, R.F. Baggaley, R. Maddren, C.Vegvari (2020), 'Covid-19 spread in the UK', *Lancet*, 396(10251): 587–590, 3 August.

Baker, S. (2020) 'Close to tears, libertarian Tory approves Boris Johnson's measures, bill for "dystopian society"', *YouTube*, 24 March www.youtube.com/watch?v=m_51gGZKTyc. Accessed: 16 October 2020.

Beaver, K. (2020a), 'Majority of people want borders closed as fear about Covid-19 escalates', *Ipsos MORI*, 17 March www.ipsos.com/ipsos-mori/en-uk/majority-people-want-borders-closed-fear-about-covid-19-escalates. Accessed: 16 October 2020.

Beaver, K. (2020b), 'Public divided on whether isolation, travel bans prevent Covid-19 spread; border closures become more acceptable', *Ipsos MORI*, 24 March www.ipsos.com/ipsos-mori/en-uk/public-divided-whether-isolation-travel-bans-prevent-covid-19-spread-border-closures-more-acceptable. Accessed: 16 October 2020.

Blair, T. (2002), 'Speech on welfare reform', *Guardian*, 10 June.

Bridge-Wilkinson, A. (2020), 'Committee criticizes lack of planning for economic impact of Covid-19 pandemic', *Parliamentary Review*, 23 July www.theparliamentaryreview.co.uk/news/committee-criticises-lack-of-planning-for-economic-impact-of-covid-19-pandemic. Accessed: 16 October 2020.

Brogan, B. (2020), 'Boris Johnson interview', *Telegraph*, 29 April.

Burke, E. (1909–14), *Reflections on the Revolution in France* [1790], New York, P.F. Collier.

Campbell, A. and S. Caul (2020a), 'Deaths involving Covid-19, England and Wales deaths occurring in March 2020', *Office of National Statistics* [*ONS*], 16 April www.ons.gov.uk/peoplepopulationandcommunity/birthsdeathsandmarriages/deaths/bulletins/deathsinvolvingcovid19englandandwales/deathsoccurringinmarch2020. Accessed: 16 October 2020.

Campbell, A. and S. Caul (2020b), 'Deaths involving Covid-19, England and Wales deaths occurring in June 2020', *ONS*, 17 July www.ons.gov.uk/peoplepopulationandcommunity/birthsdeathsandmarriages/deaths/bulletins/deathsinvolvingcovid19englandandwales/deathsoccurringinjune2020. Accessed: 16 October 2020.

Crouch, C. (2020a), *Post-Democracy After the Crises.* Cambridge: Polity.

Crouch, C. (2020b), 'Democracy and the Coronavirus', *Compass*, 11 May www.compassonline.org.uk/democracy-and-the-coronavirus/. Accessed: 16 October 2020.

Demianyk, G. (2020), 'Boris Johnson ignored plea from government's scientific advisers for two week national lockdown', *Huffington Post*, 12 October.

Dixon, J. (2020), 'Public Health England', *Prospect*, 25 August.

Donnelly, L. and A. Mikhailova (2020), 'Chief Nurse says she was dropped from Downing Street briefing during Dominic Cummings controversy', *Telegraph*, 20 July.

Draper, P. (2020), 'Pandemic ready?' *NHS Confederation*, 26 June www.nhsconfed.org/resources/2020/06/bha-briefing-pandemic-ready-managing-another-coronavirus. Accessed: 16 October 2020.

Dunn, P., L. Allen, G. Cameron, and H. Alderwick (2020), 'Covid-19 policy tracker', *Health Foundation*, 6 August www.health.org.uk/news-and-comment/charts-and-infographics/covid-19-policy-tracker. Accessed: 16 October 2020.

Forrest, A. (2020), 'WHO condemns idea of herd immunity for Covid-19 as "dangerous"', *Independent*, 12 May.

Gallagher, James (2020), 'Are we still listening to the science?', *BBC News*, 13 October.

Genschel, P. and L. Seelkopf (2015), 'Competition State', in S. Leibfried, E. Huber, M. Lange, J.D. Levy, F. Nullmeier, and J.D. Stephens, *Oxford Handbook of the Transformations of the State*. Oxford: Oxford University Press, pp. 237–52.

Hakimi Zapata, N. (2020), 'How Brexit infected Britain's Coronavirus response', *Nation*, 20 April.

Home Affairs Committee (2020), 'Home Office preparedness for Covid-19', *UK Parliament*, 5 August https://publications.parliament.uk/pa/cm5801/cmselect/cmhaff/563/56302.htm. Accessed: 16 October 2020.

Honeycombe-Foster, M. (2020) 'Boris Johnson says he's ditched 'libertarian' position on obesity after coronavirus battle', *PoliticsHome*, 29 June www.politicshome.com/news/article/boris-johnson-says-hes-ditched-libertarian-position-on-obesity-after-coronavirus-battle. Accessed: 16 October 2020.

Hopkins, J. (2020) 'Brexit thinking poisoned the government's response to Covid-19', *LSE Blogs*, 9 June https://blogs.lse.ac.uk/brexit/2020/06/09/brexit-thinking-poisoned-the-governments-response-to-covid-19/. Accessed: 16 October 2020.

Ipsos MORI (2020), 'Britain's view of Covid-19 as "high threat" to their business jumps 19 points in a week', *Ipsos MORI*, 26 March www.ipsos.com/ipsos-mori/en-uk/britains-view-covid-19-high-threat-their-business-jumps-19-points-week. Accessed: 16 October 2020.

Johnson, B. (2014), *Churchill Factor*. London: Hodder and Stoughton.

Johnson, B. (2020a), 'Boris Johnson says "there really is such a thing as society" in self-isolation update – video', *Guardian*, 29 March.

Johnson, B. (2020b), 'PM Economy Speech', *Gov.UK*, 30 June www.gov.uk/government/speeches/pm-economy-speech-30-june-2020. Accessed: 16 October 2020.

Johnson, B. (2020c), 'PM Commons statement on coronavirus', *Gov.UK*, 12 October www.gov.uk/government/speeches/pm-commons-statement-on-coronavirus-12-october-2020. Accessed: 16 October 2020.

Klos, F. (2016), 'Boris Johnson's Abuse of Churchill', *History Today*, 1 June.

Mance, H. (2016) 'Britain has had enough of experts', *Financial Times*, 3 June.

Marmot, M. (2015), *Health Gap*. London: Bloomsbury.

Marmot, M. (2020), 'Why did England have Europe's worst Covid figures?', *Guardian*, 10 August.

Mason, P. (2020), 'How his "Brexit" project explains Johnson's dithering on Covid-19', *Social Europe*, 6 April www.socialeurope.eu/how-his-brexit-project-explains-johnsons-dithering-on-covid-19. Accessed: 16 October 2020.

McKinstry, L. (2020), 'Boris Johnson needs to unleash his inner Churchill in our war against coronavirus', *Telegraph*, 2 April.

Nuki, P. (2020), 'Whitehall's systemic failure exposed', *Telegraph*, 15 August.

O'Donoghue, D. (2020), 'Boris Johnson refuses to rule out lock-down to stop spread of outbreak', *Press and Journal*, 18 March. Oxford University (continuing), 'Coronavirus Government Response Tracker', Oxford University, www.bsg.ox.ac.uk/research/research-projects/coronavirus-government-response-tracker. Accessed: 16 October 2020.

Parker, G. and D. Strauss (2020), 'Pressure grows on Rishi Sunak to extend UK furlough scheme', *Financial Times*, 7 August.

Parliamentary Committees and Public Enquiries (2020), 'Employment and Covid-19 inquiry launched by Lords Economic Affairs Committee', Parliamentary Committees and Public Enquiries, 3 August www.wired-gov.net/wg/news.nsf/articles/Employment+and+Covid19+inquiry+launched+by+Lords+Economic+Affairs+Committee+03082020161500?open. Accessed: 16 October 2020.

Payne, S. and L. Hughes (2020), 'Senior Tories express anger over Johnson policy U-Turns', *Financial Times*, 26 August.

Power, M., B. Doherty, K. Pybus, and K. Pickett (2020), 'How Covid-19 has exposed inequalities in the UK food system [version 2]', *Emerald Open Res*, 2:11 https://emeraldopenresearch.com/articles/2-11/v2. Accessed: 16 October 2020.

Reuters Institute/University of Oxford (n.d.), 'UK Covid-19 news and information project', *Reuters Institute/University of Oxford*, https://reutersinstitute.politics.ox.ac.uk/UK-Covid-19-news-and-information-project. Accessed: 16 October 2020.

Roberts, A. (2019), 'This is your "Churchill moment" Boris – if you have what it takes', *Telegraph*, 29 June.

Ross, T. (2016), 'Boris Johnson interview', *Telegraph*, 14 May.

Saradna, S. (2020), 'UK economic recovery is running out of steam', *Business Insider*, 9 October.

Saunders, R. (2020), 'There is such a thing as society', *New Statesman*, 31 March.

Savage, M. (2020), 'Cross-party MPs to sue UK government for details of Covid PPE contracts', *Observer*, 23 August.

Scruton, J. (2020), 'GDP first quarterly estimate, UK', *ONS*, 3 August www.ons.gov.uk/economy/grossdomesticproductgdp/bulletins/gdpfirstquarterlyestimateuk/apriltojune2020. Accessed: 16 October 2020.

Smith, A. (2020), 'Johnson's libertarian views behind hesitancy to lock down Britain', *NBC News*, 20 March www.nbcnews.com/news/world/coronavirus-johnson-s-libertarian-views-behind-hesitancy-lock-down-britain-n1164786. Accessed: 16 October 2020.

Smith, M. (2019), 'Four more discoveries from the Conservative member survey', *YouGov*, 18 June https://yougov.co.uk/topics/politics/articles-reports/2019/06/18/four-more-discoveries-our-conservative-member-surv. Accessed: 16 October 2020.

Sunak, R. (2020a), 'Chancellor Rishi Sunak provides an updated statement on coronavirus', *Gov.UK,* 20 March www.gov.uk/government/speeches/the-chancellor-rishi-sunak-provides-an-updated-statement-on-coronavirus. Accessed: 16 October 2020.

Sunak, R. (2020b), 'Rishi Sunak', *Conservatives*, 5 October 2020 www.conservatives.com/news/rishi-sunak-read-the-chancellors-keynote-speech-in-full. Accessed: 16 October 2020.

Sylvester, R. (2020), 'How right wing is Boris Johnson?' *Prospect*, 7 January.

Thatcher, M. (1987), 'Interview for *Woman's Own*', *Margaret Thatcher Foundation*, 23 September www.margaretthatcher.org/document/106689. Accessed: 16 October 2020.

Tyler, C. (2017), *Common Good Politics*. London: Palgrave MacMillan.

Tyler, C. (2020), 'Brexit: Hatred, lies and UK democracy', *Dialogi polityczne/Political Dialogues*, 27, 63–81.

What UK Thinks (2020), 'In hindsight, do you think Britain was right or wrong to vote to leave the EU?' *NatCen Social Research*, 25 August https://whatukthinks.org/eu/questions/in-highsight-do-you-think-britain-was-right-or-wrong-to-vote-to-leave-the-eu/. Accessed: 16 October 2020.

Wheatcroft, G. (2020), 'Johnson as Churchill?' *Guardian*, 20 March.

White, C. and V. Natfilyan (2020), 'Coronavirus (Covid-19) related deaths by ethnic group, England and Wales', *ONS*, 7 May www.ons.gov.uk/peoplepopulationandcommunity/birthsdeathsandmarriages/deaths/articles/coronavirusrelateddeathsbyethnicgroupenglandandwales/2march2020to10april2020. Accessed: 16 October 2020.

Wilkinson, R. and K. Pickett (2018), *Inner Level*, London: Allen Lane.

Wood, V. (2019), 'Boris Johnson not remotely like Winston Churchill, says wartime PM's secretary', *Independent*, 25 September.

11

SPAIN AND COVID-19

Mariah Miller

Spain suffered serious consequences from Covid-19 early on in the pandemic. In May 2020, Spain was the coordinated market economy (CME) with the highest number of Covid-19 cases. It had the fourth highest total cases in the world, behind the US, Russia and Brazil, and one of the highest rates of Covid-19 infection and fatalities per capita (Johns Hopkins, 2020; New York Times, 2020). The entire country was under a state of alarm from March 14 to June 21 with a strict lockdown that brought the first wave to an end. Spain's experience during this period provides insight into crisis response in a CME.

Spain is a CME in which the state plays a strong role (Fainshmidt et al., 2018). Article 7 of the Spanish constitution establishes unions and employers' associations as social partners forming an essential part of a healthy democracy (Spanish Government, 1978). During the transition to democracy, the state supported the development of coordinating institutions (Royo, 2008). Under the Spanish process of social concertation, the government and the social partners negotiate pacts on working conditions and salary ranges. Due to this process and the underlying culture and social structure, Spain and other coordinated market economies have much stronger welfare states and more generous social protections than liberal market economies (LMEs) (Schröder, 2013). LMEs' welfare states are based on the principle of reliance on the market to solve social problems (Schröder, 2013).

Elements of the welfare state, such as unemployment benefits, public healthcare systems and elderly care facilities, have been key factors in the Covid-19 pandemic in many countries.[1] As expected for a CME, Spain provided strong social support during the Covid-19 pandemic through the existing welfare institutions. The institutions facilitating bargaining and collaboration aided Spain's government in responding to the needs of those involved in social concertation: the unions and the employer's associations, and the workers and owners they represent. During the first wave, the social partners met frequently with the government and were consulted on the pandemic response and the policies adopted had strong protection for businesses and workers.

The social partners do not represent Spain's most vulnerable residents, who still haven't recovered from the 2008 financial crisis. Their needs fall outside the scope of social concertation, yet the precarious nature of their situations often put them at high risk for the coronavirus. Civil society agents of the welfare state found in the social economy are more likely to understand and represent these needs. Although some of their demands to protect the vulnerable were implemented, the social economy institutions do not have an equivalent institutionalized role in policy development and had to demand the right just to participate in policy discussions. By the end of the first wave, non-profits on the verge of collapse from providing essential services in a time of great social need were faced with plans that would substantially cut their funding.

This chapter reviewed the official documents and press releases on the websites of both employers' associations, both unions and the main associations representing the social economy on a national level[2] from January through June 2020. Their recommendations for state responses to the evolving Covid crisis were then compared with official responses in public policies, official statements and media reports.

Overview of first wave of Covid-19 in Spain (March–June 2020)

Before signs of Covid in Spain, the government had already established a Covid task force, which included representatives of the autonomous communities and took into consideration the guidance of international organizations, cooperation within the EU and scientific advice. A Covid plan based on previous pandemic responses was distributed to emergency rooms. The government and health authorities delivered calm statements that Spain was prepared and the outbreak there wouldn't be serious.

The impact of Covid reached Spain before the virus. By early February, Chinese communities were already experiencing xenophobic acts and pharmacies sold out of masks and hand sanitizer. By mid-February, the economic impacts of the pandemic began to be felt. Major international events, such as the Mobile World Congress, were canceled and tourism began to fall as well. Spanish ports recorded decreased traffic and factories had supply chain problems that led to the first temporary layoffs. The last week of February was the worst week for the Spanish stock market in a decade.

While the pandemic control response, including testing, screening and information, originally focused on travel to and from Asia, the first cases were brought by European tourists. The first outbreaks were related to a funeral, skiing trips, a businessman on holiday, soccer matches and, later, the Women's Day marches held on March 8. The outbreaks occurred in areas with stronger economies, that is, Madrid, the Basque Country and later Catalonia. Each region adopted response measures at will following national guidance. The government worked to have a coordinated, inclusive response. Achieving this meant attending to ongoing tensions in the coalition government between Spanish Socialist Workers' Party (PSOE) and Podemos, unprecedented calls between the socialist President and conservative party, and all parties temporarily putting aside the issue of Catalan independence.

On March 14, the President declared a state of national emergency for only the second time. The state of emergency was in place for two weeks, with additional two-week periods approved continuously until late June. All non-essential businesses were ordered to close their physical locations. Adults were only allowed to leave the home to work in essential services and buy supplies. Children were not allowed outside at all. The private healthcare system was placed under the authority of the public healthcare system. All businesses had 48 hours to turn in any protective gear or medical supplies to the government.

On March 17, the government announced a social shield (*escudo social*) supported by the largest allocation of public money in the history of Spain. The social shield included support for businesses and workers, scientific research and vulnerable families. This included rental assistance for individuals who had lost work and small businesses with lost income. It prohibited utility companies from cutting electricity, gas, water and electronic communications during the state of emergency. It provided funds to continue serving school lunches and for elderly and dependent care. For the first time, care workers were made eligible for unemployment benefits.

Nevertheless, the social impact of the virus began to be felt with the state of emergency, continued throughout and afterward. Although economic and social assistance had been approved, systems to register for it collapsed. Residents of elderly care homes received inadequate care, and many died. Calls to domestic violence centers rose. Parents across the country began to clamor for the right of their children to go outside to protect their mental health. Non-profits reported much higher demand for their services and asked for provisions responding to the needs of their specific group of beneficiaries.

Despite forming and working with reoccurring tensions to maintain a coordinated response, enlisting the public and private healthcare system, military hospitals and the army, the healthcare system was under great stress. There was a lack of beds, medical professionals, protective gear and tests. Emergency numbers crashed. However, the strict lockdown brought the spread of the virus under control. By the end of April, the government had approved the Transition Plan toward a New Normal (*Plan de Transición hacia una Nueva Normalidad*) with four two-week phases. On June 21, the coronavirus was declared defeated and the entire country was allowed out of lockdown.

There is no simple explanation for the size of the Covid outbreak in Spain. Until May 10th, Spain reported confirmed and probable cases using all possible forms of testing, which may have caused Spain's reported cases to be higher than other countries. Since then Spain has only been reporting cases confirmed with a PCR test. The Ministry of Health stated that data reported prior to May 25 were invalid, though these numbers continue to be used as revised numbers have not yet been released. Numerical data from Spain should be considered provisional, but differences between data collected in Spain and other countries does not appear to fully explain the high levels of infection, deaths confirmed to be due to Covid or the excess mortality rate, especially through the summer and in the start of the second wave.

A study on the diffusion of Covid during the first wave found that higher case rates in an autonomous community corresponded with the percentage of healthcare workers infected, the percentage of elderly living in nursing homes and risks related to travel internal to Spain, especially connections with Madrid and the Basque Country (Instituto de Salud Carlos III, 2020). This study did not evaluate causality and it did not include social factors such as poverty rates. In August, a group of epidemiologists raised concerns about why Spain has had such a serious outbreak given that it has one of the world's best healthcare systems and called for an independent investigation taking into consideration 'governance and decision making, scientific and technical advice, and operational capacity' along with social inequalities (García-Basteiro et al., 2020).

Role of social partners – protecting employers and workers

The social partners are the two main unions, CCOO and UGT, and the two main employers' associations, Spanish Confederation of Employers' Organizations (CEOE) and the Spanish Confederation of Small and Medium-Sized Enterprises (CEPYME). The social partners have guaranteed participation in councils in many government ministries and on the Economic and Social Council (ESC), which advises the government on socioeconomic and labor issues. The ESC's membership comprises 20 representatives of unions, 20 representatives of employers' associations and 20 other representatives, including the agricultural sector, fishing sector, the Consumers' and Users' Board and the social economy.

The institutionalized nature of the social partners' role gave them voice and opportunity to participate in crisis response. When the Ministry of Labor and Social Economy released a plan for business response to Covid-19 without consulting the social partners, there was a strong backlash. The Ministry Labor and Social Economy lost power over the Covid response and the social partners were guaranteed daily meetings with government ministries. The social partners met with Prime Minister Pedro Sanchez on March 12 when he was deciding whether to implement the stay-at-home order and the conditions of this order; this meeting had already been scheduled for another matter.

The social partners published joint proposals on March 12 focused on layoffs, protection of workers with discontinuous contracts, responding to workers' illness or quarantine needs, how to respond to closed schools, day centers and travel restrictions and remote working. They had made earlier calls for action driven by supply chain problems (fashion, automobiles), sectors suffering from cancelations (hotels, travel agencies, conference facilities and organizers) and protection of workers in healthcare and airports.

The employers' associations argued for special provisions that would transfer the cost of the temporary layoffs to the government and streamlined provisions to implement them quickly. CEOE[3] asked the government for practical mechanisms to guarantee liquidity, simplify layoffs, suspend social security contributions by companies and the self-employed, facilitate legal remote work, promote automatic and interest-free deferrals and partial tax payments, enable access to credit through public guarantees and to pay its own suppliers' invoices quickly.

The unions aimed to ensure that using social security entitlements during the pandemic would not reduce workers' accumulated rights. They requested provisions to make it more difficult and expensive to fire employees and guarantees that employment would be maintained in companies receiving state support. They lobbied for better protections for those with vulnerable employment situations, including immigrants who might lose visas; the unemployed, fieldworkers, domestic workers and others without unemployment benefits; job seekers with no social payments; people who left their jobs to take care of youth or elderly dependents; people requesting subsidies and people with difficulties paying rent. CCOO announced support for government actions protecting victims of domestic violence, deferring evictions, prohibiting cutting off utilities and paying a universal basic income.

Social concertation was used for the initial response, extensions, and two decree-laws.[4] Though Spanish GDP fell by 5.2 percent during the first quarter of 2020 and 17.8 percent in the second quarter, Spanish companies were able to stay open. Corporate bankruptcies were lower and fewer trading companies closed during the first and second quarters of 2020 than the previous year. Companies responded by laying off workers with the national emergency process instead. The currently available data show 3,778,135 workers requested social security payments for a full or partial layoff in March, April and May 2020, which is equivalent to 20 percent of the registered active workforce at the end of February 2020.[5] In contrast, unemployment in Spain only increased by 1.55 percentage points in the first two quarters of 2020 to 15.33 percent. In inter-annual comparison, total unemployment was 1.31 percentage points higher, male unemployment 1.6 percentage points higher and female unemployment 0.9 percentage points higher than in second quarter 2019 (Spanish National Statistics Institute, 2020). The government's Covid response did transfer the cost of these temporary layoffs to the government without employees losing their accumulated social security entitlements. The mechanisms of the CME were able to provide protection to those participating in the process.

The social concertation system has not been able to protect Spanish businesses or workers from many impacts of Covid. The actual delivery of the services suffered from the strain on the system. Support numbers were flooded, and the online application system was not straightforward. In some cases, payments were made to some employees, but not others in the same company. Matters originating outside of Spain, primarily supply chain interruptions, cancelation of international events, cancelation of international travel and travel prohibitions, have had a devastating effect on the economy.

Role of the social economy – working collectively and serving the marginalized

The social economy contributes 10 percent of Spanish GDP and employs 12.5 percent of the workforce (CEPES, 2020). There are strong institutions representing the third sector, cooperatives and the social economy nationally and many more active on a regional level.[6] The social economy does not have political voice within the CME bargaining process as they do not have employees and owners.[7] It also has much less institutionalized participation in policy making. For example, the social economy is entitled to 6 percent of the Economic and Social Council, which can be compared with 33 percent each for the unions' and employers' associations. All four seats are held by CEPES, the main representative of the social economy. Furthermore, while the employer's association is represented on numerous councils in nine different national ministries (CEOE, 2020), the social economy generally does not have guaranteed participation on this level. Unlike the social partners, these institutions do not have extensive representation on government councils or an equivalent role in social policy making.[8]

The social economy made five types of demands during the first wave of Covid-19: to be given financial protection for workers and organizations similar to those granted to other businesses; to be provided with personal protective equipment so that they could continue essential services; to be provided with resources to provide new kinds of support suddenly needed in the pandemic; to be involved in planning the pandemic response and recovery through meetings with government and participation in the planning committees; and the adoption of specific measures needed by their beneficiaries. The government did approve provisions similar to those extended to businesses and their employees. This was the main demand of associations representing social economy organizations that work collectively, but do not specifically provide social services.

The social economy is a significant part of the provision of social services in Spain, primarily though third sector organizations.[9] Third sector associations, including the European Anti-Poverty Network Spain, the Platform of the Third Sector and the Spanish Committee of Representatives of Disabled Persons, made all five demands. Their documents identified in advance groups that would be adversely affected by Covid and the lockdown, highlighted how the current crisis worsened existing social inequalities and challenges, suggested solutions to use during the lockdown and called for a plan of action for coming out of the lockdown and moving forward to avoid further fallout from the crisis. In addition to highlighting issues that the government incorporated into policy responses, the third sector highlighted weaknesses and omissions from the social shield. Their calls for support for groups such as women, gypsies, the disabled and families without internet access were made after the social shield was announced, indicating that these needs were still not being met.

Demand for social services increased during the first wave of Covid-19. While businesses experiencing decreased demand were being subsidized for losses, the third sector asked the government to pay its outstanding debts to third sector organizations and to honor existing contracts so that they could meet demand for ongoing and new services. By the end of the first wave, many third sector organizations were on the verge of economic collapse and the government was proposing to reduce one of their main sources of funding, the automatic contribution of 0.7 percent of personal income taxes for social causes.

The social economy also demanded a participative role in developing the Covid response and in developing social policy moving forward. Some organizations were able to meet with Ministers and some were given a seat at the table during the Covid crisis, especially on a regional level. This could be a step toward institution-building.

Discussion

The Spanish response to the Covid crisis reflects the fragmented nature of the Spanish welfare state. The Spanish welfare state is unequal by sector and by autonomous community. There are strong differences between those inside and outside of the system's coverage. It is not designed to create an equal society for all, but to maintain social stability by ensuring the benefits to existing social groupings (Schröder, 2013). These differences parallel differences in the Covid response for the workforce, represented by the unions, and other citizens.

The size, type and development social economy also vary by autonomous community and some types of social economy organizations are subject to different laws in each. The social economy has an especially strong presence in the Basque Country, Catalonia and Andalusia. This variation may also be reflected in social responses to the Covid outbreak, but the accuracy of such comparisons is limited as the autonomous communities differed in how they collected data about Covid and how quickly they reported it to the central government.

The difficulty translating plans into action showed the consequences of weakened institutions. Spanish institutions have been weakened by elite corruption and the failure of ordinary citizens to engage in the political process and hold elites to account (Royo, 2014). This institutional degradation was one of the causes of the 2008 financial crisis in Spain. A series of scandals came to light at the time of the crisis and the ruling political party, the People's Party (Partido Popular), was found to have been running a system of corrupt accounting and public concertation at least from 1989 (Jones, 2018). Austerity policies following the financial crisis further weakened Spanish institutions. Even social concertation was affected by the financial crisis, making agreements between the unions, employers' associations and government challenging or at times impossible, though the commitment to the process continued (Royo, 2013).

The most significant institution to have been weakened by austerity was the public healthcare system. The reduction in spending on the healthcare system was proportionally higher than overall budget cuts made by the austerity policies following the 2008 crisis. Healthcare spending was reduced 14 percent between 2009 and 2013 and absolute investment in healthcare decreased, including spending on personnel and supplies (Lopez-Valcarcel and Barber, 2017). Austerity cuts meant lower salaries, more working hours and a higher percentage of insecure contracts for healthcare employees (Lopez-Valcarcel and Barber, 2017). This also increased the differences between the autonomous communities (Lopez-Valcarcel and Barber, 2017). During the first wave, Spain reincorporated retired doctors, hired doctors who passed their exams without high enough scores to get a job, and accelerated graduation for current medical students. Facing the second wave, with medical professionals exhausted, they are again facing a shortage of medical professionals.

Going into the Covid-19 crisis, Spain's existing social support was already insufficient. A UN mission raised the alarm about poverty levels in Spain just before the Covid outbreak (Jones, 2020). The United Nations Special Rapporteur on extreme poverty and human rights, Philip Alston, who led the mission, is now highlighting the country's failure to address marginalized individuals during the pandemic, making poverty worse. He has also praised the response of the third sector (Alston, 2020). It is unfortunate that the problems of poverty and inequality highlighted by the third sector went largely unaddressed, were exacerbated by the crisis and most likely contributed to its spread.

The austerity policies also generated widespread public protest, including the *indignados* movement which led to the founding of the political party, Podemos. As a key part of Unidas Podemos, a group of left-wing political parties, Podemos and the PSOE comprised the coalition government in power during the Covid pandemic. As an anti-austerity party sensitive to the needs of vulnerable communities, Podemos included a universal basic income payment as part of the agreement to form a coalition with the Socialists. Covid was the stimulus to actually bring the policy into effect. This policy has the potential to help Spain's most impoverished families. In the absence of a roll for the third sector in the bargaining process, the interests of the vulnerable are represented by government, but supportive politics at the present time do not ensure attention to marginalized groups in a future crisis. Despite aiming for a united front, the government response in this crisis has struggled with party and regional tensions. Ultimately, the plans for reconstruction, approved in July, did not include the social provisions proposed jointly by many social economy associations.[10]

A stronger civil society is needed in Spain to balance 'rent-seeking activities by organized interest groups' (Royo, 2014). Marginalized groups would be better insured by institutionalized participation of the third sector giving them similar voice and role to the unions and business associations. This might be accomplished with better representation of the existing civil society organizations in the political system through the development of long-lasting institutions that guarantees them voice and participation in crisis response even in an unfavorable political climate.

Conclusion

Spain's experience responding to Covid-19 demonstrates the importance of thinking globally. In the prevention phase, they did not consider the movement of the virus in relation to multidimensional global flows but focused exclusively on the risk of contagion from the initial outbreak point. The integration of the Spanish economy into the global economy meant that a domestic response was insufficient to protect Spanish companies from supply chain delays and fallen demand. Tourism not only brought Covid to Spain, but the drive to re-open Spain for tourism may have contributed to the second wave of outbreaks.

Spain's experience also demonstrates which issues and, importantly, *whose* issues are not addressed through the CME system, and shows the relevance of considering which institutions participate in the bargaining process and which are not included. Building institutions to represent the social economy could be complex to achieve due to diversity within the social economy. These institutions might have a different character as the social economy's proposals are complex, multiple and often addressed at long-term structural change. Nevertheless, in moments of crisis like the Covid-19 pandemic, all of society could benefit from their participation.

Notes

1 Of course, other variables, such as population density, standards for recording Covid-19 cases, surplus or deficit economy, and regional politics, could also affect the response.
2 The unions were CCOO and UGT. The employers' associations were CEOE and CEPYME. The social economy organizations were Confederación Española de Empresas de Economía Social, Confederación de Cooperativas de Viviendas de España, Confederación Española de Cooperativas de Consumidores y Usuarios, La Confederación Española de Cooperativas de Trabajo Asociado, La Confederación Española de Mutualidades, Cooperativas Agro-alimentarias, Federación de Asociaciones Empresariales de Empresas de Inserción, Federación Empresarial Española de Asociaciones de Centros Especiales de Empleo, Federación Nacional Cofradías de Pescadores, Grupo Social ONCE, Unión Española de Cooperativas de Enseñanza, Plataforma Tercer Sector, Fundación Espriu, Plataforma de ONG de Acción Social, Plataforma de infancia España, Comité Español de Representantes de Personas con Discapacidad, Red de redes de economía alternativa y solidaria, Plataforma de voluntariado de España and European Anti-Poverty Network España.
3 Cepyme is itself a member of CEOE and many of the statements were issued jointly.
4 Decree-law 18/2020, of May 12, on social measures in defense of employment and Decree-law 24/2020, of June 26, on social measures for the reactivation of employment, protection of the self-employed and competitiveness of the industrial sector.
5 Final data on the total number of workers affected by layoffs during the COVID period was not yet available from the Spanish Ministry of Labor and Social Security at the time of writing.
6 Including the social and solidarity economy which has not yet developed effective national representation.
7 The exception is employees of social economy organizations who are represented by unions.
8 Another example is the State Council for Social Action NGOs, but there was no mention of this council being active in forming the Covid response in any of the sources consulted.
9 The third sector is the sector of the economy comprising non-profit organizations.
10 Participating associations were the Plataforma del Tercer Sector, la Plataforma de Infancia, ONCE, Cáritas, CERMI and the European Anti-Poverty Network Spain.

References

Alston, P. (United Nations Special Rapporteur on extreme poverty and human rights), 2020. Covid-19 exposed deep flaws in Spain's poverty programs, press release, Center for Human Rights and Global Justice, NYU School of Law.

CEOE. 2020. Presencia en Organismos Nacionales. www.ceoe.es/es/contenido/Sobre-CEOE/que-hacemos/presencia-en-organismos-nacionales, accessed on September 7, 2020.

Fainshmidt, S., Judge, W.Q., Aguilera, R.V. and Smith, A. 2016 Varieties of institutional systems: A contextual taxonomy of understudied countries, *Journal of World Business* 53, 3: 307–322.

García-Basteiro, A., Alvarez-Dardet, C., Arenas, A., Bengoa, R., Borrell, C., Del Val, M., Franco, M., Gea-Sánchez, M., Otero, J.J.G., Valcárcel, B.G.L., Hernández, I., March, J.C., Martin-Moreno, J.M., Menéndez, C., Minué, S., Muntaner, C., Porta, M., Prieto-Alhambra, D., Vives-Cases, C. and Legido-Quigley, H. 2020. The need for an independent evaluation of the Covid-19 response in Spain. *The Lancet* 396, 529–530. https://doi.org/10.1016/S0140-6736 (20)31713-X.

Johns Hopkins University & Medicine, Coronavirus Dashboard, viewed on May 30, 2020 https://coronavirus.jhu.edu/map.html.

Jones, S. 2018. Court finds Spain's ruling party benefited from bribery scheme. The Guardian. www.theguardian.com/world/2018/may/24/court-finds-spain-ruling-party-pp-benefited-bribery-luis-barcenas, accessed on October 26, 2020.

Jones, S. 2020. Spain abandoning the poor despite economic recovery, says UN envoy. Special rapporteur says urgent action is needed to tackle 'appallingly high' poverty rates. *The Guardian*. www.theguardian.com/world/2020/feb/07/spain-abandoning-poor-despite-economic-recovery-un-envoy-philip-alston, accessed on September 7, 2020.

Instituto de Salud Carlos III, Factores de difusión Covid 19 en España, COV20-00881, viewed October 26, 2020 from https://portalcne.isciii.es/fdd/.

Lopez-Valcarcel, B.G. and Barber, P. 2017. Economic Crisis, Austerity Policies, Health and Fairness: Lessons Learned in Spain. *Applied Health Economics and Health Policy* 15, 13–21. https://doi.org/10.1007/s40258-016-0263-0.

New York Times, Coronavirus Map: Tracking the Global Outbreak, viewed on May 30, 2020 from www.nytimes.com/interactive/2020/world/coronavirus-maps.html, accessed on May 30, 2020.

Royo, S. 2014. Institutional Degeneration and the Economic Crisis in Spain. *American Behavioral Scientist* 58, 1568–1591. https://doi.org/10.1177/0002764214534664.

Royo, S. 2008. *Varieties of Capitalism in Spain Remaking the Spanish Economy for the New Century*. Palgrave Macmillan: New York.

Schröder, M. 2013. Welfare State Research and Varieties of Capitalism, in: Schröder, M. (Ed.), *Integrating Varieties of Capitalism and Welfare State Research: A Unified Typology of Capitalisms, Work and Welfare in Europe*. Palgrave Macmillan UK: London, pp. 5–30. https://doi.org/10.1057/9781137310309_2.

Spanish Government. 1978. The Spanish Constitution.

Spanish National Statistics Institute (INE). 2020. www.ine.es, accessed on September 7, 2020.

Spanish Social Economy Employers' Confederation (CEPES). 2020. www.cepes.es/cifra,s accessed on September 7, 2020.

12

GERMANY AND COVID-19

Markus S. Schulz

Among the European Union's larger countries, Germany had the lowest rates of Covid-19 infections, hospitalizations, and deaths.[1] Social distancing and lock-down measures were widely accepted. The largest budgetary amendment in the country's history was passed to contain the economic fall-out. There was broad national and international praise for the government's crisis management. How did this happen, and what does it reveal about the country's governance, its medical system, political-economic model, and institutional interventions? To address these questions, this chapter will survey first how the virus entered Germany and how institutions responded. On this basis and through contrasting comparisons with other countries, it will then examine how the health and governance systems shaped the response, paying special attention to intersectional consequences. The conclusion will discuss the institutional strengths and weaknesses, along with recommendations for improvements.

How the virus entered Germany

SARS-CoV-2 emerged in Germany at the end of January 2020. The first infections were reported at an automotive supplier in Starnberg, near Munich, with ties to China. Federal Minister of Health Jens Spahn declared that Germany was 'well prepared' (SZ 2020). A few days earlier, Spahn had maintained that its course would be 'even much milder' than in the case of the flu (Spahn 2020). It took him a full month until February 26 to acknowledge that the epidemic had spread to Germany and to ask the state health ministers to activate their pandemic plans (Geil, Iser, and Gökkayaie 2020).

While this first known contagion cluster was swiftly traced and successfully isolated, several other chains of contagions started to spread. As was discovered later, numerous tourists brought the virus from the Austrian ski town of Ischgl, where local authorities covered up the outbreak over worries about the economic impact of a curtailed vacation season. By the end of February, a first German hotspot emerged in the district of Heinsberg (North Rhine Westphalia), where the local spread was traced to an indoor carnival event. It took only until March 8 for Germany to cross the 1,000 mark of known infections and then merely two more days for this number to double. With an exponential rise taking off, the federal government went into full crisis mode.

Institutional responses

Germany's economic model of *soziale Marktwirtschaft* grounded its legitimacy in the idea that a well-coordinated social market economy with a strong welfare state would bring the greatest benefits to its citizens by harnessing market dynamics for the common good while protecting against market failures, thereby pacifying class conflicts (cf. Müller-Armack 1956; Abelshäuser 2009; Enquete-Kommission 2013). The neoliberal reforms under successive governments from Kohl (1982–98) to Schröder (1998–2005) to Merkel (since 2005) tilted the model toward corporate interests but did not dismantle the underlying historical compromise. This allowed a relatively robust response.

Concerned that the pandemic could exceed the health system's surge capacity, Federal Chancellor Angela Merkel coordinated on March 12 a meeting with the heads of the federal states. With the number of known infections having climbed to 3,000, they agreed to cancel mass events and to close schools. A shutdown of non-essential stores, gastronomic and other types of businesses and institutions was announced for March 18. Hospitals were incentivized to cancel elective procedures and to increase intensive care capacities. The population was asked to maintain social distancing of at least 1.50 meters in public. Several of the federal states closed their borders and imposed for several weeks restrictions on going out except for a 'compelling reason', which included exercise or walk.

Organizations from businesses to universities rushed to update contingency plans. Large research universities were among the first to proactively cancel non-essential travel and meetings, postpone the semester start, and switch to online instruction. Globally interlinked businesses started to notice the disruption of supply chains and drops in demand.

With the specter of a spreading virus and looming quarantines, the demand for storable food supplies spiked but did not exceed restocking capacities. What was sold out for several weeks, however, were disinfectants and protective gear. Facemasks became available to the wider public only when local tailors started producing them, though they still lacked the effectiveness of basic surgical masks made from non-woven fabric and melt-blown material.

The major German broadcast media had begun to report about a 'mysterious lung disease' in Wuhan as early as January 6, 2020, emphasizing the World Health Organization's alertness and the many uncertainties about the actual risk, including the absence of a 'clear proof' of human-to-human contagion (ARD 2020). By mid-March, the coverage about the spread of the virus turned dramatic with grim footage from Northern Italy about overwhelmed hospitals, mounting casualties, and army trucks hauling corpses. The 'new coronavirus' became the main story of the nightly news and the subject of special documentaries and talk shows.

On March 11, Chancellor Merkel called for 'solidarity' at a press conference, and explained that she based her policy on advice from scientists and experts, that knowledge about the virus was to remain highly dynamic, and that in absence of a vaccine or remedies the goal of measures was to slow the spread of the virus (Bundesregierung 2020). A week later, on March 18, Merkel took the rare step to address the nation in a live broadcast, watched by 25 million viewers (Tagesspiegel 2020).

The drastic reduction of economic activity[2] prompted state intervention. On March 25, the German Parliament passed by large majority a supplementary budget that removed balance requirements (*Schwarze Null*) and authorized deficit spending to strengthen the health system and to assist businesses and workers with income shortfalls caused by the crisis. An otherwise balanced budget and low debt provided little hesitation to respond to the crisis with a Keynesian spending package that provided social protections and corporate subsidies. The expansion of the *Kurzarbeitergeld* program nationalized payroll for work shortages to prevent permanent lay-offs. The administrative structures to process quickly millions of claims were already in place. In line with the longstanding model of its coordinated social market economy, the government alleviated liquidity concerns with its 'Corona Protection Shield', the largest rescue package in Germany's history with a finance volume of 350 billion Euro and further state guarantees of 820 billion Euro aimed at economic stabilization. In addition, it provided exemptions from insolvency rules and three months legal protections against evictions or utility shut-offs.

Like other European states, Germany acted largely on its own before developing plans for coordinated measures. In line with European Treaties, health policies were national matters, though Schengen states closed also borders between themselves, in several instances over weeks, until an EU agreement was negotiated. Over the five weeks since March 17, Germany's Foreign Ministry brought back over 240,000 stranded tourists from around the world, many of them on special charter flights.

Getting ready for her upcoming turn to take over the revolving presidency of the European Council, Merkel proposed in May, together with French President Macron, an EU Recovery Fund of 750 billion Euro. By comparison, the 7.5 billion that were raised in support of the Global South for vaccines and treatment at the initiative of the EU Commission under Ursula von der Leyen at a donor conference in May appeared rather too little and under unclear terms.

Germany's health system: strengths and weaknesses

Despite neoliberal reforms, Germany retained a relatively strong health system.[3] A comparative study just prior to the pandemic recognized Germany's health system, along those of the Netherlands, Norway, and Taiwan, as the best in the world (Emanuel 2020). It had per capita more hospital beds, intensive care units, ventilators, and medical personnel than other OECD countries,[4] yet elective procedures were canceled for months to create pandemic surge capacity. The corporatist mode of Germany's dual system of public and private insurers gave ample room to the specialized expertise of various stakeholders but also to vested interests. While health insurance coverage in Germany was nearly universal, the pandemic highlighted unmet needs of undocumented immigrants. Neoliberal politics of austerity prevented over decades increases to the public health budget high enough to meet the rising demands of an aging population and expanded treatment opportunities.[5] Publically insured patients experienced the imposition of cost containment measures in the form of lengthy waits for medical appointments or procedures, rushed interactions with physicians and care personnel, and diminished quality of overall service. The low compensation and stressful workloads for nurses had become obstacles for recruitment and retention. The pandemic revealed striking shortcomings, especially the lack of a strategic stockpile of protective equipment for health care workers, which led the government to scout for supplies on a tightened world market at inflated cost and compromised quality (Trappe 2020).

Beyond the lock-down and social distancing, testing and tracing were the main components of Germany's strategy for containment. A team of the Deutsches Zentrum für Infektionsforschung (DZIF) around Christian Drosten at the Charité Berlin was worldwide the first when it announced on January 16 a test specific to the new virus and shared freely its protocol (Charité 2020). As SARS-CoV-2 spread, competing companies raced to meet the demand for massive testing, which could be taken at any licensed physician's office or special test centers. This early availability of testing helped contain the first wave and thus reduce the number of fatalities.

German's parastatal public health agency, the world-renowned Robert Koch Institute (RKI) monitored infections at the national level, liaised with its scientific counterparts worldwide, and drew up policy advice. Like the Center for Disease Control (CDC) in the US, it served as the government's central scientific institution in the field of biomedicine, but unlike its American counterpart, it did not face overt pressure during the pandemic to bend its messaging to political campaign objectives. RKI developed in collaboration with the US-based commercial corporations Apple and Google a Corona Tracing App. Its 18 million downloads made it the most successful voluntary tracing app worldwide. Yet, it still suffered from malfunctions and a lack of trust in data privacy assurances. The longstanding failure in regulating predatory data practices by conglomerates limited a broader adaptation.

The nationwide network of *Gesundheitsämter* (health authorities) operated at the district level, in charge of local tracing and monitoring the compliance with quarantine requirements. Reinforced by quickly hired tracing assistants, the Gesundheitsämter were able to handle much of the caseload in conjunction with federal support for specific hotspots. The process was far from flawless. While chronic staff shortages led the Gesundheitsämter to fall short on many tasks during the best of times, the pandemic prevented fulfillment of even basic duties such as mandatory school enrollment health examinations, dental services, or consultations. The lack of civilian surge capacities for infection tracing was so severe that Bundeswehr soldiers were deployed to assist, thus creating dangerous precedents of re-normalizing the military after past lessons of dictatorship and World Wars.

Despite the health system's shortcomings and stress on personnel, the pandemic strategy succeeded in flattening the curve of infections to an extent that the hospitals' life-saving capacities were never near exhaustion (as of August 2020). The quickly built extra surge capacities allowed them even to fly in patients from neighboring France and Italy for treatment. German vaccine research companies and university hospitals with strong research departments joined the race to develop vaccines, with experts fostering hopes that it could become available in 2021, but also warning that it could remain an elusive goal.

Germany's governance system: strengths and weaknesses

The pattern of Covid-19 spread in Germany exposed strengths and weaknesses of a complex governance system. The decisions of reasoned leaders can make a difference, can save human lives or doom a nation. Yet, an institutional structure can enable or restrain a leader's contingent decisions. Institutional structures tend to last longer than the terms of a particular office holder. Institutional structures may become obstacles to change, but they may also secure a democracy through checks and balances. Ultimately, a viable democracy depends on the deliberative quality of a public sphere and on the cohesion, habits, trust, and values of a sustaining political culture.

What difference did leadership make during the Covid-19 crisis in Germany? Trained as scientist with a doctorate in quantum chemistry, the Chancellor was able to understand pandemic modeling and the threat of exponential spread. She mobilized federal resources, coordinated policies with the federal states, and deployed her authority to promote to public compliance with safer practices. She seemed to follow expert guidance for crisis communication in a pandemic, that is, to build trust through transparency, including the admittance of uncertainties, and to solicit collaboration by appealing to solidarity. Her leadership stood in striking contrast to the President of the United States who largely abdicated responsibility to the individual states, played down the threat of the virus, and undermined countermeasures.

How did Germany's institutional setup shape its Corona response? Serving as Chancellor since 2005, Merkel relied since 2013 on a 'grand coalition' of the Christian (CDU, CSU) and Social Democratic (SPD) parties, at least one of which had always been in power since the end of World War II. Informed by the fate of the Weimar Republic, the constitutional design of Germany's parliamentary-representative democracy included enhanced checks and balances. It accorded the President a mainly ceremonial role, while the power to define policy was vested in the Chancellor, who could be replaced by parliamentary majority through a constructive vote of no confidence. To maintain enough support, Merkel had to negotiate pragmatic compromises among the different wings of her coalition. The containment and economic protection policies had to balance major interests of business and labor. The Green (Grüne), Left (Linke), and libertarian (FDP) opposition parties criticized the government's policies mainly regarding their effects on the environment, social equity, or regulatory matters. Fundamental opposition came only from the AFD (Alternative für Deutschland), a far-right party with neo-fascist tendencies that had won seats in Parliament in 2017 and organized also extra-parliamentary protests to channel discontent with pandemic restrictions.

Germany's federal structure yielded advantages and disadvantages during the Covid-19 crisis. Its cooperative multi-level system of governance has been criticized for requiring often-lengthy negotiations yielding to the smallest common denominator. Federal states were prone to make quick decisions on their own that led often to a patchwork of differing rules. During the pandemic's early spread, the state of Mecklenburg-Vorpommern closed its borders and barred even nationals with vacation properties from entering. On the other hand, coordinated by Chancellor Merkel and under the pressure of a looming disaster, the heads of the states sprang into joint action at their March 12 meeting with quick and quite drastic agreements. Yet, once the pressure from high infection rates subsided, new disagreements emerged and competition over re-opening schools and businesses ensued. The pandemic's uneven prevalence and specific circumstances such as divergent vacation periods demanded regionally and locally adjusted responses. It had thus advantages that the federal system allowed regionally fine-tuned responses in accordance with infection rates, population density, and statewide demands.

Germany's federal government had considered the risk of a pandemic for many years but did not develop anticipatory capacity commensurate with the challenge. Prior warnings from the highest sources had circulated for many years (e.g. WHO 2007). The official security report had pointed to heightened pandemic risks (BMV 2006). RKI's study of how a respiratory pandemic could overwhelm its health system was shared with Parliament (BMI 2012). As host of the G-20 health ministers meeting in Berlin, Chancellor Merkel (2017) invoked the President of the World Bank, Kim, for making the point that if the Spanish Flu of 1918–20 were to break out today, 'we would probably not be adequately prepared for it'. Revised in 2017, Germany's National Pandemic Plan incorporated insights from the SARS pandemic in 2002–03 and the global spread of H5N1. Among its many recommendations to hospitals and nursing homes was advice for 'the stocking or management concept for quick procurement' of personal protective equipment, including masks (RKI 2017). Warnings continued up to the eve of the Covid-19 pandemic. The Global Preparedness Monitoring Board (GPMB 2019) pointed out in its report of September 2019 the lack of preparedness in the case of a pandemic, specifically of a SARS-type spread through respiration. The Health Security-Index (GHS-Index) ranked Germany only 14th, well below the UK, USA and many other European countries (Cameron, Nuzzo, and Bell 2019). Covid-19 exposed a lack of action on the part of government to heed such warnings.

The Covid-19 crisis highlighted also the importance of institutional structures for quality journalism. Well-researched information and a diversity of juxtaposed opinions served as an antidote to the flood of unfounded rumors, wrong facts, and conspiracy theories circulating on social media. The tension in the media system between trustworthiness through solid reporting and attention maximization through sensationalism became particularly problematic during the pandemic. The news tickers of newspaper websites ran alerts about infection increases even at times that the rate of new infections was declining. Newspapers faced the dilemma that such sensationalist tactics in competing for attention could lead to crisis fatigue and undermine credibility. Institutional safeguards for quality journalism became most visible during infractions. When the yellow press paper Bild-Zeitung accused Drosten in front-page headlines of malpractice while misrepresenting his very words, the Press Council, a well-esteemed voluntary association of German publishers, issued a public reprimand, admonishing the paper for 'grave violations' of journalistic standards of due diligence (Deutscher Presserat 2020).

Although much of the television coverage was in typical fashion emotionally charged, there was also solid reporting and reasoned debate. The public channels had maintained public trust and dominance in ratings over the less respected, often shallower and more sensationalist, advertising-saturated commercial providers, which were allowed to operate since the introduction of the dual broadcasting system in 1984. The nightly news and special documentaries on the public channels provided often in-depth background on the pandemic, including educational content on fundamental aspects of microbiology and epidemiology. In accordance with the principle of balanced coverage, a typical public TV talk show had a mix of invitees from the parties in Parliament and major civil society sectors. The public channels' content reflected a broad spectrum of mainstream perspectives and power in society, thus contributing—for better or worse—to social stabilization.

The pandemic turned a spotlight on the values of care, responsibility, and solidarity, just as much as on self-preservation or greed. Civil society responded to the outbreak of the pandemic with numerous individual acts of kindness, which ranged from bringing elderly neighbors food to engagement in charitable organizations. Yet, there was also hoarding of goods deemed in critical supply. The tension between individualistic and collectivist orientations increased with the rise of neoliberalism. While fear for oneself and concern for others were arguably motivators for compliance with distancing and hygiene rule, the internalized self-discipline of a rule-abiding civic culture helped to maintain it, especially when the infection rate sank. The custom to admonish rule breakers in public was another mechanism in which civil society exercised social control. However, since the wearing of facemasks had never been common, like in East Asia, this practice did not take hold easily, leading to increased calls for enforcement.

Protests against restrictive pandemic control measures were initially very small but grew by August into mobilizations estimated at tens of thousands. Among the protesters were concerned libertarians, pandemic skeptics and denialists, esoteric spiritualists, conspiracy theorists, and activists of the extreme right who tried to channel discontent. The group Querdenken invoked frequently QAnon, a conspiracy movement, which originated in the United States well before the pandemic but became especially popular among Covid-19 skeptics. On August 29, following claims about a secret arrival of US President Trump, hundreds of protesters gained broad mass media attention by storming the stairs of the historic Reichstag building, the seat of Parliament, with several of them waving the Reich flag popular among Neonazis. However, the strategy of these groups to mobilize discontent remained limited.

Polls suggested strong trust in the government's pandemic policies. A representative survey undertaken April to June saw a clear majority across different social groups satisfied with the government's crisis management and the democratic institutions (Kühne et al. 2020). A late August survey by the Mannheim Forschungsgruppe Wahlen found 60 percent fully agreeing with the existing measures and 28 percent demanding yet stronger control measures (Politbarometer 2020). As decreased infection and fatality rates indicated containment, the feeling of collective accomplishment appeared to strengthen social cohesion in Germany, quite in contrast to the US with its intensified polarization. Also in contrast to the US were general expectations for government to protect society and not leave crisis management to markets.

Uneven impact

Germany's State and health system demonstrated their capacity to contain the crisis but burdens were unevenly distributed. The responsivity of its political systems had longstanding bias in favor of the wealthy and against the poor, as studies showed for the period 1998–2013 (Elsässser/Hense/Schäfer 2017). The management of the Covid-19 crisis created winners and losers. The spiked demand for deliveries directed record profits to corporations such as Amazon. Among the hardest hit were the hotel, gastronomy, tourism, and culture industries. The national carrier Lufthansa used its lobbying power for state support. Recipients of state subsidies retained the ability to distribute future dividends to shareholders, that is, while risks were socialized, profits were to remain private. After its deep plunge in March 2020, the German Stock Index DAX recouped most of losses within months and climbed to a new 12-month high. Other businesses, organizations, and individuals responded to the crisis with innovations, accelerated digitization, video-conferencing, and home office. The country's socio-economic inequality assigned different segments of society varying levels of resources to adapt to the crisis.

Workers were impacted by the crisis in varying ways, depending on the economic sector, type of work, corporate policies, and regulatory oversight. Essential workers faced the highest risks of infection, especially in the health sector, but also in other parts of the service and in the manufacturing industries where protections were inadequate. Since essential workers were often also among the least remunerated, their burden was compounded.

The border closures led to an outcry from the agrarian industry whose operational design depended on low-wage seasonal labor from Eastern Europe for the harvest. The government created swift exemptions to allow 40,000 seasonal workers to be flown in by special charter flights. Subsequent scrutiny exposed an exploitative system with gross violations of minimum wage and safety provisions (Maurin 2020).

Infection hotspots in Germany's highly concentrated, 40-billion Euro meatpacking industry drew attention to unsafe work and living conditions, abusive contracting practices, weak regulatory and enforcement provisions, and a breakdown of oversight (DGB 2020). The media coverage of conditions at Tönnies, Europe's largest slaughterhouse, the Bundeswehr deployment at its quarantine quarters, and the prospect of locking down the entire district of Gütersloh drew attention and spurned the Ministry of Labor into reform action (Neuhaus and Leber 2020).

Another major divide appeared between workers with or without options to work remotely. This depended on the nature of the job, technological means, and varying other issues such as availability of childcare, which for many weeks was reserved for essential workers only.

By August 2020, Germany's number of unemployed reached almost 3 million, and was thus over 636,000 higher than in the same month of the previous year (BfA 2020). A steeper rise was arguably prevented by the quick expansion of the federal *Kurzarbeitsgeld* program that incentivized companies to keep employees on their job while covering salary gaps from shortened work hours. The extension of regular unemployment benefits by three months provided immediate relief but were to fall short for more prolonged economic contraction. Hardest hit were households with lower income, which had typically also less assets to buffer temporary income shortfalls.

Policies mandating sheltering in place meant entirely different things depending on a domicile's size, features, location, and occupancy. Staying in the convenience of a spacious mansion a garden contrasted sharply with being squeezed into a dormitory or crowded apartment without a balcony or window. Proximity and mode of transport options to work and shopping influenced the risk of infection. Germany's digital divide shaped opportunities for both remote work and social interaction. The impact of living conditions was compounded by intersecting inequalities and vulnerabilities. The elderly were the most vulnerable age group to be affected by the virus, but the actual risk of infection depended largely on whether one could afford a protected residence or had to stay in a neglected nursing home. Risks of domestic violence were exacerbated during the lock-down by the closure of women's shelters and the delayed public rental of hotels (Hecht 2020). Children from economically poorer families faced higher obstacles to online learning such as shortcoming in hardware, software, Internet bandwidth, ergonomic furniture, paces conducive to concentration, and household members for encouragement and mentoring. The school lock-down exacerbated these longstanding inequalities.

While the fatality risks of those infected increased by age, those with specific pre-existing conditions suffered the greatest risks, and these conditions closely correlated with access to healthy food and medical care and protection from environmental pollutants at home or work—all factors that were linked to financial resources and socio-economic status.

Germany's institutional structures produced unequal consequences. Its economic system subjected large numbers of workers, poor and discriminated groups not only to lesser comforts but also to significantly higher infection and fatality rates than others. And, so far, the pandemic's socio-economic impact appeared bound to further increase inequalities.

Conclusion

The global spread of Covid-19 exposed institutional strengths and weaknesses of existing modes of governance at all levels. The world's fragmented system of nation-states proved incapable to prevent the global spread of the virus. Nation-states focused their efforts within their borders, next came commitments to regional blocs such as the EU, and only after that global coordination. In Germany, the state and the health system demonstrated their capacity to keep overall fatality rates lower than other major Western countries but burdens were shared unevenly. Its differential impact and its infection and lethality patterns were consequences of governance. As discussed above, it resulted from the institutional setup of the federal-corporatist governance structure of the coordinated social market economy, mass media, political culture, and leadership.

Assessment depends on a standard. There were clearly shortcomings that could have been avoided to save lives. Yet, in comparative terms, Germany fared much better than most other countries on a number of criteria. The fact that in Germany almost 10,000 people died with Covid-19 and a quarter million got infected between the first known outbreak in January until the end of August 2020 was by many not perceived as a disastrous failure but rather as a relative success. Because other major European countries did much worse, Germany's performance was largely lauded. A nuanced assessment can thus benefit from comparisons with a theoretical standard and peer performance.

Geography, timing, leadership, and institutional structures shaped how the virus spread, the responses to it, and the consequences. As an intensely connected country with a central position in global trade and travel flows, it is no surprise that the virus entered Germany early in its global diffusion. Yet, the already available test and tracing capacity stopped the spread from the first detected case at the end of January, and bought crucial time. The shocking images from the overwhelmed hospitals and morgues in Lombardy were alarm signals. They convinced the government and public of the need to improve preparations and to take drastic steps of containment just at the moment the virus had found numerous entry routes with returning vacationers and super-spreading opportunities in carnival events. The country's political leadership followed scientific expert advice from epidemiologists and virologists. Over time, the medical systems gained experience in how to treat patients and how to better protect especially the vulnerable elderly in nursing homes.

When comparing the role of leadership in the federal systems of Germany and the US, a strong contrast emerged between Merkel's mobilization of federal resources and active coordination with the Bundesländer, on the one side, and Trump's abdication of responsibility to the individual states, which had to compete at times over scarce equipment, on the other. That Germany achieved better containment outcomes than highly centralized France suggested that leadership and well-timed policy choices could override the potential disadvantages of a federal system even in such a sudden crisis of widest scope.

Germany's institutional pandemic preparedness was uneven. It had an excellent research sector that delivered the world's first test for the virus. Despite austerity measures, it maintained one of the best health care systems with the worldwide highest per capita counts of hospital beds and intensive care units. The government had institutionally recognized the heightened risk of a respiratory pandemic. Yet, it had failed to follow WHO advice for stockpiling enough masks and personal protective equipment. In ordinary times, the global supply chains had always delivered enough in time at a lower cost than if they were produced domestically. The Covid-19 crisis revealed a breakdown of this model. Due to the shortage, the wearing of masks became mandatory only in April after 6,000 Covid-19 deaths. The network of Gesundheitsämter was already in place for the contact tracing of infection cases but budget cuts had led to an understaffing that compromised its capacity.

The pandemic exposed the vulnerability of Germany's export dependence when international demand collapsed. It brought also to light the problematic reliance on complex global supply chains for just-in-time production. Their sudden disruption brought manufacturing to a halt and prompted a rethinking of priorities.

Germany's coordinated social market economy, which balanced capitalist relations of production with a strong welfare state, had come under the pressure of neoliberal reform during consecutive governments, but not as severely as in Anglo-Saxon countries. The Kurzarbeit law and administrative structures to process quickly millions of claims were already in place. An otherwise balanced budget and low debt eased hesitation to respond to the crisis with a Keynesian package that provided social protections and corporate subsidies. Yet, the stimulus package lacked the long-term vision to use such unprecedented financial means for a profound, ecologically sound transformation.

Large majorities of the population trusted government and accepted the containment measures as meaningful. Germany's media system played a stabilizing role during the pandemic. Strong public programming provided airtime for quality journalism, investigative reporting, expert interviews, and talk shows with representatives from the full range of parliamentary parties and established interest groups. This limited the influence of disinformation spread via social media, which, for example, intensified polarization in the United States.

The Covid-19 crisis is, at the time of writing, far from over. Much is still unknown about the virus itself. Many deep uncertainties remain, among which are even most basic issues such as whether and when there might be an effective vaccine or remedies. Yet, the contradictions in the existing institutional frameworks and modes of governance demand timely debate.

The pandemic provided important lessons that have begun to yield change. Government and business leaders began to balance the paradigm of short-term cost efficiency with a greater concern for resilience against disruption. To modernize its hospital system in the wake of the pandemic, the German government planned to invest three billion Euro in enhanced emergency capacities and digitalization (*Krankenhauszukunftsgesetz*). A long-delayed digitalization initiative for schools appeared to near implementation.

Yet more institutional learning is needed. The government's advisory bodies included primarily epidemiologists and economists but lacked broader social science participation. The latter is needed to understand the differential impact of policies and design more equitable measures. The shortcomings in preparedness call for a strengthening of anticipatory capacities, including institutional re-design for enhanced follow-up, adaptive resilience, and flexible responses. Considering that the fall-out from the Covid-19 pandemic may still be small compared to the challenges from climate change make this an urgent task.

Notes

1 Germany had 249,063 total known cases; 249 daily new cases; 9,399 total deaths; 224,600 total recovered; 15,064 active cases; 223 serious, critical; 2,971 total cases per 1 million population; 112 deaths per 1 million population; 12,383,035 total tests; 147,713 per 1 million population; 83,831,702 population, as of the end of August 2020 (Worldometer, www.worldometers.info/coronavirus/, accessed September 4, 2020). Germany had thus a fifth of the Covid-19 fatality rate of the USA, Italy, or Brazil, or a quarter of that of France. A relatively high per capita rate of tests limited the undercount of infection cases in Germany more than in countries with less testing.

2 The retraction in the first quarter of 2020 was with almost 10 percent almost double as severe as in the worst quarter of the financial crises in 2008 (Destatis 2020).

3 Like in most wealthy countries, Germany's health system constituted a major economic sector. In 2018, health expenditure amounted to 390.6 billion Euro, that is, 4,712 Euro per capita, or 11.7 percent of GDP (GBE 2020).

4 In 2017, Germany counted six hospital beds (acute care) per 1,000 inhabitants across its 1,300 hospitals (OECD 2020).

5 The federal budget for health rose since 1992 both in absolute nominal and in per capita terms consistently year over year, exact for a small dip in 2004, while the percentage of BIP increased by 2.3 points (GBE 2020).

References

Abelshauser, Werner. 2009. *Des Kaisers neue Kleider? Wandlungen der Sozialen Marktwirtschaft*. Munich: Roman Herzog Institut.

ARD. 2020. 'Rätselhafte Lungenkrankheit in China: WHO ist alarmiert,' *Tagesschau*, January 6.
BfA (Bundesagentur für Arbeit). 2020. Auswirkungen der Coronakrise auf den Arbeitsmarkt. Nuremberg: BfA. https://statistik.arbeitsagentur.de (Downloaded August 28, 2020).
BMI (Bundesministerium des Innern). 2012. Bericht zur Risikoanalyse im Bevölkerungsschutz. Deutscher Bundestag, Drucksache 17/12051.
BMV (Bundesministerium der Verteidigung). 2006. Weißbuch 2006: Zur Sicherheitspolitik Deutschlands und zur Zukunft der Bundeswehr. Berlin: BMV.
Bundesregierung. 2020. Pressekonferenz. Mitschrift, March 11.
Cameron EE, Nuzzo, JB, and Bell JA. 2019. Global Health Security-Index (GHS-Index). Center for Health Security/Johns Hopkins University, Nuclear Threat Initiative (NTI), and Economist Intelligence Unit (EIU): www.ghsindex.org/, accessed August 28, 2020.
Charité. 2020. Pressemitteilung, January 16.
Destatis (Statistisches Bundesamt). 2020. Statistik Dossier, no. 14 (August).
Deutscher Presserat. 2020. *Pressemitteilung*, September 11.
DGB (Deutscher Gewerkschaftsbund). 2020. *Für faire Arbeitsbedingungen in der Fleischindustrie.* Berlin: DGB.
Elsässer L, Hense S, and Schäfer A. 2017. "Dem Deutschen Volke?' Die ungleiche Responsivität des Bundestags,' *Zeitschrift für Politikwissenschaft*, Vol. 27, pp. 161–180.
Emanuel EJ. 2020. *Which Country Has the World's Best Health Care?* New York: Public Affairs.
Enquete-Kommission. 2013. Schlussbericht der Enquete-Kommission `Wachstum, Wohlstand, Lebensqualität – Wege zu nachhaltigem Wirtschaften und gesellschaftlichem Fortschritt in der Sozialen Marktwirtschaft, Deutscher Bundestag, Drucksache 17/13300.
GBE (Gesundheitsberichterstattung des Bundes). 2020. Informationssystem der Gesundheitsberichterstattung des Bundes. www.gbe-bund.de, accessed August 28, 2020.
Geil K, Iser JC, and Gökkayaie H. 2020. 'Spahn: Deutschland "am Beginn einer Coronavirus-Epidemie"', *Die Zeit*, February 27.
GPMB (Global Preparedness Monitoring Board). 2019. World at Risk: Annual Report on Global Preparedness for Health Emergencies. Geneva: WHO.
Hecht P. 2020. 'Häusliche Gewalt und Corona: Eine doppelte Bedrohung,' taz, May 17.
Kühne S, Kroh M, Liebig S, Rees J, Zick A, Entringer T, Goebel J, Grabka MM, Graeber D, Kröger H, Schröder C, Schupp J, Seebauer J, and Zinn S. 2020. 'Gesellschaftlicher Zusammenhalt in Zeiten von Corona: Eine Chance in der Krise?' DIW: SOEP Papers on Multidisciplinary Panel Data Research, no. 1091.
Maurin J. 2020. 'Vorwürfe gegen Gemüsehof in Bayern: 250mal Corona, 6 Euro Stundenlohn,' taz, August 13.
Merkel A. 2017. 'Rede von Bundeskanzlerin Merkel bei der Eröffnung des G20-Gesundheitsministertreffens am 19. Mai 2017 in Berlin,' Berlin: G20 Germany.
Müller-Armack, Alfred. 1956. 'Soziale Marktwirtschaft.' In: Handwörterbuch der Sozialwissenschaften, Vol. 9. Stuttgart: Fischer/Tübingen: Mohr/Göttinger: Vandenhoeck & Ruprecht, pp. 390ff.
Neuhaus C and Leber S. 2020. 'Mehr als 650 Corona-Infizierte bei Tönnies: Wie Europas größte Fleischfabrik zum Hotspot wurde,' taz, June 17.
OECD (Organization for Economic Cooperation and Development). 2020. Beyond Containment: Health Systems Responses to Covid-19 in the OECD. Paris: OECD.
Politbarometer. 2020. 'Mehrheit für stärkere Corona-Kontrollen,' *ZDF*, August 28.
RKI (Robert Koch Institute). 2017. *Nationaler Pandemieplan*. Berlin: RKI.
Spahn J. 2020. Interview mit Gesundheitsminister Spahn. *Tagesschau*, January 23.
SZ (Süddeutsche Zeitung). 2020. 'Spahn nach Coronavirus-Fall in Bayern: Sind gut vorbereitet.' *SZ*, January 28.

Tagesspiegel. 2020. '25 Millionen Zuschauer sehen Ansprache der Bundeskanzlerin,' *Tagesspiegel*, March 19.

Trappe T. 2020. 'Chaotische Maskenbestellungen: Jens Spahn muss sich vor dem Kartellamt verantworten,' *Tagespiegel*, July 28.

WHO (World Health Organization). 2007. A Safer Future: Global Public Health Security in the 21st Century. The World Health Report 2007. Geneva: WHO.

13

TURKEY AND COVID-19

Facing a global crisis during a domestic crisis

Sarp Kurgan

The coronavirus crisis has instantly become the biggest global crisis of the century. Like all major crises, it may lead to fundamental structural changes at global, regional, and national levels. It also reveals much about the character of political-economic governance. Questions regarding effective struggles against the pandemic and its relation to institutional strength and state capacity have come to the forefront.

While government policies ultimately impact how the pandemic unfolds at the domestic level, political-economic regime types and their corresponding institutions have an undeniable impact on how governments determine their policies. Yet, regime types and institutions are not fixed but constantly transform, sometimes through such major crises. National responses to the pandemic will impact how these transformations unfold. Further authoritarianism, neoliberalism and isolationism stand as likely but not inevitable outcomes.[1]

This chapter analyzes the Covid-19 response of Turkey's AKP (*Adalet ve Kalkınma Partisi*, Justice and Development Party) government, which has been in power since 2002 and confronts the crisis amidst increasing monopolization of power by President Recep Tayyip Erdoğan, an ongoing economic crisis, and an unprecedented institutional decay. In other words, Turkey faces the pandemic during a domestic crisis.

The chapter is divided into four parts. The first offers an overview of Turkey's initial steps against the pandemic. The second part analyzes the response through the lens of state-affiliated institutions, while the next part deals with institutions outside the AKP's direct tutelage. The last section analyzes the pandemic's economic impact.

In recent years Erdoğan's government drove decisively towards neo-populist authoritarianism through executive centralization, emergency policies, control over judiciary and legislative apparatuses, and crackdowns on varied sources of opposition.[2] Economically, Turkey has a long history of state-led capitalism, regardless of its political regime or development model.[3] The AKP's neoliberalism did not reduce the state's agency on economic governance. On the contrary, it used state funds to create a new bourgeoisie stratum firmly allied to the new government. This trend has shifted Turkey from state-led towards crony capitalism.[4]

Neither of these two processes could have been possible without a conscious attack on institutions. Since its early years in power, the AKP has sought greater control over political, social, judicial, and economic institutions that need to be autonomous in order to be effective. Loyalty instead of merit gradually became the main criteria in all state-affiliated institutions, while the AKP effectively marginalized any non-state institution that it could not bring under its tutelage. Institutional decay has been both a tool and a symptom of AKP's monopolization of power. In practice, this means Turkey's institutions can neither pressure the government on specific issues, nor can they override or check and balance its decisions.

Authoritarianism, institutional decay, and crony capitalism emerge as the key factors in the making of Turkey's domestic crisis prior to the pandemic. This chapter argues that these trends have played the determining role in shaping the government's response. Rather than revealing something hitherto unknown, the pandemic has accelerated ongoing trends in Turkey's political-economic governance.

Turkey, of course, is not alone experiencing these trends. Multiple countries across the globe sharing little in terms of political-economic governance and/or sociocultural traits such as the US, the UK, Venezuela, Brazil, Hungary, Poland, Iran, Egypt, Israel, Russia, India, and the Philippines have witnessed similar processes at varying degrees during the 2010s. Sociopolitical polarization, distrust in official institutions, increasing inequality, and the emergence of 'strong leaders', among others, have been common traits. An analysis of the impact of institutions and governance in confronting Covid-19 in Turkey could help us better evaluate their significance against major crises.

Overview of Turkey's Covid-19 response

This part offers a brief analysis of how Turkey responded to the crisis. Relying on political attitude towards the crisis, enforcement of measures to slow the spread, and safe normalization as the three evaluation criteria, I claim that the AKP prioritized the economy over public health, and campaigned more than it governed, especially during the normalization process.

An important note is that relying on official data in assessing Turkey's pandemic management would be inaccurate. Officially, as of mid-October, Turkey has reported 4,177 cases, 112 deaths, and 15,0787 tests per 1 million people, while the total death toll is around 9,500 (Worldometer). Yet this is not reliable as the government has consistently refused accountable and transparent data sharing. In late-September, Health Minister Fahrettin Koca was forced to admit that Turkey was hiding its true statistics both from the public and the WHO for concerns over 'national interests' and admitted that Turkey had only been publishing symptomatic cases.[5] Testing criteria was also not transparent.[6] Additionally, Turkey did not report coronavirus-related deaths in accordance with the WHO guidelines either.[7] Some studies have shown that Turkey's confirmed case numbers were 10 to 20 times higher, and the total coronavirus-related deaths were two to three times higher than announced.[8]

Turkey announced its first Covid-19 case on March 11. Over the following weeks, the government announced several measures to slow the spread such as closing bars and night-clubs on March 15; cafes, restaurants, gyms, schools, and universities on March 16; mosques on March 19; implementing a stay-at-home order for people over 65 on March 21; mandatory masks, travel restrictions, and stay-at-home order for people under 20 on April 3; and weekend lockdowns from April 10 to early June. Moreover, the government declared Covid-19 treatment to be free in private hospitals, although there were significant problems in practice.[9] Some of these steps were efficient in slowing the spread, and ramped up the health sector, indicating that the government initially took the crisis seriously.

One timely and accurate step was the formation of the Science Board under the Health Ministry in February, consisting of medical, public health, and epidemiology experts. Officials often emphasized that they implemented measures based on the Board's suggestions. However, the Board was a consultative committee with no decision-making authority and their suggestions were not made public. Some scientists within the Board hinted that the government often ignored their pleas (TTB 5.14.2020: 38).

It became quickly obvious that Turkey was not prepared for the crisis. At the initial phases, there were significant PPE deficiencies.[10] Turkey did not implement its own pandemic protocols created in 2006 and recently revised them in 2019 (TTB 5.14.2020: 28). Turkey also did not implement quarantine measures properly for foreign travelers. The biggest mistake was not quarantining many of the returning Umrah pilgrims. In late March, when Turkey had carried only 28,000 tests, Fahrettin Koca confirmed that Turkey sold 500,000 tests to the US.[11] The private sector self-implemented closures in various sectors such as shopping malls or factories without any government initiative. The government constantly ignored pleas for stricter measures from the opposition, medical experts, unions, or civil society organizations such as the Turkish Medical Association (*Türk Tabipleri Birliği*, TTB). Economic concerns seem to be at the top of the government's agenda for not ordering a total lockdown.[12]

Despite these negative elements, however, Turkey managed to keep the pandemic relatively under control until the normalization steps. Several factors were important such as Turkey's historically strong medical sector, the high number of intensive care beds, extremely altruistic efforts of health care workers, young population,[13] late arrival of the pandemic, and several accurate and timely decisions by the Science Board. These factors were also crucial in keeping the mortality rate relatively low.

After stagnation in daily case numbers, Turkey initiated normalization steps in May. The process has fully exposed how the government prioritized campaigning over governance and economy over public health. The AKP sought to turn its pandemic response into political gains, propagandizing an epic success story. Simultaneously it launched attacks on the opposition. Political parties, opposition municipalities, professional associations (including doctors), unions, media, Kurds, feminists, and LGBTQs frequently became targets.[14]

The government prioritized saving certain economic sectors, most notably construction, tourism, manufacturing, and retail. Shopping malls reopened in mid-May when parks were still closed. Travel restrictions to major tourism hubs were lifted in May. The government also held university and high school entry exams, forcing more than 4.5 million students into schools. The exam date, which had been pushed to late-July at the initial outbreak, was moved back to early June to boost tourism, angering many students. The government turned a blind eye to construction and manufacturing industries as Covid-19 spread rapidly among workers. Informal, women and refugee workers were more severely affected.[15]

The impact of uncontrolled and rapid normalization became apparent after July. Hospitals became overwhelmed and exhaustion spread among medical workers. Major inconsistencies made official data completely irrelevant.[16] Hospitals started refusing new patients due to a lack of available beds, causing preventable deaths. As the government cut payments for Covid-19 treatment in private hospitals, they refused to admit patients to intensive care units, further overwhelming public hospitals.[17]

Overall, the AKP's response to the pandemic showed patterns with its traditional governance that considers moments of crises not as issues to be solved through efficient and rational governance but as potential political gains.

AKP authoritarianism and Covid-19: confusion and disarray

The pandemic was a test for Erdoğan's novel presidential system, which has effectively implemented a one-man regime.[18] For years, the AKP has argued that a more centralized and powerful executive branch with minimum checks and balances would increase government efficiency and would work particularly well in times of crisis. I claim that Turkey's pandemic response proves otherwise. Erdoğan's regime was not only unprepared for the crisis but it was also confused, irrelevant, and contradictory in its response. Moreover, the AKP avoided taking initiative and put the responsibility on the public. Despite being discursively obsessed with 'strong state', the government kept itself outside the pandemic as much as possible. The crisis did also not change the AKP's traditional political strategy of polarization.

The AKP's disarray became quickly obvious following March 10. Erdoğan, who during normal times would give multiple speeches on a daily basis and be broadcast live by almost every TV station, was nowhere to be found until March 18, when he announced Turkey's initial measures against the pandemic. His announcements and measures taken in the following days showed the government's unprepared and reactive response. Many measures were inconsistent and meaningless. For example, Erdoğan announced the government would distribute masks and sanitizer to people over 65, only to be followed by a stay-at-home order for the very same people days later. Reducing taxes on domestic flights or hotel accommodation was meaningless, which was followed by a ban on flights. After making masks mandatory in markets and public transport, Erdoğan promised that the government would distribute masks for free to everyone and prohibited mask sales. The result was a failure. Most people got neither government-sponsored masks, nor could they buy masks at their own expense. The government changed mask distribution plans six times in two months. Ultimately, it re-allowed mask sales.

Delayed and reactionary responses caused problems. Some examples include keeping mosques open until March 19, not quarantining many of the returning pilgrims, and not closing the land border to Iran, the epicenter of the disease in the Middle East, until March 24. Another problem was the lack of coordination between ministries. The clearest example was the announcement of weekend lockdown by the Interior Ministry on April 10, announced only two hours before it would begin. At least 250,000 people rushed to markets to buy necessities, forming huge queues without any social distancing.[19] Municipalities, the Health Ministry, and the Science Board were not informed of the decision. A similar event occurred on June 5, when the Health Minister announced there would be no weekend lockdown, followed by the Interior Minister's announcement declaring there would be a lockdown, followed by Erdoğan's announcement via Twitter that he had lifted the lockdown because 'his heart did not allow it'.[20]

Erdoğan remained unwilling to implement stricter measures. The AKP did not effectively use its vast executive powers. Furthermore, how pandemic response decisions were taken further exemplified institutional decay. All lockdown decisions were implemented through Interior Ministry Notices, while it was Health Ministry Notices that implemented data collecting apps. Legally, only Presidential Decrees can implement them. An important sign on the AKP's attitude towards the crisis is its refusal to declare a state of emergency, despite Turkey having a long – and problematic – history of states of emergencies. Following the coup attempt in 2016, the AKP declared a state of emergency for two years, using it to oppress the opposition and amend the constitution. During the pandemic, the AKP officials asked the people to 'declare their personal states of emergencies'.[21] This signals that a state of emergency in Turkey's political-economic system is a tool to protect the state against its citizens, not to protect citizens against a crisis.

This relates to the government's refusal to take more initiative during the crisis. The AKP's pandemic motto, 'caution – cleanliness – distance' is an example of how the government has put the responsibility on the public while it simultaneously has incentivized people to normalize. Another example is the relatively small size of rescue packages to Turkey's GDP. The 'Economic Stability Shield' announced by the AKP was worth of 200 billion TRY, most of which were loans, and made up less than 5 percent of Turkey's GDP.[22] Many critics argued that actual crisis-related government spending, loans or otherwise, was significantly lower.

Mismanaging the crisis forced the AKP to manage people's perceptions. Demonizing the opposition and aggressive sociopolitical polarization has been Erdoğan's standard practice. Uniting its base around symbols and/or Erdoğan's personality against enemies, such as foreign interest groups and their domestic allies, has been a longtime crisis recipe for the AKP. This tactic might be effective for political purposes. Yet, sociopolitical polarization, non-inclusive governance and political feuds are counterproductive during a pandemic. This is especially so for Turkey where political efficacy is already damaged by widespread public normlessness and distrust.[23]

Its pandemic response has exposed the AKP to be more confused and irrelevant than ever. The lack of a capable, meritocratic, and rational bureaucracy – a by-product of AKP's authoritarianism – also became exposed with the pandemic. Turkey's political institutions were reactive, incapable, uncoordinated, and often counterproductive. Turkey's 'strong' government, fully in control of the state apparatus, avoided taking responsibility in the biggest global crisis of the century. Hence, the Turkish example debunks authoritarian effectiveness claims. Instead of providing effective governance, AKP's authoritarianism led to a more incapable response.

Institutions outside AKP direct tutelage: sidelining and marginalization

The AKP has maintained its historical attitude towards institutions during the pandemic. The main reason behind this was that institutions with relative autonomy such as opposition municipalities have performed duties that the AKP failed, especially in terms of social policy. Furthermore, civil society organizations such as unions or professional associations have exposed the AKP's failures.

The pandemic has shown that autonomous civil society organizations can play major roles during the crisis, especially when they work in coordination with the state or when they can freely expose policy mistakes. Throughout the pandemic, the AKP has continuously ignored the TTB, Turkey's largest medical association, and launched investigations against its members for 'spreading misinformation'.[24] By September, ultranationalists and Islamists within the AKP's governing coalition started demanding TTB's closure. The AKP's attitude towards unions has been more hostile. For years, the AKP has been marginalizing autonomous unions while promoting pro-government yellow syndicates. Even with government-sponsored unions, however, Turkey's unionization rate is only 12 percent.[25] Unorganized labor is the key reason why the wage earners suffer most in economic and public health crises. With the outbreak, the government banned all union activities. Workers, who complained of or exposed working conditions, faced firing and in some cases arrest. Faced between virus and unemployment, most workers had to choose employment.[26] Some companies went as far as building 'labor-camps' with the government's tacit approval, forcing workers to stay at isolated manufacturing facilities to continue production, even as Covid-19 spread among workers (Toker 7.31.2020).

Local governance can also play major roles in a pandemic. Even in Turkey, where local governments are historically weak against the central authority, municipalities performed major duties during the crisis, especially in filling the gaps left by the state's social security policies. The AKP has a contradictory legacy in social policy that combines its neoliberalism, populism, and Islamic charity.[27] The AKP has extended health, retirement, and insurance benefits to include informal, urban poor segments and initiated a policy of conditional cash transfers to the poorest classes. These measures helped the AKP to gain the support of the urban poor. Yet such policies incorporated labor into the financial markets, eroded the idea of social support as a citizenship right, and instead promoted Islamic charity notions that articulated it as a privilege. These social policy measures were already crumbling under the pressure of Turkey's deepening economic crisis. As a result, the poorest segments in Turkey found close to nothing in the government's rescue programs.

The metropolitan municipalities, which the opposition won in 2019, started filling these gaps through multiple aid and social solidarity policies that included cash and food aids, rent and bill relief, and housing for the homeless. The AKP, however, disrupted these efforts by confiscating municipality funds, launching slander campaigns, and even banning aids.[28] While the AKP's attitude towards the main opposition party CHP (*Cumhuriyet Halk Partisi*, Republican People's Party) municipalities was counterproductive, its attitude towards the pro-Kurdish, socialist-oriented HDP (*Halkların Demokratik Partisi*, People's Democratic Party) municipalities was blatantly antagonistic. The AKP continued its policy of confiscating the HDP municipalities illegally through trustees and many HDP politicians and activists were arrested during the pandemic.[29]

The AKP's response against institutions outside its tutelage during the pandemic showed continuity with its previous policies, although its attempts to disrupt their efforts became more blatant. The AKP's lethargic pandemic response has left the vulnerable segments without any meaningful protection. The opposition municipalities, by filling these gaps, threatened to break the link between the AKP and the urban poor. Moreover, they constituted an alternative to the AKP's ineffective response, which explains its increasing pressure. This could also explain why Erdoğan increasingly pursues socio-politically polarizing policies since they help to mobilize his base around ideology and identity when he cannot mobilize them around material benefits.

Crony capitalism, economic crisis, and Covid-19

Covid-19 is likely to create the biggest recession in modern history. Disruptions in supply chains, bankruptcies, unemployment, increasing poverty, and economic uncertainty will have long-term effects on the global economy, with harder impacts on the developing countries. The standard financial response in rich countries has been to ensure macroeconomic stability by creating public debt through central banks. This policy will not work for the poorer countries that neither possess the financial capacity nor a globally exchangeable currency.

Additionally, Turkey faces the pandemic in the midst of a deep economic crisis, caused by the AKP's neoliberal-oriented crony capitalism, as well as mismanagement, corruption, and institutional decay, especially in the legal and financial systems. Although restricted, the AKP still had to implement rescue packages to confront pandemic's economic impact. I claim that they reflect the AKP's class politics, oriented to protect cronies and big business at the expense of wage earners.

Turkish economy is in a deep economic crisis as it has been shrinking gradually since 2013. Per capita GDP has shrunk from $12.519 in 2013 to $9.042 in 2019, while the US Dollar-Turkish Lira ratio has risen from 1.8 in 2013 to 7.9 in 2020. Foreign investment and Central Bank reserves have been declining over the past years; while trade deficit, unemployment, public and private debt, and inflation have been rising. The longevity of the crisis is due to policy mistakes. For years, Erdoğan stood behind his 'unorthodox theory' that inflation would not go down if interest rates were high. He forced the Central Bank to artificially reduce interests below the inflation rate, which jeopardized the Bank's autonomy and further reduced the Lira's value. Mismanagement of public funds, corruption, and bureaucratic extravagance were additional contributing factors.

Because Turkey's major economic crises have historically resulted in major political changes (Öniş 2010), the AKP had much to fear. Like most governments, the AKP aimed at maintaining employment and purchasing power while preventing bankruptcies. Big business, among which AKP's cronies, construction, manufacturing, and tourism being heavily prioritized, benefited from tax remissions and reduced labor costs. Small and medium-sized businesses that had long benefited from the AKP's policies received cheap credit and tax deferral. Yet many businesses had trouble with receiving these credits.[30]

Maintaining employment rate, which was already low with 45 percent in 2019,[31] was a major challenge for the AKP. Despite the economic crisis, Turkey could afford income/salary support while partly compensating the negative impacts of the crisis, using only 4 percent of its GDP (Taymaz 4.8.2020). The government could also rely on Unemployment Insurance controlled by the Treasury and Finance Ministry which on paper had funds to provide a minimum wage for 15 million workers (60 percent of Turkey's employed) for four months.[32]

Instead, the AKP developed a short time working and unpaid leave scheme. The government banned firings during the pandemic but allowed employers to cut hours or send their workers to unpaid leave with income support of less than half of the minimum wage. The income support came from the Unemployment Fund at the expense of workers' insurance, which means that if they actually get fired after the government's ban expires, they will have sharply reduced benefits, if any. Employers' right to send someone to unpaid leave would be permanent, giving major long-term leverage to employers. Moreover, it is difficult to receive income support for formal employees, while it does not cover the informal sector at all. Out of 3.5 million applications, only 1 million received unpaid leave support.[33]

Despite steps toward rapid normalization and curtailing unemployment, labor participation decreased drastically. Employment loss due to the pandemic reached 9.4 million people, while broad unemployment reached 17.2 million. People who were neither employed nor in education within the 15–29 age group reached an unprecedented 32.8 percent, excluding those on reduced hours or unpaid leave.[34]

The AKP's macroeconomic response to the pandemic has been in line with its previous economic policies. It aimed to increase demand by offering cheap credits through public banks while reducing interest rates below inflation. These credits incentivized spending in the tourism and construction sectors, signaling that the AKP has no real plan against the crisis. In the absence of foreign exchange, the AKP continued to sell reserves to stabilize the Lira, which hit -$33 billion in August.[35] As a result, the USD/TRY ratio increased from 6.85 to 7.95 in early October. With currency losing value, Central Bank losing credibility, declining employment numbers, declining foreign investment, and mismanagement, it would be fair to say that Turkey faces the biggest crisis in its history. Once again, the wage earners will be paying the price.

Regardless of the magnitude of the crisis, the AKP's policies showed continuity. It had to save the big business and cronies because they constitute the most fundamental and loyal supporters of the regime and they are less likely to be convinced by ideology or identity. Prioritizing cronies and big business over wage earners, and ultimately over public health and welfare, reflect the class character of Turkey's state-led capitalism.

Conclusion

The pandemic has immediately worsened socioeconomic inequalities. The crisis is also likely to widen the global inequalities between richer and poorer nations. The economic impact will be much more severe for Turkey than in other developing countries.

Regardless, Turkey does have the necessary means to ensure food, employment (or income), and health security for all during a crisis. This was hardly how Turkey responded to the crisis. It requires an efficient state apparatus and political will that prioritizes public health and welfare over political gains. Globally, the pandemic has become a test on governance. State capacity, inclusive governance, public trust in institutions and officials emerged as key factors in the pandemic response. After years of institutional decay and political-economic governance prioritizing regime survival before all, it is not an accident that the AKP, like other populist-nationalist governments and their 'strong' leaders, failed to respond adequately.

I have argued that authoritarianism, institutional decay and crony capitalism, as defining features of the AKP regime, have determined the AKP's response to the crisis. The crisis has also incentivized the AKP to accelerate these processes. Yet the crisis might also bring existing but marginalized ideas to the forefront. Demands for food, health, employment, as well as housing and education securities, and an accountable, transparent, democratic order backed by meritocratic, reliable institutions, already constitute social pressure on the government. With organized, collective masses behind them, these demands might ultimately lead to a political-economic alternative to AKP's crony capitalist authoritarianism.

Notes

1 For discussions on pandemic-related transformations see Harari 2020; Acemoglu 2020; Diamond 2020; Fukuyama 2020.
2 For discussions on AKP's authoritarian turn, see Esen and Gümüşçü 2016; Tansel 2018; Yılmaz and Turner 2019; Arat and Pamuk 2019; Somer 2016.
3 For the history of Turkey's state-led capitalism, see Keyder 1987; Buğra 1994; Pamuk 2014; Boratav 2018.
4 For relations on the AKP and the new bourgeoisie, see: Buğra and Savaşkan 2014.
5 See TTB 5.14.2020; *Reuters* 9.30.2020 and *BirGün* 10.01.2020.
6 Critics argued that political factors took precedence over contact tracing, as regime elites had easy and frequent access to testing while many frontline medical workers or people with clear symptoms could not get a test. Moreover, the health ministry has contracted only one company, an affiliate of the government, for PCR tests. By July, several researchers claimed that Turkey's PCR test accuracy was 40 percent (*DW Türkçe* 07.25.2020).
7 For a death to be reported as Covid-19 related, the person must test positive in her/his very last test (TTB 5.14.2020: 141). Thereby, the Health Ministry has prevented hospitals to report people who died without ever being tested and people whose test results were falsely negative, or died in hospital receiving Covid-19 treatment but tested negative in their last test (even if they had tested positive in previous tests) as Covid-19 related deaths. See *Diken* 04.09.2020.
8 Erzurumluoğlu and Şaylan (2020) calculated that the excess deaths in Istanbul from mid-March to mid-August are twice higher than official Covid-19 death toll in Istanbul. *BBC Türkçe*'s report on 09.24.2020 on excess deaths in 11 cites that make up one-third of Turkey's population shows that there has been over 11,000 excess deaths.
9 See for example TTB 07.10.2020: 57.
10 See for example TTB 03.23.2020.
11 See *BirGün* 3.25.2020.
12 Despite government's concerns over the economy, two studies (Taymaz 7.9.2020; Çakmaklı et al. 2020) found that if the government had implemented a total lockdown instead of unplanned, partial, and reactive measures, the death toll would be significantly lower while the economic impact would not be different.
13 People over 65 constitute 9 percent of Turkey's population.
14 In late July, Erdoğan went as far as holding a mass prayer-rally, attended by 350,000, as he transformed historic Hagia Sophia from a museum to a mosque, destructing a major symbol of Turkey's secularism and fueling sociopolitical polarization.
15 For reports on working conditions during Covid-19, see: DİSK 4.20.2020; DİSK 5.14.2020; DİSK 6.20.2020; *BBC Türkçe* 6.20.2020.
16 In some cases, the daily case number or death toll for one city announced by its governor or mayor surpassed the national daily case number or death toll announced by the Health Ministry. Also see TTB 8.14.2020: 6.
17 See *BirGün* 8.19.2020.
18 Turkey's political system prior to the AKP was already prone to authoritarianism. The 1982 Constitution, implemented by the military junta, prioritized protecting the state against its citizens by crippling individual and sociopolitical rights and liberties while strengthening the executive branch against judicial and legislative branches (Özbudun 2001: 31–44). The AKP found little institutional checks and balances in its drive towards authoritarianism.
19 See *Diken* 4.11.2020.

20 See *DW Türkçe* 6.5.2020.
21 See *Diken* 3.25.2020.
22 See *AA* 4.28.2020.
23 See for example Çarkoğlu and Kalaycıoğlu 2009: 43–46.
24 See TTB 7.3.2020.
25 See DİSK 4.8.2020.
26 See Delen and Peksan 2020; DİSK 4.27.2020.
27 For AKP's social security policies, see Akçay 2018; Buğra and Candaş 2011; Aytaç 2013; Çarkoğlu and Aytaç 2014; Buğra 2008; Bozkurt 2013.
28 See *Diken* 03.29.2020; *Diken* 03.31.2020.
29 See *T24* 07.15.2020.
30 See Soydan 6.25.2020.
31 Source: Turkstat.
32 See DİSK 3.28.2020: 6–7.
33 See DİSK 7.11.2020.
34 See DİSK 7.11.2020; DİSK 8.10.2020; Genç İşsizler Platformu 8.10.2020.
35 Demiralp 8.10.2020.

References

'20 Haziran Dünya Mülteci Günü: 'Türkiye'deki Mültecilerin Yüzde 70'i Pandemi Sürecinde İşini Kaybetti.' *BBC Türkçe*, 20 June 2020.

Acemoglu, Daron. 'The Post-COVID State.' *Project Syndicate*, 5 June 2020.

Akçay, Ümit. 'Neoliberal Populism in Turkey and Its Crisis.' *Institute for International Political Economy Berlin Working Paper, No. 100/2018*, 2018, www.ipe-berlin.org/fileadmin/institut-ipe/Dokumente/Working_Papers/IPE_WP_100.pdf.

Arat, Yeşim, and Şevket Pamuk. *Turkey between Democracy and Authoritarianism*. Cambridge University Press, 2019.

Aytaç, S. Erdem. 'Distributive Politics in a Multiparty System: The Conditional Cash Transfer Program in Turkey.' *Comparative Political Studies*, vol. 47, no. 9, 2013, pp. 1211–1237. doi:10.1177/0010414013495357.

Boratav, Korkut. *Türkiye İktisat Tarihi: 1908–2015*. Imge Kitabevi, 2018.

Bozkurt, Umut. 'Neoliberalism with a Human Face: Making Sense of the Justice and Development Party's Neoliberal Populism in Turkey.' *Science & Society*, vol. 77, no. 3, 2013, pp. 372–396., doi:10.1521/siso.2013.77.3.372.

Buğra, Ayse. *State and Business in Modern Turkey: A Comparative Study*. State University of New York Press, 1994.

Buğra, Ayşe. *Kapitalizm, Yoksulluk ve Türkiye'de Sosyal Politika*. Iletişim Yayınları, 2008.

Buğra, Ayşe, and Osman Savaşkan. *New Capitalism in Turkey: The Relationship between Politics, Religion and Business*. Edward Elgar, 2014.

Buğra, Ayşe, and Ayşen Candaş. 'Change and Continuity under an Eclectic Social Security Regime: The Case of Turkey.' *Middle Eastern Studies*, vol. 47, no. 3, 2011, pp. 515–528. doi:10.1080/00263206.2011.565145.

'Cumhurbaşkanı Erdoğan: Ekonomik İstikrar Kalkanı ile açıkladığımız desteklerin tutarı 200 milyar lira.' *AA (Anadolu Ajansı)*, 28 Apr. 2020.

Çakmaklı, Cem, Selva Demiralp, Şebnem Kalemli Özcan, Sevcan Yeşiltaş, and Muhammed Ali Yıldırım. 'COVID-19 and Emerging Markets: The Case of Turkey.' *Koç University-TÜSİAD Economic Research Forum Working Paper Series No: 2011*, Apr. 2020.

Çarkoğlu, Ali, and Ersin Kalaycıoğlu. *The Rising Tide of Conservatism in Turkey*. Palgrave-Macmillan, 2009.

Çarkoğlu, Ali, and S. Erdem Aytaç. 'Who Gets Targeted for Vote-Buying? Evidence from an Augmented List Experiment in Turkey.' *European Political Science Review*, vol. 7, no. 4, 2014, pp. 547–566. doi:10.1017/s1755773914000320.

Delen, Meltem Güngör, and Selcan Peksan. 'COVID-19 ve İşçiler: Salgının İlk Döneminde Sanayi İşletmelerinde Çalışan Sendikalı İşçiler (Mavi Yakalılar).' *İstanbul Üniversitesi İktisat Fakültesi İnsan Kaynakları Araştırma Merkezi*, July 2020.

Demiralp, Selva. 'Money for Nothing: Currency Crisis in Turkey.' *Yetkin Report*, 10 Aug. 2020, www.yetkinreport.com/en/2020/08/10/money-for-nothing-currency-crisis-in-turkey/.

Diamond, Larry. 'Democracy versus the Pandemic.' *Foreign Affairs*, 13 June 2020.

DİSK (Devrimci İşçi Sendikaları Konfedarasyonu). 'COVID-19 Ile Mücadele Ve İşsizlik Sigortası Fonu.' 28 Mar. 2020.

DİSK (Devrimci İşçi Sendikaları Konfedarasyonu). 'Covid-19 Ve Sonrasında DİSK'in Çalışma Yaşamı Yol Haritası.' 14 May 2020.

DİSK (Devrimci İşçi Sendikaları Konfedarasyonu). 'DİSK-AR Covid-19 Döneminde Kadın İşgücünün Görünümü Raporu.' 20 June 2020.

DİSK (Devrimci İşçi Sendikaları Konfedarasyonu). 'DİSK-AR Covid-19 DİSK Raporu 2.' 20 Apr. 2020.

DİSK (Devrimci İşçi Sendikaları Konfedarasyonu). 'DİSK-AR Covid-19 DİSK Raporu 3.' 27 Apr. 2020.

DİSK (Devrimci İşçi Sendikaları Konfedarasyonu). 'DİSK-AR Covid-19 Salgın Günlerinde Türkiye'de Sendikalaşmanın Durumu Araştırması.' 8 Apr. 2020.

DİSK (Devrimci İşçi Sendikaları Konfedarasyonu). 'İşsizlik Ve İstihdamın Görünümü Raporu.' 10 Aug. 2020.

DİSK (Devrimci İşçi Sendikaları Konfedarasyonu). 'İşsizlik Ve İstihdamın Görünümü Raporu.' 11 July 2020.

'Erdoğan Sokağa Çıkma Yasağını İptal Etti.' *DW Türkçe*, 5 June 2020.

Erzurumluoğlu, Mesut, and Defne Üçer Şaylan. 'İstanbul'da Haftalık Vefat Sayıları.' *Sarkaç*, 10 Aug. 2020.

Esen, Berk, and Şebnem Gümüşçü. 'Rising Competitive Authoritarianism in Turkey.' *Third World Quarterly*, vol. 37, no. 9, 19 Feb. 2016, pp. 1581–1606. doi:10.1080/01436597.2015.1135732.

'Fahrettin Koca: ABD'ye 500 Bin Adet Tespit Kiti Satıldığı Doğru.' *BirGün*, 25 Mar. 2020.

Fukuyama, Francis. 'The Pandemic and Political Order: It Takes a State.' *Foreign Affairs*, 3 Aug. 2020.

Genç İşsizler Platformu, 'Genç İşsizlik Bülteni.' 10 Aug. 2020.

'Gündem 'Corona': CHP ile AKP'nin 'Kalabalık Otobüs' Polemiği.' *Diken*, 29 Mar. 2020.

Harari, Yuval Noah. 'The World after Coronavirus.' *Financial Times*, 20 Mar. 2020.

'HDP'den 'Salgın Döneminde Kürt Düşmanlığı' Raporu: Kayyım, Gözaltı ve İşkence Vakalarında Artış Gözlendi.' *T24*, 15 July 2020.

'Kamu Covid-19 Hastalarını Tedavi Etsin: Özel Parasına Baksın.' *BirGün*, 19 Aug. 2020.

Keyder, Çağlar. *State and Class in Turkey: A Study in Capitalist Development*. Verso, 1987.

'Koca itiraf etti: Koronavirüs verileri 'ulusal çıkarlar' için gizlenmiş!' *BirGün*, 1 Oct. 2020.

'Koronavirüs: BBC Türkçe'nin araştırmasına göre 11 ilde 8 ayda yaklaşık 11 bin ek ölüm var, artış beklenenin üzerinde' *BBC Türkçe*, 24 Sep. 2020.

Öniş, Ziya. 'Crises and Transformations in Turkish Political Economy.' *Turkish Policy Quarterly*, vol. 9, no. 3, Jan. 2010, pp. 45–61.

Özbudun, Ergun. *Türk Anayasa Hukuku*. Yetkin Yayınları, 2001.

Pamuk Şevket. *Türkiye'nin 200 Yıllık İktisadi Tarihi: Büyüme, Kurumlar ve Bölüşüm*. Türkiye Iş Bankası Kültür Yayınları, 2014.
Somer, Murat. 'Understanding Turkey's Democratic Breakdown: Old vs. New and Indigenous vs. Global Authoritarianism.' *Southeast European and Black Sea Studies*. Nov. 2016. doi:10.1080/14683857.2016.1246548.
Soydan, Barış. "Restoran-Kafe Destek Kredisi' Gerçeği: Bir Avuç Büyük Tesisten Başkası Alamıyor.' *T24*, 25 June 2020.
'Soylu: Erken Saatte Yasağı Açıklasaydık, Marketlere Akın Olsaydı Daha Mı Iyi Olurdu?' *Diken*, 11 Apr. 2020.
'Soylu: Vatandaş Kendi OHAL'ini İlan Ederse Üst Tedbire Şimdilik Gerek Olmayabilir.' *Diken*, 25 Mar. 2020.
Tansel, Cemal Burak. 'Authoritarian Neoliberalism and Democratic Backsliding in Turkey: Beyond the Narratives of Progress.' *South European Society and Politics*, vol. 23, no. 2, 3 June 2018, pp. 197–217. doi:10.1080/13608746.2018.1479945.
Taymaz, Erol. 'Covid-19 Tedbirlerinin Türkiye Ekonomisine Etkisi ve Çözüm Önerileri.' *Sarkaç*, 8 Apr. 2020.
Taymaz, Erol. 'Salgın Devam Ederken Ekonomi Düzelebilir Mi? – Bir Mikrosimülasyon Analizi.' *Sarkaç*, 9 July 2020.
Toker, Çiğdem. 'Köleliğin Yeni Adı: Kapalı Devre Çalışma.' *Sözcü*, 31 July 2020.
'TTB: Sağlık Bakanlığı 'Corona' Ölümlerini DSÖ Kodlarına Göre Raporlamıyor.' *Diken*, 9 Apr. 2020.
TTB (Türk Tabipler Birliği). 'COVID-19 İzleme Kurulu COVID-19 Pandemisi 2. Ay Değerlendirme Raporu.' 14 May 2020.
TTB (Türk Tabipler Birliği). 'COVID-19 İzleme Kurulu COVID-19 Pandemisi 4. Ay Değerlendirme Raporu.' 10 July 2020.
TTB (Türk Tabipler Birliği). 'TTB COVID-19 İzleme Kurulu Üyesi Halk Sağlığı Uzmanı Prof. Dr. Kayıhan Pala'ya Bilimsel Açıklamalarından Dolayı Soruşturma Açıldı!' 3 July 2020.
TTB (Türk Tabipler Birliği). 'TTB'den Sağlık Bakanlığı'na: Sağlık Çalışanlarının Koruyucu Malzeme Eksiklikleri Hızla Giderilmelidir.' *TTB*, 23 Mar. 2020. www.ttb.org.tr/kollar/COVID19/haber_goster.php?Guid=b181ff1a-6ce1-11ea-a219-c213173be5c8.
TTB (Türk Tabipler Birliği). 'Türk Tabipleri Birliği COVID-19 İzleme Kurulu 5. Ay Değerlendirmesi: Salgın Kontrol Altına Alınamıyor, Sağlıkçılar Tükeniyor!' 14 Aug. 2020.
'Turkey has only been publishing symptomatic coronavirus cases – minister.' *Reuters*. 30 Sep. 2020.
Turkstat (Turkish Statistical Institute), 'Population by Labor Force Status.' June 2020.
'Yavaş: Yardım Hesaplarımız Genelge Sonrası Bloke Edildi.' *Diken*, 31 Mar. 2020.
'Yerli Test Kiti Tartışması: Testler Ne Kadar Güvenilir?' *DW Türkçe*, 25 July 2020.
Yılmaz, Zafer, and Bryan S. Turner. 'Turkey's Deepening Authoritarianism and the Fall of Electoral Democracy.' *British Journal of Middle Eastern Studies*, vol. 46, no. 5, 11 July 2019, pp. 691–698. doi:10.1080/13530194.2019.1642662.

Americas

14

THE US, SOUTH KOREA, AND COVID-19

Governance

Hyug Baeg Im

The performance of the US and South Korea in responding to coronavirus disease 2019 (Covid-19) presents a striking contrast. As of August 9, 2020, according to Worldometer Covid-19 data, the US has recorded 5,441,647 confirmed cases and 170,952 deaths—both of which are the highest numbers of any country in the world. In contrast, the numbers of cases and deaths in South Korea have remained stable at around 15,000 cases and 300 deaths. South Korea has recorded a death rate of six persons per million population, which is one of the lowest death rates among OECD countries. Among the seven large industrial democracies with more than 50 million population and a GDP per capita of at least 30,000 dollars (the US, Japan, Germany, UK, France, Italy, South Korea), South Korea has the lowest numbers of both cases and deaths. The US and South Korea are exemplars of countries that have failed and succeeded, respectively, in responding to the Covid-19 pandemic among large industrial democracies. Therefore, comparing the US and South Korean management of Covid-19 is a useful lens through which to explore the virtues and vices, strengths and weaknesses, resilience and fragility of liberal market economy (LME) and coordinated market economy (CME) approaches to the governance of large industrial democracies in responding to the Covid-19 crisis.

In comparing the two countries' responses to Covid-19, I will focus more on endogenous sources of difference such as institutional governance and the virtues and vices of political leaders than on exogenous factors, such as pre-existing economic conditions, the international regime, environmental challenges, and climate change. The analysis of these two countries' responses to Covid-19 is based on the premise that 'institutions matter'—that is, institutions influence norms, beliefs and actions, and therefore they shape outcomes (Hall and Soskice 2001: 1–68; Przeworski 2004: 192). In explaining the different responses to Covid-19 of the US and South Korea, I will compare five aspects of institutional governance: (1) the healthcare system, (2) the disease control and prevention system, (3) central and local government relations, (4) state and civil society relations, and (5) governance of new forms of labor in the era of the fourth industrial revolution. Then, deficiencies and lacunae in the institutional governance-based explanation of Covid-19 crisis management will be complemented by an analysis of virtues and vices of political leaders of the two countries in responding to Covid-19.

The disastrous response of the US is essentially an institutional failure. The US is a typical LME that, compared to CMEs, puts 'economy over society' and 'profit over people', minimizes the role and responsibility of the state in dealing with epidemic disease, has an underdeveloped and privatized healthcare and welfare system, and overexploits the environment for the sake of profits (Unnikrishnan, 2020). These neoliberal institutions are responsible for the worse management of the Covid-19 crisis in comparison to the institutions of CMEs, which put 'society first over the economy', assign a more active role and responsibility to the state, maintain a more robust public health system and welfare state, and create a sustainable environment (Saad-Filho 2020).

The American LME places the primary responsibility on the market to provide public goods and services such as health, education, sanitation, and environmental protection. However, public services—and health services in particular—are typical services that are prone to recurring market failures. If the market is responsible for the provision of health services, these services will be undersupplied because the market does not supply health services to those in need, but instead to those who can pay for those services. The conservative Reagan and Bush administrations extensively privatized public services, including health services and education, shrunk the safety net for the disadvantaged, and lifted regulations on banks and stock exchanges for the sake of letting market forces operate freely (Avineri 2020).

As public health services have become privatized and commodified, the provision of health services by profit-seeking private health industries has overwhelmed public healthcare. When Covid-19 expanded throughout the cities and countryside of America, the US government was not prepared to control the pandemic. The US had neither facilities and personnel for Covid-19 testing and treatment, nor an effective pandemic prevention and control system capable of protecting citizens from Covid-19. The neoliberal response rendered the American people unprotected from Covid-19, as evidenced by the fact that the number of deaths in the US by Covid-19 exceeded the combined number of US deaths in the Vietnam War, Korean War, and wars in the Middle East. It has become clear that the urban poor, homeless, and irregular workers have been more vulnerable to Covid-19 than the middle and upper class and regular workers. The neoliberal US provides unequal access to testing and treatment by gender, class, and ethnicity, thereby increasing gender, class, and ethnic inequalities (Alsbrook 2020).

Adding to these institutional failures, the US has shown extremely poor leadership of any global government, as it has failed to lead and coordinate the various actors engaged in pandemic prevention, detection, treatment, and recovery. The Trump administration has been responsible for medical supply shortages (including kits, masks, gloves, gowns, and ventilators), testing delays and failures to implement social distancing and self-isolation. Trump's response was inadequate because he prioritized the impact of Covid-19 on his reelection prospects in November 2020 over listening to the opinions of medical, hygiene, and healthcare experts about overcoming the Covid-19 crisis.

Unlike the US, South Korea has a state-led CME that emphasizes the governmental coordination of actions, policies, and strategies among the market, civil society, and local governments. South Korea, which has a long, centralized statist tradition, has established embedded autonomy in both the civil and economic society. Equipped with embedded autonomy, the central government can establish close coordination and cooperation among the central and local governments, as well as medical institutions and civil society, to build a system for pandemic prevention, case detection, and treatment, and to elicit followership from the people. Collectively, these factors enabled voluntary social compliance with the counter-Covid-19 measures of the government. As a consequence, South Korea has emerged as a model country that has succeeded in defending its people from the Covid-19 pandemic through coordination and cooperation among civil, economic, and medical actors.

For-profit healthcare in the US versus public universal healthcare in South Korea

US: private for-profit health system

The US is the only high-income, advanced, industrially developed country that does not operate a universal healthcare system. As a result, 8 percent of the population has no health insurance coverage of any kind (2019). The 2010 Affordable Care Act, often referred to as 'Obamacare', was praised as the first step to universal healthcare in the US, but has been derailed by Donald Trump, who repealed the individual mandate of obligatory participation in the health insurance system.

The US health system is a mix of public-private sources, in which private insurance accounts for two-thirds of the market and the remaining one-third of the people are covered by public insurance plans, including Medicare, Medicaid, and veterans' programs. Medicaid covers vulnerable groups and Medicare covers people over 65 years old and those with disabilities (Maizland and Felter 2020).

Healthcare in the US is unimaginably overpriced and has a low accommodation capacity. Even though the citizens pay 17 percent of the GDP for health services as of 2018, which is the highest rate among advanced industrial countries, the US provides extremely low-quality and unequal health services for the elderly, the infirm, and those with a low income. The US healthcare system is not a public system but a 'private for-profit system' (Reich 2020). The US system prioritizes profits of the health industry over public health. The privatization of health services has transformed hospitals and medical institutions into 'medical industries', which maximize their profits from medical services and healthcare. The neoliberal government withdrew from healthcare and public pharmaceutical provision. The privatization of health services has limited the ability of many Americans to access affordable healthcare.

When the Covid-19 outbreak took place, American facilities, personnel, and organizations were revealed as far from sufficient to deal with the crisis. Medical and health facilities were not fully operational and the production and supply of medical kits, masks, gowns and ventilators did not increase immediately. In sum, the US was not prepared to contain and mitigate the coronavirus, even though the Global Health Care Index in 2019 evaluated that 'the US is number one in Health Security, with a score of 83.5' and concluded that the US would be 'the most well-prepared country to combat a pandemic disease'. The evaluation of the Index in 2019 was proven wrong in 2020.

Faced with Covid-19, the market-oriented medical system has not responded to the needs of Covid-19 patients but instead has provided medical services only for those who can pay it. Under these circumstances, the groups at the highest risk for coronavirus infection, such as the old, the infirm, the low-income, immigrants, and single-parent families, are less likely to seek treatment and more likely to die from the virus. As 44 million Americans do not have health insurance and 38 million do not have adequate health insurance, they must pay very high costs to receive tests and treatment. Covid-19 once again revealed that in neoliberal America, healthcare is not seen as a right of people, but as a commodity to buy privately. The absence of universal healthcare has rendered economically poor workers with neither paid-sick leave nor medical coverage extremely vulnerable to Covid-19 because they had to work even though they were infected.

South Korea: universally accessible, responsive, and efficient public-private health system

The health service system in South Korea is a mixture of a public and private health system. Both public medical institutions and private hospitals participate in Korean healthcare and both public and private institutions provide medical services under legally equal conditions. While private medical institutions treat most patients, the universal National Health Insurance Service (NHIS) pays most of the expenses. As of 2006, about 96.3 percent of the total population was covered through the NHIS (57.7 percent were employee insured, 38.9 percent self-employed insured), while the remaining 3.7 percent was covered by the Medical Aid program (Song 2009). The coverage of the NHIS has expanded to emergency treatment, medicines, medical supplies, and dental treatment. Therefore, the Korean healthcare system can be described as a universal healthcare system with a balance between public insurance system and private medical institutions.

The public-private balance in Korean healthcare system has enabled universal access to healthcare, secured abundant resources for healthcare, and enhanced the reaction capability for containing and mitigating Covid-19. The *de facto* universal healthcare system in South Korea has minimized the medical costs of Covid-19 patients and has facilitated free testing for coronavirus. The Korean healthcare system has been rated very high by international medical agencies. For instance, the Korean system was rated the best in universal access, the highest in patient satisfaction, and the fourth-highest in efficiency in the OECD (OECD 2015; Lu 2016).

The National Health Insurance (NHI) is the mandatory public health insurance system that Koreans must subscribe to throughout their lifetime. Koreans can add private insurance to NHI coverage. The main features of NHI are mandatory subscription, income-based premiums, and equal benefits. For efficient operation of the NHI, the Health Insurance Review and Assessment Service (HIRA) reviews medical expenses, while the NHIS reimburses them. In 2008, the HIRA established a highly digitalized health care information system by adding a comprehensive pharmaceutical information service, a drug utilization review, and a medical billing portal. In 2018, more advanced IT systems were added, such as a mobile service system, a healthcare big data hub, and a national healthcare portal (NRC and STEPI 2020). With the aid of the HIRA, the Korean government has been able to establish an efficient and effective supply and distribution system of masks for the public through highly accessible pharmacies throughout the nation and has implemented advanced digitalization of healthcare information.

Politicized CDC in the US versus institutionalized KCDC in South Korea

Both countries have a national institute for disease control and prevention, the Centers for Disease Control and Prevention (CDC) in the US and the Korea Centers for Disease Control and Prevention (KCDC). While the KCDC initiated, led and enforced policies of disease prevention, testing, treatment, tracing, and quarantine, the CDC in the US only set guidelines for disease control and allowed local governments to implement pandemic control policies as they deemed appropriate, with or without consultation of local public health departments. The decentralized disease control system in the US resulted in ineffective, non-comprehensive and inconsistent efforts to control the pandemic crisis.

Politicized CDC in the US

Politicians in the US, President Trump in particular, politicized and meddled with the pandemic control and prevention efforts, prohibiting experts and scientists in the CDC from implementing effective pandemic control policies based on scientific information and knowledge.

Since it opened in 1946 in Atlanta, the CDC has played core roles in beating back epidemic disease threats. However, when the nationwide Covid-19 outbreak took place, CDC experts and scientists were sidelined, and their prevention guidelines were never adopted. The Trump administration took control of clearing CDC communications about the coronavirus and rejected CDC doctors' recommendations for surveillance, social distancing, and safe reopening of schools. The CDC adopted a hands-off approach regarding the reopening of states, and thus, more states arbitrarily lifted lockdowns (*The Japan Times* 2020). Political interference and top-down bureaucratic regulations blocked initiatives and innovations at the CDC, and thus prevented the CDC from renewing its organizational power and authority to develop vaccines and diagnostic tests, to build a CDC-run surveillance system, and to develop guidelines for quarantines and social distancing. President Trump placed strict limits on the CDC's advisory capacity, reduced the scope of CDC activities by cutting 15 percent of the CDC's 2021 budget on February 10, 2020, and moved the responsibility for Covid-19 control and prevention from CDC to the White House Coronavirus Task Force (*The Japan Times* 2020). As a consequence, the CDC director has kept a low profile, experts and scientists in the CDC have been sidelined, and politicians and bureaucrats have disseminated politically massaged information and guidance for Covid-19 control and prevention.

Institutionalized KCDC and the TRUST strategy in South Korea

In contrast to US political leaders, Korean political leaders respected the expertise of scientists and officials in the KCDC and delegated authority for controlling and preventing the Covid-19 pandemic.

The development of the KCDC furnishes an excellent case study exemplifying the theory of historical path dependency, which explains how an institution created in the past has persisted and developed in certain ways over time (Thelen 1999). The KCDC was built for preventing and controlling an epidemic like severe acute respiratory syndrome (SARS) in 2004, and by 2015 it had developed into a more autonomous institution capable of preventing and controlling an epidemic like Middle East respiratory syndrome (MERS) (Kim 2020).

The KCDC succeeded in preemptively preventing the spread of SARS in its early stages by strengthening quarantine inspections for those entering from high-risk areas. After controlling SARS, the Korean government enhanced the capacity of the KCDC to implement a specialized and systematic response to epidemics, and specifically took steps 1) to reinforce quarantine, 2) to enforce R&D capabilities for diagnostic technologies and vaccines, and 3) to integrate inspections and quarantines by transferring policy coordination power from the Ministry of Health and Welfare (MOHW) to the KCDC (KCDC 2005) After the outbreak of MERS, South Korean government strengthened the power of the KCDC by establishing the Reform of National Quarantine System, which granted full authority to the KCDC and restructured the KCDC into an independent policy-coordinating body for national infection control and quarantine. The restructuring made the KCDC the leading agency for national quarantine policies, with other agencies, including the Prime Minister's office, the Ministry of Health and Welfare, and the Ministry of Public Safety and Security, playing a supportive role (NRC and STEPI 2020). When South Korea confronted Covid-19, the KCDC had already evolved into a more autonomous and stronger institution that was capable of containing and mitigating the pandemic. With its accumulated know-how, information networks, technologies, and legal mechanisms, the KCDC so far has performed excellently in preventing, detecting, and treating Covid-19, as well as implementing social distancing and quarantine measures.

The keys to successful prevention and control of the pandemic by the KCDC are open information and transparency, mass testing, tracing, social distancing, and self-isolation. First, the provision of open information and transparency contributed to the success of the KCDC. The KCDC chief, Jung Eun Kyeong, has held regular public briefings twice per day and shared information about Covid-19 with the Korean people, and governors and mayors have also briefed, shared information, and communicated with their local residents. Second, mass testing and transparent information-sharing have contributed to effective social distancing. Third, a comprehensive telemedicine network and contact-tracing enabled effective monitoring in self-isolation. Contact-tracing involves tracing the route of patients who test positive and their contacts through GPS, smartphones, credit cards, and video surveillance equipment. In addition, the KCDC developed an innovative drive-through testing method that is capable of simultaneous and quick mass testing. The KCDC and Moon Jae In's government have managed to prevent and control Covid-19 without a lockdown.

The strategy through which the KCDC succeeded in preventing and controlling Covid-19 is called the TRUST strategy, which stands for Transparency, Robust screening and quarantine, Unique but universally applicable testing, Strict control, and Treatment for pandemic control and prevention (Klinger 2020).

New Federalism in the US versus a centralized state and coordinated center-periphery system in South Korea

New Federalism in the US

Federalism in the US is a decentralized system of distributing rights and powers between federal and state governments, which sometimes inhibits the federal government from implementing coherent and comprehensive policies for the whole country. In addition, with the rise of 'New Federalism', which was proposed by President Ronald Reagan and combines neoliberalism and federalism, the federal government has returned the responsibility for domestic policies to state governments, giving states more discretionary power in implementing 'block grants' (Conlan 1998).

President Trump, succeeding Reagan's New Federalism, has abandoned federal leadership and responsibility for pandemic control and left states to fend off Covid-19 for themselves. Trump's New Federalism has deepened and worsened interstate inequalities. Under New Federalism, as the federal government has compelled state and local governments to implement balanced budget requirements, a number of local governments have faced a budget squeeze forcing them to make public employee pay cuts and layoffs, which have led to downsized employment and reduced services. As a consequence, state and local governments are overburdened in controlling the pandemic and attempting to restore local economies with a reduced budget. Trump's abandonment of federal responsibilities caused states to vie over precious resources, to the point of virtually dissolving the union into 50 component parts. The weakening of New Deal Federalism and the disappearance of the civic federalism of Tocqueville would likely increase the possibility of turning toward autocratic solutions and discretionary decisions by federal leaders (Kreitner 2020) and of rising 'emergency politics', which rule with the state of emergency outside of the usual and accepted rule of law (Teskey 2020).

Centralized state with a coordinated center-periphery system in South Korea

South Korea has maintained a centralized state and local government relationship. Even though the autonomy of local governments has increased through recent decentralization reforms, local governments are not sufficiently independent from the central government, especially with regards to budget and personnel. Thus, compared with the US federal government, the Korean central government has more power to implement comprehensive and consistent policies on pandemic disease control and prevention.

The Moon Jae In government, however, has not monopolized the power to control Covid-19, but devolved authority and transferred disaster relief funds to local governments, and established a system of coordination between central and local governments. The coordination system of central and local governments in Korea comprises the KCDC as the control tower of Covid-19 pandemic, the Central Disaster Countermeasure Headquarters (Prime Minister's office) as the nationwide support and control tower between central and local governments, and the Government Support Headquarters (Ministry of the Interior and Safety) as the center for coordination and cooperation between central and local governments, and Local Disease and Safety Countermeasure Headquarters (local governments across the nation). These control and coordination institutions in central and local governments have built a nationwide system of close cooperation and policy coordination to manage an unprecedented Covid-19 crisis (NRC and STEPI 2020).

Fractured civil society in the US versus voluntary civil followership in South Korea

Since the outbreak of Covid-19, the power and authority of the government have increased in both the US and South Korea, but the behavior and role of civil society in the two countries show major discrepancies. While Korean civil society has shown strong support for governmental efforts to test, trace, and treat the disease, civil society in the US has often rejected testing and tracing without a warrant and not allowed the government to intrude on privacy through the collection of personal data. Extreme libertarianism and advocacy for privacy have obstructed the state from effectively testing, tracing, and treating Covid-19.

Fractured civil society in the US

American civil society has become more fractured, contentious, plural, and diverse than the civil society in the 1830s when Tocqueville observed that American civil society was characterized by voluntary, mutual, and self-help civil societies. As US society has become more unequal and polarized due to neoliberal globalization, voluntary civil society with an emphasis on civic virtue based on a strong prosperous middle class has been disappearing. When Covid-19 spread throughout America, mutual aid associations did not come out to volunteer because they were too fragile economically to help Americans in need and too busy earning living expenses to make time for mutual help. As the neoliberal government, without a nationwide program for containing Covid-19, let individuals, family, schools and local governments take responsibility for preventing the spread of coronavirus, local governments have engaged in bidding wars to buy masks, testing kits, medical gowns, and ventilators. When the federal government devolved the power and authority of controlling the pandemic to states and local governments, American civil associations did not step forward to voluntarily help the overloaded states and local governments because they did not have enough time and money.

Voluntary civil followership in South Korea

In contrast, Koreans have a strong community consciousness, allowing the state to enforce self and social isolation. Some Koreans voluntarily submitted to social isolation and distancing, even closing stores before the government advised them to do so. A Korean resident told reporters that 'social distancing has been the main weapon of mass protection … It's less about protecting ourselves, and more (that) we don't want to spread this throughout the community' (Jo 2020). Most Koreans have voluntarily participated in efforts to prevent the spread of Covid-19. Many volunteer doctors, nurses, and medical workers rushed to Daegu when coronavirus exploded in the city. Later, volunteering has gradually expanded to companies, lessors, and the general public. During the period of intensive social distancing, more than 90 percent of citizens faithfully observed preventive guidelines, such as the use of masks and social distancing. The voluntary cooperation of Korean citizens allowed the government to avoid draconian lockdowns, roadblocks, and restrictions on movement and assembly and to maintain a delicate balance between public safety and civil liberties (Jo 2020). When off-line civil participations, surveillance, and street demonstrations became almost impossible due to Covid-19, Korean civil society organized itself online to cooperate with the government's measures for pandemic prevention and social distancing, and contributed to guarding democracy in Korea by cooperating with the National Election Commission (NEC) to hold the general election on April 15, 2020 safely and fairly amidst Covid-19 turbulence.

Moreover, Korean citizens proactively shared innovative ideas for combatting Covid-19, such as drive-through and walk-through screening stations, and the local and central government accepted these ideas and distributed guidelines on the screening stations. Drive-through screening stations are a good example of public-private partnership (NRC and STEPI 2020).

Unprotected precariat labor in the US versus precariat workers with social welfare in South Korea

The neoliberal economy in both the US and South Korea has produced a massive class of precarious and low-income workers called the 'precariat'. The ongoing fourth industrial revolution and the outbreak of Covid-19 have accelerated the transition to the post-capitalist society based on a shared economy, platform economy, and online-based non-contact economy. This economic transformation has shifted the mainstream of labor from regularly paid industrial workers to part-time, unprotected, temporary gig workers. The working conditions of gig workers such as freelancers, day workers, and informal workers are precarious and unprotected by health and unemployment insurance. Thus, gig workers, care workers, the poor elderly, immigrants, and homeless people in neoliberal America are the most vulnerable to Covid-19 pandemic (Komlik 2020).

Unprotected precariat workers in neoliberal America

US gig workers have become 'precaritized'. Precarious and low-income temporary workers are especially vulnerable to Covid-19 because of their low income, low savings, inadequate housing, poor sanitation, and bad nutrition. Gig workers in the US are more fragile than those in South Korea because American gig workers are not protected by universal healthcare nor by other social safety nets. The disproportionally high spread of coronavirus among socially unprotected workers in neoliberal America shows that the response to Covid-19 has been unequal among classes, and thus has worsened class inequality. It has been very difficult to organize precariat workers in the US collectively and to establish protections for collective actions from firms and the state. Platform-based companies and the state in neoliberal America have refused to provide precariat workers with basic social protections, such as employee insurance, health insurance, and industrial safety insurance; instead, they have ruthlessly exploited these workers to maximize profits.

Precariat workers with social welfare in the CME of Korea

Even though the gig economy and untact (non-contact) economy have grown explosively in South Korea, the inequality between regular workers and gig workers is much less severe than that in the US. The lower inequality in South Korea can be explained by the ethnic homogeneity of South Korean society, which is one of the most homogeneous societies in the world. The high degree of ethnic homogeneity may explain why Korean society discriminates against precariat workers less than is the case in ethnically heterogeneous American society. It is surprising that discrimination toward the recently increasing immigrant workforce has been remained low in South Korea. The Korean government has provided precariat workers with comprehensive welfare such as universal healthcare, a social safety net, and basic income. Therefore, gig workers with welfare protections in South Korea are less vulnerable to Covid-19 than those in the US. The Korean CME has proven to be superior to the American LME in protecting less privileged workers from the vagaries of the market and the Covid-19 pandemic.

Leadership matters: virtue and vice in US and Korean leaders' response to Covid-19

Marx wrote in 1852 that 'Men make their own history, but … they do not make it under circumstances chosen by themselves, but under the circumstances directly encountered, given and transmitted from the past' (Marx 1852). Marx taught us that both actors' choice and institutional governance are important in explaining history. So far, I have based this exposition on the premise that 'institutions matter'. Nonetheless, 'leadership, too, matters' in explaining the contrasting responses of the two countries to Covid-19. The leadership differences between the leaders of these two countries have also contributed to the failure and success of the two countries' responses to Covid-19.

Trump's failed leadership in responding to Covid-19

Trump's failed leadership contributed to the disastrous response to Covid-19. First, Trump does not show 'listening leadership', as shown by the fact that he hates to receive bad news and spreads fake news, leading to communication failures that obstruct the effective response to Covid-19 (Lopez 2020). Second, Trump has preferred personal over institutional leadership (Neumann 1941). He downplayed the role of institutions in preventing the spread of coronavirus by weakening the CDC and hamstringing public health agencies, and, instead, acted on his personal and political judgment in responding to Covid-19. Third, Trump's nationalist, isolationist, and 'America First' leadership prevented the US from cooperating internationally to contain the Covid-19 pandemic (Fried 2020; Myre 2020; Shea 2020). The failed US response to Covid-19 has been caused partly by Trump's leadership failure.

Moon Jae In's democratic and international leadership

Unlike President Trump, President Moon Jae In and political leaders in South Korea did an excellent job in mobilizing voluntary civil cooperation for mass testing and social distancing. Compared to Trump's leadership, President Moon Jae In's leadership is democratic, international, and empathetic. First, President Moon has shown democratic leadership by transferring power and authority to the KCDC, an institution of experts focusing on epidemic prevention, by communicating tirelessly with experts, representatives of various industries, and members of the public about pandemic prevention and control, and by encouraging cooperation between central and local government, as well as between the state and civil society. Second, President Moon displayed international leadership in pandemic prevention and control by building a global and regional pandemic prevention system based on the 'K-Pandemic' prevention system.

References

Alsbrook, Jamille Fields (2020). 'The Coronavirus Crisis Confirms that the US Health Care System Fails Women,' A Center for American Progress report. www. americanprogress. org/issues/women/ reports/2020/04/23/483828/coronavirus.

Avineri, Shiomo (2020). 'Coronavirus Has Killed Neoliberalism. Even Trump Knows That,' HAARETZ.com. www.haaretz.com/misc/article-print-page/.premium-coronavirus-has-killed-neoliberalism.

Conlan, Timothy (1998). *From New Federalism to Devolution*. Washington, DC: Brookings Institution.

Fried, Daniel (2020). 'The Ugly, Bad, and Good of America's Coronavirus Response,' *New Atlanticist*, March 17.

Hall, Peter A. and David Soskice (2001). 'An Introduction to Varieties of Capitalism,' in Hall and Soskice, eds., *Varieties of Capitalism: The Institutional Foundation of Comparative Advantage*. Oxford: Oxford University Press.

Japan Times (2020). 'Experts Worry US is Sidelined in Coronavirus Response,' May 8.

Jo, Eun A (2020). 'A Democratic Response to Coronavirus: Lessons from South Korea,' *The Diplomat*, March 30.

Kim, Hyun Jung (2020). 'South Korea Learned Its Successful Covid-19 Strategy from a Previous Coronavirus Outbreak: MERS,' *Bulletin of Atomic Scientists*, March 20.

Klinger, Bruce (2020). 'South Korea Provides Lessons, Good or Bad, on Coronavirus Response,' Commentary Asia, *Heritage Foundation*, March 28.

Komlik, Oleg (2020). 'Neoliberalism, Varieties of Capitalism, and Coronavirus,' *Economic Sociology and Political Economy*, March 10. https://economicsociology.org /2020/03/10/ bb-neoliberalism-corona-and-virus-pandemic.

Kreitner, Richard (2020). 'When Confronting the Coronavirus, Federalism Is Part of the Problem,' *The Nation*, April 1.

Lopez, Linette (2020). 'Trump Is Blowing the US Response to Corona Virus Because He Can't Handle Bad News,' *Business Insider*, April 2.

Lu, Wei (2016). 'US Health-care System Ranks as One of the Least-efficient,' *Bloomberg*, September 29.

Marx, Karl (1852). *The Eighteenth Brumaire of Louis Bonaparte*. New York: International Publishers, printing edition, 1973, p. 15.

Maizland, Lindasay and Claire Felter (2020). 'Comparing Six Healthcare Systems in a Pandemic,' A background paper, Council on Foreign Relations.

Myre, Greg (2020). 'Pandemic Fuels Debate: Trump's "America First" versus US global leadership,' www.witf.org/2020/04/30/ pandemic-fuels-debate-trumps-areica-first-versu-us-global-leadership.

Neumann, Sigmund (1941). 'Leadership: Institutional and Personal,' *Journal of Politics*, 3(2), 133–153.

NRC (National Research Council for Economics, Humanities, and Social Sciences) and STEPI (Science and Technology Policy Institute) (2020). *Korea Report No. 1: South Korea's Response to Covid-19: Factors Behind*. Seoul: NRC.

OECD. (2015). 'Health Glance 2015.' www.keepeek.com/Digital-Asset-Management/oecd/social-issues-migration-health/health-at-a-glance-2015_health_glance 2015-en#page26.

Przewoski, Adam (2004). 'Institutions Matter?' *Government and Opposition*, 39(4), 192.

Reich, Robert (2020). 'America Has No Real Public Health System: Coronavirus Has a Clear Run,' *The Guardian*, March 15.

Saad-Filho, Alfredo (2020). 'Coronavirus, Crisis and the End of Neoliberalism,' *Socialist Project-The Bullet*, April 18. http://mtonline.org/2020/04/18/coronavirus-crisis-and-of-neoliberalism/.

Shea, Jamie (2020). 'Missing in Action: US Leadership is the Biggest Casualty in the Coronavirus,' *Friends of Europe*, April 22. www.friendsofeurope.org/insights/missing-in-actioon-us-leadership-is-the-biggest-casualty-in-the-coronavirus.

Song, Young Joo (2009). 'The South Korean Health Care System', *International Medical Community*, JMAJ (Japan Medical Association Journal), 52(3), 206–209.

Teskey, Graham (2020). 'The Worry of Governance: Coronavirus and Emergency Politics,' *Governance and Development Soapbox*, April 3.

Thelen, Kathalen (1999). 'Historical Institutionalism in Comparative Politics,' *Annual Review of Political Science*, 2, 387–401.

Unnikrishnan, Ramlai (2020). 'Politics of Pandemic: The Failed Neoliberal Response to Coronavirus.' countercurrents.org. www.hamptonthink.org/read/politics-of the pandemic-the failed neoliberal response to coronavirus.

15

THE UNITED STATES AND COVID-19

Hairpin turns

Jan Nederveen Pieterse

With 4 percent of the world population the US has 25 percent of cases and 22 percent of the world's Covid-19 deaths. Worldometer data for the US are 14,983,425 cases, 287,825 deaths and climbing (12.5.2020). November and December see the US' highest number of additional daily cases across the country, also in the rural states. American deaths per million of population (870) place the US in the neighborhood of the UK (897), Mexico (845), Spain (989), Brazil (828), and Peru (1,091).

In December 2020 the US is still at square one: no agreement on basics, no plan, no organization. No hammer, no dance. Cases and deaths are rising fast. Eight months after Covid-19 was acknowledged, the US still doesn't come near the threshold of planning, testing, and tracing that most countries passed eight or nine months ago. The federal government is in disarray and state and local governments are improvising amid contradictory pressures.

An iconic power center, the White House doesn't practice social distancing, holds indoor gatherings without use of masks, and hosts super spreader events. White House staff, secret service personnel, chief of staff Mark Meadows, and members of the Trump family have tested positive. The public conversation is mired in mixed messages.

A large advanced economy, a model society by some accounts, in a state of confusion and impasse. What explains this tragic failure? Many blame Donald Trump. Trump is responsible for inept policies and disinformation on a mass scale. But Trump is not to blame for American healthcare being geared to profitable private care, not public health. Trump is not to blame for the limitations of federal government, a weakness by design that goes back decades. This is a society that JK Galbraith described decades ago as a society of 'private opulence and public squalor' (1958). American society and economy tilting towards private, not public services has deep roots. They match conservative moorings that are entrenched in American governance. Hence, this chapter considers three themes: governance, American capitalism, and the GOP as hairpin turns in the United States' forward motion.

Governance

Late 18th-century institutions in a combination known as the constitution form the bedrock of American governance. The institutions served to secure the representation of states in the governance of the American Union. From the outset, the constitution was a compromise between the northern states and the Southern plantation slaveholding states, with the new capital Washington in-between. To secure the union, the Southern states were given in-built guarantees: each state in the union is represented by two senators; the president is chosen by an Electoral College of state delegates; the president and senate appoint federal judges. According to the Second Amendment, the right to bear arms, the states can call on armed militias to guard against a tyrannical government. *Changing the constitution* requires the approval of two-thirds of both the representatives and the senate as well as three-quarters of the states. This 1788 compromise and some later adjustments embed conservatism in the American Union. The objective was to keep states together, not people.

At the time, the union consisted of four million people who were mostly farmers. Now it means that North Dakota and South Dakota with a combined population of 1.5 million are represented in congress by four senators while California with 39.5 million people is represented by two senators. Wyoming with 600,000 people is also represented by two senators. A country where 82 percent of people live in cities is governed by a senate whose majority represent thinly populated states with a mostly rural population. While cities account for well over 90 percent of US economic growth they function under the veto power of rural majority states, most of whose elected officials are conservative in outlook.

The American senate is not like the first chamber of European parliaments or the House of Lords in Westminster, whose role is to provide counsel and amendments to legislation. In contrast, the American senate has evolved as the powerhouse of politics. The senate decides on passing legislation, cabinet appointments, appointments to head government departments and to the Supreme Court. According to the filibuster rule, it takes 60 senators, out of 100, to pass votes, another legacy of bygone times. The senate can block legislation, appointments, international treaties, or withhold ratification of agreements adopted by the White House or the Representatives. Even basic international agreements such as nuclear non-proliferation, covenants to counter violence against women or environmental regulation can remain without senate ratification; hence, the senate is the bottleneck of the United States and the bottleneck of the world (Nederveen Pieterse 2008). In the words of law professor Sanford Levinson, 'The US Senate is an affirmative action program for white, rural, Christian conservatives, who have an increasingly powerful veto over America' (in Luce 2020).

In this setting, even though national elections are major media spectacles every two years, electoral shifts have limited impact. Even if the opposition party gains a senate majority, it takes 60 senators to pass a bill. Even if a bill is passed it can be overruled in another round. This explains why decades of social struggle have had limited impact.

The Electoral College means that voters choosing a presidential candidate are actually casting a vote for an elector. All states, except two, use the 'winner-take-all' method in which all electoral votes are awarded to the winner of the popular vote in that state, no matter the margin of victory. The Electoral College means that millions of votes are counted but don't count. It means that the presidential election is decided by a handful of states; 'swing states' decide (Wegman 2020).

> Over the past 20 years, Republicans have won the popular vote just once yet have had the presidency for 12 of those years. Because of the skewed apportionment of Electoral College vote numbers in favour of the thinly populated and rural states, a vote in California is worth less than a third of one cast in Wyoming.
>
> (Schama 2020)

Fundamental constraints also apply to the American legal system: 'the American judiciary is … the most potent force for conservatism in America, especially since the end of the civil rights era as it became dominated by big money ideological think tanks' (Lanza 2020). The Supreme Court is not part of the constitution but derives from early 19th-century dispute settlements (Rasmus 2020). The Supreme Court is another bulwark of conservatism. The ideology of originalism—stay with the original texts—that is held by the conservative Federalist Society and conservative judges, parallels the 'fundamentalism' of 1920s American Protestants (stay with the original Bible text) and is about as relevant; in effect, it serves as a pretext for archconservative interpretations of law (Rennix and Nimni 2018).

According to the Second Amendment, states can call on armed militias as recourse against tyrannical government. Part of the definition of the state is the monopoly on the legitimate means of violence; armed militias are legitimate, so in this sense the United States is not a state. Guns in wide circulation, increasingly military grade firearms, have long contributed to the escalation of violence and the militarization of policing. The US leads the world in gun deaths. The response to any crisis is to buy more guns and ammunition. In 2020 in response to the pandemic and Black Lives Matter protests, Americans have bought 17 million guns (Beckett 2020).

Institutional reforms are possible in times of crisis. The Civil War produced the Declaration of Emancipation; the Great Depression led to the New Deal; segregation in the South produced civil rights legislation; Vietnam War protests led to the end of the draft. Yet in-built conservative leverage is such that over time conservatives can claw back many progressive gains.

Time and again the US has seen powerful social movements, movements that have inspired people worldwide; worker movements, the civil rights movement, women's movements, peace movements, LGBT, and environmental movements.

Decades hence, where are the achievements? The unionization rate of American workers in the private sector is 7.2 percent. Black American living standards remain a fraction of that of whites.Voter restrictions and gerrymandering in Republican-led states are severe. Police kill blacks with impunity nearly on a weekly basis. Women in the workplace face sexual harassment and nondisclosure contracts, and abortion rights may be rolled back. The Pentagon and the national security apparatus are larger than ever with a combined annual budget in the order of a trillion dollars.

American police are equipped like an occupying army. Their training of 12 to 16 weeks mostly deals with how to use their equipment. In Germany and Scandinavia it takes two years of education to become a policeman; in Japan it takes four years. Because of cuts in local government budgets, the police are given more and more tasks, such as dealing with domestic disputes, mental health, poverty and homelessness, but are not trained or equipped to deal with them.

Rural support is the foundation of authoritarian rule worldwide. In Europe it was the basis of support of aristocracy and church, fascism, and Nazism. Rural votes sustain conservative parties the world over. In Malaysia, the UMNO party has ruled since independence for 61 years (with an interruption in 2018) largely on the basis of the kampong vote.

Also the world's largest economy and mightiest military power is governed by conservative rural power. Their power is ensconced in the senate, the Electoral College, the courts, the Supreme Court, and states' rights, all of which safeguard conservative power. In contrast to the national rhetoric of democracy, together these institutions ensure a society that is structurally conservative. The talk is of democracy but other leading institutions—corporations and the armed forces—are not democratic institutions either. As world hegemon, the US aims to promote democracy worldwide and wages wars to 'bring democracy to the Middle East', while in international rankings of democracies the US ranks only 25th. In 2017 the US was downgraded from a 'full democracy' to a 'flawed democracy' in the annual Democracy Index report of the Economist Intelligence Unit (2017, 2018). Ranking criteria include an underdeveloped political culture, low levels of participation in politics, and issues in the functioning of governance, which doesn't even take into account the institutional fundamentals discussed above.

Dixie capitalism, the revenge of the Confederacy

The Confederacy lost the Civil War. 'The Confederate States of America was defeated, definitively defeated, politically and militarily' (McCurry 2013). Yet the compromises with the Southern states made at the outset have given them lasting political heft (cf. McCurry 2012, Lepore 2019). The South lost with the Emancipation Declaration and regained ground with Jim Crow, lost with civil rights legislation and regained ground in the Reagan era.

The South had been in competition with the industrial North through the 19th century; the Civil War was a contest between the plantation economy of manual labor (and slavery) and the industrial economy of mechanical labor, and the

South lost (Davis 1984). However, upon the profit squeeze of the late 1970s, the industrial North found recourse in the plantation capitalism policy package of the South—low taxes, low wages, low services, no unions. When the Reagan era recast Dixie capitalism as a winning formula of growth, the South finally won the economic contest with the industrial North. Rollback government, deregulation and tax cuts became keywords ever since. Plantation capitalism, that is, labor without rights or with minimal rights (no unions), refurbished as the free market is the revenge of the Confederacy (discussed in detail in Nederveen Pieterse 2004). The policies deployed by the South to undo Reconstruction were repackaged under fresh headings (supply-side economics, monetarism, the Chicago school, the Laffer curve). When the poorest states of the US became the new standard, the US took a path of steadily growing inequality. The Reagan era dialed back many achievements of the New Deal. It reversed progressive taxation and the financial sector that had been reined in after the crash of 1929 was deregulated and made a comeback. New Deal social market capitalism gave way to high-exploitation capitalism, Walmart capitalism, capitalism without a moral compass. Stagnant wages, rising cost of living, rising productivity, rising inequality combined with corporate deregulation, efficiency, and cost benefit analysis as societal beacons. Ronald Reagan's 1980 and 1984 election victories established the new pact. Sunbelt Republicans (Goldwater, Nixon, Reagan) replaced East coast Republicans (Rockefeller and GHW Bush). Republicans embracing the Southern strategy and becoming the Confederate party (Frank 2004, Blight 2020) solved many dilemmas.

You want more democracy? The free market will keep you busy. 'Get government off our backs'? Welcome corporations on your backs. 'Starve the beast' (the beast of federal government social spending)? There go the GI bill, labor unions, social protection, the American dream, the Great Society. Here come industries without unions, deindustrialization without a safety net, and down the road are crystal meth in rural towns, the opioid crisis and 'deaths of despair' (Case and Deaton 2019). New Democrats of the Clinton brand add gender rights and identity politics to the mix while rolling back social rights, from the welfare to the workfare state, in the shiny new combination of 'progressive neoliberalism' (Fraser 2017).

The American Covid-19 failure, according to Rana Foroohar, is 'Fifty years of policy come home to roost': 'Decades of bad choices have relentlessly favoured the interests of the private sector in the US' (2020). American healthcare is geared to profitable private care, not public health. Each hospital is a profit center. The failures are basic: 'Broken data system stymies hospitals' (Evans and Berzon 2020). Consider a report on nursing homes in the US:

> Across the country, nursing homes are looking to get rid of unprofitable patients—primarily those who are poor and require extra care—and pouncing on minor outbursts to justify evicting them to emergency rooms or psychiatric hospitals. After the hospitals discharge the patients, often within hours, the nursing homes refuse them re-entry, according to court filings.
>
> (Silver-Greenberg and Abrams 2020)

Seventy percent of US nursing homes are for profit. Nursing homes have been a major site of Covid-19 deaths, also among nurses and staff (Editorial 2020). Hospitals and medicines for profit, both at exorbitant rates, are part of the picture. Hospitals can put indigent patients on the street. In the name of efficiency, hospitals don't have surge capacity and are unable to cope with a public health crisis. Extrapolate the profit principle to every sector of society, media and social media, prisons, detention centers for undocumented migrants, higher education, and so forth. Student loan debt affects 30 million people and stands at $1.6 trillion, at interest rates of 7 percent, higher than anywhere in the world (in the UK they are capped at 2.75 percent).

Neoliberalism is plantation capitalism. It means, in short, capitalism without benefits, capitalism stripped of social cost, permissive capitalism. It means promote corporations, neglect and denigrate government agencies and institution, and ignore or sideline social forces, such as labor unions, consumer rights, and communities. Implementing this over four decades yields underfunded, dysfunctional government agencies that lag behind the corporate sector in organization, efficiency, and prestige. Under the neoliberal banner, government itself becomes anti-government government. Neoliberalism comes with several distortions. The 'free market' gradually turns into corporate monopolies. Deregulation with the adroit aid of lobbies and corporate lawyers becomes regulation that benefits the strongest corporate players. Shrink government by cutting taxes means cutting social government while increasing security and law and order spending. Cost/benefit analysis and the profit principle are applied across society while underfunding public services in the name of efficiency. Prisons for profit, elderly care and nursing homes for profit, healthcare for profit become organizing motifs. Corporate media must be profitable. Funding for public broadcasting is marginal ($3 per person per year is absurdly low by international standards). Hence, the public sphere is a corporate sphere and is short of reflection.

The Covid-19 failure is part of the harvest of decades—defund social services, fund security spending. Rollback government is justified as a rejection of 'big government'. However, actual government size and spending don't shrink but just change composition, from service and social government to security and law and order government.

The casualty isn't just public health. Many government agencies have suffered major cuts and loss of purpose, such as the Food and Drug Administration (which enabled the opioid crisis), the Federal Aviation Authority (Boeing crisis), bank regulation (Wells Fargo scams), environmental regulation, the Immigration Service, and the Internal Revenue Service (functioning at half capacity). The new normal has come with a dumbing down of the public sphere. Media for profit (ratings) means adult public conversation is scarce and collective learning, also learning from other societies, has long been stagnant. The right to be stupid is institutionalized. Denial of Covid-19 and resistance to containment measures are more widespread in the US than in any advanced country. Thus, the American Covid-19 tragedy is part of a wider societal drama.

Peeling Trump and the GOP

The top layer of Donald Trump, on display for all to see, is a media blitz of nonstop lies, distortions, and self-promotion, pettiness on a grandiose scale. Features that characterize Trump's conduct throughout, notes a commentator, are authoritarianism, chaos, and incompetence (Douthat 2020). Plant this in the White House and these attributes spillover across all domains. In campaigning, these features make up a contrarian popular style, in governance, they produce erratic outcomes, and applied to a public health crisis, they spell disaster. Poo-pooing Covid-19, disavowing responsibility, promoting alt-science and politicizing mask wearing add up to a devastating record that is extensively documented. The leader of the world's most advanced and powerful country advised people to try disinfectants as a cure. It is national news when the president agrees with scientists of his government institutions. The result is headlines that are unusual for most heads of state:

> Passing off virus burden, White House fueled crisis
>
> (New York Times, *July 19 2020)*

> For health agencies, the rock is the pandemic, the hard place is Trump
>
> (New York Times, *September 13, 2020)*

> Study finds 'single largest driver' of coronavirus misinformation: Trump
>
> (New York Times, *September 30, 2020)*

> To be near Trump is toxic
>
> (Financial Times, *October 10–11, 2020)*

Layer two is the con, 'the art of the deal'. Economic success is a mirage: job growth built on the Obama administration legacy and the stock market high was a result of interest rates that were kept low: 'The real driver, of course, of many of the S&P 500's gains under Trump is the Federal Reserve' (Mackenzie 2020). Make America Great Again? There was no infrastructure investment and no industrial reinvestment to speak of either (high-tech investments bear no relation to Trump policies). Trade war with China didn't lower US trade deficits and came at the expense of corporations and farmers. In foreign policy, America First is America Alone, besides tea time with dictators.

Attitude and bluster consume more public oxygen. White grievance, white supremacy and law and order are GOP refrains, but Trump turned dog whistle into bullhorn. Repurpose or disable government agencies by appointing cronies and opponents of agencies to head agencies (environment, energy, education, justice, national security, postal service) syncs with the GOP tradition of anti-government government.

The top layer, the Trump reality TV show, is what garnered his 2016 election campaign billions of dollars of free air time—bombastic lowbrow entertainment in the tradition of the American con man is good for ratings. Destroying democracy can be good for ratings too. Network media and social media thrive on polarization theater. The presidency as reality TV, nonstop performance of bad taste, an entourage of con men and grifters, and a cascade of political gossip keep media busy, a morally exhausting assault on standards and values. Conspiracy clouds pass overhead (such as the Trump administration as 'a transnational crime syndicate masquerading as a government', Kendzior 2020).

Yet, backstage is where the action is. Fox Business News and the Wall Street Journal are matter of fact. Maria Bartiromo and Freeman (2020) argue, just skip the lowbrow entertainment, Trump's policies are tax cuts and deregulation. Trump is longer on politics than policy, but tax cuts and deregulation are simply hardcore GOP, givebacks to donors, the reason why billionaires and corporations line up behind the GOP and Trump. Icing on the cake is white supremacy and appointing conservative judges to appellate courts and the Supreme Court. Trump's anti-immigration policies give demographic solace to white privilege. Arguably the task isn't peeling Trump but peeling GOP.

The GOP gained influence in the South in the wake of 1960s civil rights legislation when Southern democrats turned republican. The GOP consolidated its position by undermining federal government, the New Deal coalition and the 'Great Society'. Because aligning corporate wish lists, Wall Street and law and order may not be sufficient to sway small towns and rural counties, states' rights provide rural attraction. Teaming up with evangelicals (social conservatism and Israel), the NRA gun lobby, patriotism and populist shine close the deal. Hence, Reagan ('It's morning again in America'), neoconservatives ('Simplify, then exaggerate'), the Tea Party (freedom, courtesy of Koch brothers), Fox News (courtesy of Rupert Murdoch) and Trump (MAGA). Trump is an installment in a series: American conservatism, white supremacy, and Dixie economics.

Peel a layer further down and decades of cold war (against big government), decades of a bipolar world order consolidate binary thinking as a national bipartisan matrix—communism v capitalism, authoritarianism v democracy. Hence, the American brand of free market and democracy.

The Reagan period is often interpreted in political economy terms as corporate deregulation and tax cuts, along with social demobilization, like Thatcher in the UK. However, a more momentous accomplishment of the Reagan era is a *political realignment*. Rollback government also meant *rollback federal government* in favor of states' rights. Keep government small, keep federal government out, the vintage credo of the South (the reason why Southern states staged the rebellion that led to the Civil War) now extends to *all rural states*. This set in motion a Republican compact of the South and other rural states; the Southern strategy morphs into a *rural strategy* and brings into being a GOP block of 'red states' (20 in 2016, 21 in 2020), each with two senators. This is the Republicans' actual master move; mastering the constitution, they gain control of the cockpit of power, the senate.

In a structurally heterogeneous society a crucial variable is *social cohesion*. Emancipation, Reconstruction, the New Deal, progressive taxation, civil rights laws and the Great Society enhanced social cohesion. Jim Crow, the Reagan tax cuts, the New Federalism of states' rights, media deregulation and polarization undermined social cohesion. Just when the impact of the 2008 crisis sank in, smartphones came on the scene in 2011 and social media escalated polarization. A new motto, 'Let them eat tweets' (Hacker and Pierson 2020), set the stage for Trump, the latest populist gloss of GOP. Thus Covid-19 descends on a divided society.

Taxation, too, is a major tool of social cohesion. Next after tax cuts is tax avoidance (which is legal and a major industry of corporate law). A step further is the view that 'taxes are for suckers', a familiar notion in some circles, and a darker shade further are tax evasion (which is illegal), Swiss banks, and the Panama papers. Contrast this with another perspective. According to Kishore Mahbubani in Singapore, 'to become rich is great but to pay taxes is glorious' (2011). In his view, taxes uphold a social contract.

These polar opposite views sum up the situation in which, in short, Asia (much of Asia) succeeds in dealing with a public health crisis and the US fails. The American failure is the harvest of small government and tax cuts as leading political cults. A virus exposes tax cuts as deadly for an entire society and an economic disaster too. Even for Covid-19 tax cuts are a remedy. A headline sums up the remedy of Stephen Moore, a member of Trump's economic recovery task force: 'The best stimulus: 0% income tax'. 'Instead of collecting and spending $2 trillion, why not cut out the middleman?' (Moore 2020). In other words, who needs government?

The short story of the United States is: an urban population under a rural government. This is a drama in three acts, each of which adds hairpin turns to the way forward. First, when the constitution took shape the concern was to keep the union of states together; over time, the emphasis has shifted from political cohesion to social cohesion, from the representation of states to the representation of people. Winner-take-all systems are to the advantage of big parties and proportional representation enables small parties and the representation of minorities, yet also creates a risk of secession. A similar equation applies to the constitution of India, which also worried about Partition and also enables big party hegemony (Congress, then the BJP), which has become counterproductive over time.

Second, the Reagan administration installed Dixie capitalism as the new normal and a political alignment of the South and rural states. Corporations, banks, the South, and rural states share an interest in limiting federal government power. The constitution's emphasis on power of the states (senate, Electoral College) makes this possible. Developments from the 1960s to the 1980s generated a blend of political authoritarianism (the senate) and market authoritarianism (neoliberalism). Over time, this set the stage for figures such as Trump. The problem of course isn't Trump but the institutional ensemble that enables such figures.

Societies that rely on corporations for decades suddenly find that in the Covid-19 crisis corporations are missing in action. Societies that opt for small government for decades suddenly find that it takes big and capable government and trust in government to combat a virus. Societies that cultivate division for centuries suddenly find out that combating a virus requires social cohesion.

Many Americans take the US to be the world's most advanced nation ('the greatest') and many people abroad take it to be a place where they would like their children to study, or they would like to migrate to, that is, *until* the Covid-19 pandemic. The refrain is familiar: 'A virus has brought the world's most powerful country to its knees' (Yong 2020). 'Anglo-American brand has been humbled by a microbe' (Luce 2020b). American exceptionalism is back, but the wrong kind. The world has begun to pity Americans.

As the horizon lights up with vaccines and the new Biden administration it is dimmed by the usual problems. Small government doesn't help in organizing the distribution and delivery of vaccines, lack of coordination between federal, state, and local government and confusion prevail; senate Republicans are set to sabotage this democratic administration just as previous ones.

References

Bartiromo, M. and J. Freeman 2020 Trump has already won, whatever the election results, *Wall Street Journal*, October 31–November 1.

Beckett, L. 2020 US gun control, *The Guardian*, October 30.

Blight, D. W. 2020 Republicans: the new Confederacy, *New York Review of Books*, November 5.

Case, A. and Angus Deaton 2019 *Deaths of despair and the future of capitalism*. Princeton: Princeton University Press.

Crow, D. 2020 America's 'bad soup': Covid-19 and inequality, *Financial Times*, 6/10.

Davis, D. B. 1984 *Slavery and human progress*. New York, Oxford University Press.

Douthat, R. 2020 It's Trump's revolution, New York Times, June 14.

Economist Intelligence Unit 2017, 2018 Democracy Index Report, London.

Editorial 2020 The shameful toll of nursing homes, *New York Times*, September 6.

Evans, M. and A. Berzon 2020 Broken data system stymies hospitals, *Wall Street Journal*, October 1.

Foroohar, R. 2020 Fifty years of policy come home to roost, *Financial Times*, March 30.

Frank, T. 2004 *What's the matter with Kansas?* New York: Henry Holt.

Fraser, N. 2017 From progressive neoliberalism to Trump—and beyond, *American Affairs* I, 4: 46–64.

Galbraith, J. K. 1958 *The affluent society*. Boston: Houghton Mifflin.

Hacker, J. S. and P. Pierson 2020 *Let them eat tweets: How the right rules in an age of extreme inequality*. New York: Liveright.

Kendzior, S. 2020 *Hiding in plain sight: The invention of Donald Trump and the erosion of America*. New York: Flatiron Books.

Lanza, J. 2020 The Courts: America's most conservative institution, *Washington University Political Review*, August 3.

Lepore, J. 2019 *These Truths: A history of the United States*. New York: Norton.

Luce, E. 2020 Will America tear itself apart? *Financial Times*, October 17–18.

——— 2020b Anglo-American brand has been humbled by a microbe, *Financial Times*, July 10.

Mackenzie, M. 2020 Ignore the noise when placing bets after US election, *Financial Times*, October 17–18.

Mahbubani, K. 2011 To become rich is great but to pay taxes is glorious, *Financial Times*, October 20.

McCurry, S. 2012 *Confederate reckoning: Power and politics in the Civil War South.* Cambridge, MA: Harvard University Press.
——— 2013 Who won the Civil War? *New York Times*, July 2.
Moore, S. 2020 The best stimulus: 0% Income Tax, *Wall Street Journal*, October 7.
Nederveen Pieterse, J. 2004 *Globalization or empire?* New York: Routledge.
——— 2008 *Is there hope for Uncle Sam? Beyond the American bubble.* London: Zed Books.
Rasmus, J. 2020 Why the record vote turnout may not matter, *ZNet*, October 29.
Rennix, B. and Oren Nimni 2018 Judging the judges, *Current Affairs,* March/April.
Schama, S. 2020 The two Americas, *Financial Times*, October 31–November 1.
Silver-Greenberg, J. and R. Abrams 2020 Nursing homes seize pretexts to evict the poor, *New York Times*, September 20.
Stolberg, S. G. and N. Weiland 2020 Study finds 'single largest driver' of coronavirus misinformation: Trump, *New York Times*, September 30.
Wegman, J. 2020 *Let the people pick the president: The case for abolishing the electoral college.* New York: St Martin's Press.
Yong, E. 2020 How the pandemic defeated America, *The Atlantic*, September.

16

BRAZIL, SOUTH AMERICA AND COVID-19

Adalberto Cardoso and Thiago Peres

Covid-19 landed in Brazil and Latin America in mid-February 2020, hosted in the bodies of people from the wealthier fractions of the middle classes. In a region where, on average, about 1 in 5 people lives below 50 percent of the median income,[1] only the wealthiest portions of the population can afford international airfare, accommodation, transportation and food in the Old Continent. As a consequence, on the eve of the pandemic it was common to read that the disease was 'democratic', 'class blind' or that it would cut diagonally across the social structure irrespective of social and economic status. Reality proved it otherwise. The first fatal victim of Covid-19 in Rio de Janeiro was a domestic service woman that worked for a middle-class couple infected in Italy. The couple tested positive for Covid-19 and did not take the necessary isolation measures. Aged 63 years and with comorbidities, the lower-class woman died within two days in a public hospital.[2] The middle-class couple had only mild symptoms and were treated in a private health facility, and are still here to tell the story.

In this chapter we will present and discuss a few national institutional responses to combat the pandemic, focusing primarily on Brazil, but with an eye on selected South American countries. Country strategies were multiple and diverse. Some, like Brazilian president Jair Bolsonaro, denied the seriousness of the disease and its social consequences, while others adopted WHO protocols from the start, with other countries falling in between. Disjunctives such as save lives vs save the economy, collective vs individualized responsibilities, national vs local (or province/municipalities) coordination and governance populated the public debates and government strategies. And all South American countries had to find ways to deal with two common and persistent elements of the region's socioeconomic structure: social inequality and, most importantly, informality. Mediating the impact of the pandemic, they skewed its most dramatic consequences to the poorer strata of the population.

The chapter is organized as follows: In the next section we present a rapid analysis of the institutional responses of eight South American countries, placing them in two groups. Four of them implemented policies and models of governance that can be named collective responsibility, while the other four relied on individual responsibility. The rates of death are much higher in the second group than in the first one. The next sections analyze Brazil in more depth. First, we argue that Brazil is a transitional economy, moving from a model of state-led, quasi-welfare state to a neoliberal market economy. We then move on to present the various intertwined crisis that, beginning in the mid-2013, affected the economy and the political system, undermining the basis of the historically unstable but actually resilient pacts around the 1988 Constitution, opening the doors to an insignificant figure like Jair Bolsonaro. The following two sections show how inequality and informality skewed the incidence of the Covid-19 to the poorer and more vulnerable population, and how inefficient governance jeopardized the country's ability to combat the pandemic. The last section presents some interesting initiatives from different levels of government, and also from civil society organizations. We conclude by arguing that the death rate of 758 per million inhabitants (as of mid-October 2020) could have been worse without these initiatives, but could probably have been much lower if the federal government had decided to save lives and to coordinate the actions of the other levels of the public administration.

Institutional strategies in pandemic combat: collective vs individual responsibility

About six months after WHO declared the new coronavirus pandemic, Latin America (and especially South America) became the most affected region in the world in terms of the number of deaths.[3] One particular feature of the continent stands out as the main cause of the exponential rise in the severity of the Latin American situation: persistent labor market informality. According to the ILO standards, to be considered informal, a person must not be, in law or in practice, subject to the national labor legislation, pay income's taxes, make social security contributions or have them made by the employer, have social protection or employment benefits such as paid sick leave, paid annual leave, and so on (ILO, 2018). That is, they have little or no government support. As a result, their income is noticeably lower in comparison to formal workers, and they, more often than not, have to 'sell lunch to buy dinner'.

In the case of the pandemic, the tragedy in societies in which informality is a constituent element of life opportunities' structure is that, for the most part, people earn their income from commercial transactions or from the provision of services through direct physical contact (either on the streets, in popular markets, in small stalls of food or products, in domestic work, at neighbors' doors, etc.). The necessary social distancing policies to prevent the community transmission of the virus fatally harms informal workers' means of obtaining income.

Bearing in mind this structural constraint, in South America the most successful countries in combating the pandemic were those that adopted some sort of collective responsibility. These countries implemented institutional strategies that prioritized prevention above all, to halt or reduce the speed of community transmission of the virus. Adhesion to social isolation was to a large extent obtained by persuasion through public authorities' frequent and transparent pronouncements and official publicity campaigns on the indispensability of personal protective equipment and maintaining personal hygiene, as well as by the coordination of policies between the different levels of the executive (federal, provincial and municipal) irrespective of party affiliation of the incumbents in power. The population was *convinced* by scientifically supported statements, to voluntarily engage on the safety measures put forward by the public authorities. Countries that chose individual responsibility focused on the treatment and remediation of the most severe cases of Covid-19. With 'milder' quarantines, they concentrated on expanding the number of hospital beds to prevent the collapse of the health system, or left their citizens at the mercy of the virus without establishing coordinated strategies. In addition, the coverage of income transfer programs was worryingly timid.

Evidence of the consequences of these choices is in Table 16.1, that shows data for eight South American countries. We can see that in the four countries that chose collective responsibility (Uruguay, Argentina, Colombia and Bolivia), the number of deaths per million were lower than in the other four (Ecuador, Brazil, Chile and Peru) that chose individual responsibility. Note that the death rates in the first group are also positively correlated with informality, and seem not to be affected by the scope and reach of income transfer programs. That is, informality reduced the effectiveness of the public policies, but even the highest informal economy in the first group, Bolivia, had nearly the same number of deaths per million as the least informal country in the second group, Chile.

Uruguay is clearly the most successful case. Being the least informal economy in South America (24 percent of the occupied labor force), reported only 14.6 deaths per million (the country has 3.5 million inhabitants). On the other pole, Peru, with 33 million inhabitants and near 70 percent of informality, faced the tragic rate of 1.018 per million.

When Covid-19 landed in Argentina, poverty afflicted 35.4 percent of its population (approximately 15 million people). Shortly after the first death recorded in the country (also the first in South America), borders were closed, and the population was strictly quarantined, which was successively extended until August, with selective flexibility. Colombia followed this path and, in the first week, suspended classes, closed borders and built large-scale field hospitals to shelter patients with least severe forms of the disease, so ICU facilities could remain available to those in need of intensive care or mechanical respiration. In coordination with provincial and federal authorities, some cities adopted strict lockdowns. In both countries flexibilization measures adopted in September have not resulted in an upsurge in rates of death.

TABLE 16.1 Collective vs individual responsibility in dealing with the pandemic in selected South American countries

Country	*Deaths/1M population**	*Responsibility*	*Informality (%)*	*Income Transfer Programs (ITP)***	*Households covered by ITP (%)*	*Gini (circa 2018)*
Uruguay	14.6	Collective	23.9	0.06	5.1	39.7
Argentina	559		48.1	8.8	66.2	41.4
Colombia	559		61.4	2.6	19.3	50.4
Bolivia	717		8.,2	1.6	55.2	42.2
Ecuador	698	Individual	72.4	0.95	1.9	45.4
Chile	710		29.2	1.8	31.8	46.4
Brazil	722		41.1	29.4	43.0	53.9
Peru	1,018		68.9	0.8	2.5	41.9

Source: Multiple sources. 2014-2020. Worldometer. ILO. Euromonitor. Government websites. World Bank. Coronatracker.com. Fraschina (2020). Gentilini (2020).

*Until October (2020).

** Number of households (millions). July (2020).

In Uruguay, in addition to quarantine, one of the first institutional strategies was the cancelation of in-presence classes and the announcement of distance learning plans using computers and online tools previously provided by the Ceibal Plan ('one laptop per child').[4] Schools should remain open only to provide meals for students.[5] Bolivia quickly decreed quarantine (the violation of which could lead to imprisonment for eight hours), limiting hours of public and private transportation, establishing specific opening hours for essential services with limited use of one person per family. Subsequently, it prohibited the suspension of services such as water, electricity and internet due to default, and reduced electricity tariffs.

As to income transfer programs, the 'Ingreso Familiar de Emergencia' (IFE) in Argentina allocated U$137 to 8.8 million households and the 'Asistencia al Trabajo y la Producción' (ATP) covered about 2.3 million formal workers by making some U$2.5 billion available so firms could pay wages. Together, the programs reached two out of three Argentine households. Colombia, through the 'Ingresso Solidario', transferred approximately US$42 to 2.6 million households, covering approximately 19 percent of the total. Uruguay, which has the lowest rate of poverty in the region, provided US$28 to no more than 5.1 percent of families through a cell phone application. Those who did not have a smartphone could directly request a basic consumption basket food. Bolivia created several programs, the main one being 'Bono Familiar', which directed US$72 to families with students. One of them, 'Bono Universal' was created specifically for informal and self-employed workers and reached around 55.2 percent of families. Together they benefited approximately 3.6 million people. The result of these strategies were lower rates of deaths per 1 million people.

Chile, Ecuador, Peru and Brazil chose to direct their efforts to combat the pandemic towards individual responsibility. Chile enacted a 'dynamic lockdown' that restricted circulation only in specific neighborhoods, instead of entire municipalities. This more flexible measure contrasted immensely with the armed forces on the streets that imposed a curfew between 10 pm and 5 am. Through the 'Bono Covid-19',[6] Chile allocated about US$64 to informal workers and families who were the beneficiaries of other social programs, covering only 31.8 percent (1.8 million) of families. Low adherence to individual isolation, for many needed to keep on working, combined with the insufficient provision of new beds for hospitalization resulted in the collapse of hospitals and an increase in deaths (Bacigalupe et al., 2020).

Peru established a different isolation policy but with remarkably similar results. In the early days of the virus in its territory, an inflexible quarantine policy was established, with armed forces' barriers between municipalities, police patrol, mandatory use of masks and so on. The sudden and rigid restrictions, however, had an opposite effect in comparison to the countries that chose collective responsibility by means of persuasion. Hundreds of thousands of people were unable to return to their homes and had no money to stay in the cities they were confined to.[7] This forced a considerable number of Peruvian workers to walk in large groups for days, gathering in hostels and on the streets and roads, exposing themselves to both the virus and the army's brutality. And while the country quickly announced a series of programs aimed at the poorer populations, rural and self-employed workers, the 'Bono "Yo me quedo en casa"' reached only 2.5 percent of the Peruvian families.[8]

Ecuador suspended school classes, closed borders, made constant official pronouncements, decreed a curfew, but was unable to establish an effective social isolation policy. In addition, the country has 4.4 million people in poverty or extreme poverty and the 'Bono de Protección Familiar' covered only 950,000 Ecuadorians. As a result, the hospital system collapsed in less than a month and, with it, the funerary system. Many bodies of people killed by Covid-19 in the city of Guayaquil were plundered on the streets and parks or stayed for days at home awaiting a public authority to collect them.[9]

Different countries (states, cities and neighborhoods) are at different stages in the Covid-19 community transmission flow. The responsibility pattern adopted acts directly on this flow, intensifying or delaying it. Collective responsibility requires continuous governmental effort and society's adherence. However, with the exception of Uruguay, all countries analyzed here gave in to pressure (economic sectors, the political class, etc.) and began to relax social distancing. In Argentina, for example, the (necessary) lockdown was dubbed 'quaranternal' (wordplay with the words quarantine and eternal). The outcome could not be different: there was an explosion in the number of deaths. In July, while countries that adopted individual responsibility counted, on average, 460 deaths per million, Argentina, Colombia and Bolivia totaled 80, 203 and 262 deaths per million. In October 31, the same countries registered respectively 672, 606, 742. This shows that, while it prevailed, collective responsibility was key to avoid or delay the community transmission. On the other hand, in individual responsibility, negligence and/or low government effort cost hundreds or thousands of lives lost daily (and unnecessarily). And often, their actions seem to play in favor of the virus. As is the case in Brazil.

Brazil: a transitional market economy

Brazil must be treated as a transitional market economy. To a large extent, the governments led by the Workers Party (PT) can be read as the instantiation of the constitutional project inscribed in the 1988 Constitution, as they attempted to consolidate the welfare state implicit in that project, which an important interpreter called 'weak reformism' (Singer, 2012). Though weak, it was old-fashioned reformism, that is, aimed at building mechanisms to protect the populations that live away from their work: state investments (hitherto unprecedented in their volume and scope) in health, education, housing and urban infrastructure; income transfer programs that have lifted millions of Brazilians out of poverty; access to minimum levels of material well-being through mass consumption stimulated by improved income and cheap credit and so on, all in an environment of preservation of the privileges and guarantees to the income and wealth of the upper classes. These win-win class compromise policies were clearly foreseen in the 1988 Constitution.

Lula also halted the privatization of public companies, one of the chief F. Henrique Cardoso neoliberal strategies (from 1995 to 2002), but did not touch the pillars of macroeconomic neoliberalism: fiscal austerity, inflation targeting, open financial and capital markets, free exchange rate and so on. The PT administrations have also adopted a neo-developmentalist approach to the economy, with state-led investments in infrastructure (energy, transports, urban utilities and housing), state subsidies and loans to large companies in important value chains, from food (meat, soya) to metallurgy and oil, and the promotion of 'national champions' to compete worldwide as Brazilian multinationals.

All these were halted by the crisis starting in mid-2013, and when reelected in 2014, President Dilma Rousseff named a renowned neoliberal, a Chicago boy economist for the Ministry of the Economy, who started a strict neoliberal adjustment that the then candidate Rousseff had promised not to follow. Fiscal austerity, reform of the pension systems, reform of labor law (to flexibilize it) and many other proposed measures showed that neo-developmentalism was now (and again, as in the 1990s) out of the agenda.

Amongst an unprecedented economic and political crisis (more on which below), President Rousseff was impeached in 2016, unleashing a radical neoliberal program led by Rousseff's former vice-president Michel Temer, who proposed and the Parliament approved a draconian fiscal policy that froze the federal budget for 20 years (that is, the budget actually executed in 2016 was defined as the ceiling for the public expenditures for the ensuing 20 years, only updated by inflation), resulting in disinvestment in health, education and social policies in general, including infrastructure. A reform of the pension system was proposed that would be approved only under Bolsonaro, but Temer succeeded in passing a labor law reform in 2017 that deeply evicted labor rights and reduced the power of workers' unions, flexibilizing and individualizing work relations at an unprecedented scale, opening ways for the uberization of the labor market. All neo-developmental policies began to be discontinued, a process that was deepened under Jair Bolsonaro, guided by the Chicago-boy Paulo Guedes, who had worked for the Chilean Augusto Pinochet dictatorship.

State companies are now a minor fraction of what they used to be,[10] the oil value chain included. The labor market has been fully flexibilized, capital markets are fully opened, macroeconomic policies are fully neoliberal. The National Development Bank, the central state instrument supporting private investments during the PT administrations is now a shadow of its glorious past. Instead of loans for private investment, its resources are being requested by the Federal Treasury for fiscal reasons. Thus, Brazil is no longer a state-led, quasi-welfare market economy. It is clearly in transition to a neoliberal one.

Crisis

When the pandemic hit Brazil, the country was experiencing a set of intertwined crises, all serious and deep. An economic downturn starting in 2011, after 2014 accumulated small or zero rates of growth quarter after quarter until a GDP loss of near 7 percent in 2015 and 2016, and very low rates of growth ever since (around 1 percent annually). And although the Bolsonaro government contends that before the pandemic the economy was 'flying', the GDP growth of the four quarters ending in the first quarter of 2020 was of meager 0.9 percent.[11] That is, there was growth, but at a still very low rate.

The political crisis can be tracked back to the movements of June 2013, that unleashed social and political forces that politicized every single aspect of the sociability, opening the horizons of expectations and exponentiating demands for better public and social policies. June 2013 also brought to light a series of right and far-right movements that had been thriving unnoticed in the social media and the internet (Cardoso, 2020). These movements and virtual collectivities became hegemonic on the streets during the presidential campaign of 2014, and most particularly in the 2015–2016 mobilizations demanding the impeachment of (the just reelect) President Dilma Rousseff. She was impeached in August 2016 out of an illegal process (there was no actual crime of responsibility), which was approved by the Supreme Court in spite of the many unconstitutional decisions taken by the Parliament (Santos, 2017).

This opened a political Pandora's box, that contributed to erode the constitutional pact of 1988 and its institutions, due to an extensive judicialization of the political and social relations, also as a consequence of the Operation Car Wash against corruption, that destroyed not only large economic sectors, including infrastructure, oil and gas, naval production and heavy construction (De Paula and Moura, 2020), thus feeding the economic crisis, but also eroding the party system and the political system at large. This has put the Judicial Power and particularly the Supreme

Court at the heart of the political dynamic, and made unaccountable, idiosyncratic magistrates the central figures of the political struggle. The judicial activism of the Supreme Court was central to the erosion of the Constitution as the last instance of justice, thus virtually canceling the rule of law (Avritzer, 2018). One cannot explain the election of a far-right, politically insignificant figure like Jair Bolsonaro, with no party tradition, no visible electoral campaign,[12] without mentioning the erosion of the party system by the Operation Car Wash, supported by the Supreme Court (Cardoso, 2020).

Bolsonaro's election brought new elements to this crisis. The new power coalition's strategic plan is to bury the 1988 constitutional order once and for all. The Supreme Court started the process, it is necessary to insist, but the new government's attack on the Constitution is frontal and multidimensional, not only by trying to implement unconstitutional measures, but by proposing and implementing reforms that target the very backbone of the Constitution.

An authoritarian personality, Bolsonaro inaugurated a very conflictive way of government. Condemning 'old politics', in his view a corrupt way of governance dependent on a greedy Congress accustomed to bargain political support to the incumbent of the Executive in exchange for personal or party fiduciary gains, the apex of which had been, in Bolsonaro's view, the expelled Workers' Party, he militarized his cabinet in an unprecedented way: nine out of 22 appointed ministers were militaries from the army, including the four main posts around the president.

As a consequence, Executive x Legislative relations have been quite conflictive. Since the promulgation of the 1988 Constitution, Bolsonaro is the president with the lowest rate of approval of his legislative initiatives.[13] Of 48 Provisional Bills (Medidas Provisórias) enacted in 2019, 24 were simply not voted by the Congress and lost validity.[14] And most of the measures to alleviate the consequences of the Covid-19 pandemic were enacted as Provisional Bills, many of which still await the appreciation of Congress. This is only a symptom of a larger crisis of governance that worsened the sanitary crisis. But before we move on to this matter, a word must be said about the critical social reality of the country.

Inequality

When associated with poverty, social inequality denotes that a considerable part of the population lives under the dyad of vulnerability and precariousness, without access to basic sanitation, decent housing, potable water and whose income (often intermittent) is not enough to buy basic personal hygiene goods (including soap and alcohol), not to mention personal protective equipment.

However, Brazil has a public, Unified Health System (SUS), a notable national healthcare system that is integral, universal and free, also a product of the 1988 Constitution. As pointed out by Croda et al. (2020), SUS already had extensive expertise in combating epidemics and other respiratory diseases such as H1N1 (influenza A). The control of the Zika epidemic (2015–2016), for example, showed that Brazil was one of the world leaders in scientific research on epidemics (for correlating the infection with cases of microcephaly) and was capable of producing several laboratory inputs in its decentralized network of laboratories such as Bio-manguinhos/Fiocruz, in Rio de Janeiro, Instituto Butantan, in São Paulo, and the laboratories of the army. As a consequence, many analysts presumed that the country was in a relatively better position in terms of state capabilities to minimize the social impacts of the Covid-19 (Peci, 2020). However, this was only partly the case.

If the SUS has actually been prioritized during the first two PT administrations, its budget began to be restrained in 2013, during the first Rousseff's mandate. The economic crisis of 2015–16 resulted in further cuts, and after the impeachment of 2016, President Temer kept on restructuring the system, favoring private health companies. When the federal budget was frozen in 2017 cuts increased.[15] At the doors of the sanitary crisis, the SUS alone had lost US$5 billion (or near 20 percent) of its 2016 budget.[16] Structural deficiencies were made clearer.

In fact, before the pandemic, only 9.8 percent of Brazil's municipalities had Intensive Care Unit (ICU) beds in their hospitals.[17] And of the 50,000 available in the country, only 22,000 belonged to the SUS.[18] At this point, the weight of social inequality becomes evident, for the poorest people faced the dilemma of dying at home or in hospital queues, while private hospitals soon started to open for elective surgeries and treatments not related to Covid-19.

Table 16.2 offers a clear picture of this scenario. It shows the mortality rate of patients hospitalized due to Covid-19 from March 1 to October 5, 2020 in Brazil (in private and SUS hospitals). Years of schooling is strongly correlated with social

TABLE 16.2 Mortality rate of patients hospitalized with Covid-19 in Brazil, March 1 to October 5, 2020, according to schooling

Schooling	*N hospitalized*	*Mortality rate (in %)*
No schooling/illiterate	11.465	54.5
Up to 5 years of schooling	40.018	44.2
From 6 to 9 years	27.016	37.5
From 10 to 12	44.439	27.2
More than 12 (higher educ.)	21.101	21.4
Children	3.260	9.6
Ignored	141.799	34.2
Total	289.098	34.4

Source: Microdata of SIVEP Gripe.

This database is the most trustful in the country concerning SARS diseases, for hospitals must inform the Ministry of Health about every hospitalization due to any respiratory syndrome. The rate of mortality by Covid-19 is probably much higher than the official figures (around 160,000 in the end of October 2020). In the SIVEP database, 39 percent of the 770,000 hospitalizations from February to October 2020 due to SARS were classified as 'undetermined', with a death rate of 21 percent (compared to 34.4 percent of Covid-19). Probably the majority of these cases were actually Covid-19, which would increase the actual number of deaths by near 40 percent.

status (or class) in Brazil. Cardoso and Préteceille (2020), for instance, show that if a person has a higher education degree, s/he has 85 percent probability of figuring in a middle-class position or higher. And the death rate of the 'Ignored' category makes us hypothesize that most of them are from lower schooling strata. So moving from lower to higher education means moving up the social structure and, as can be seen, strongly reducing the chances of being killed by the Sars-Cov-2.

Even with a relatively lower informality rate than most South American countries (41.1 percent in 2019), about 42 million workers (informal wage-earners, self-employed, domestic workers) were severely impacted by Covid-19 in Brazil. These people could not get to work but in crowded public transportation. In São Paulo, the correlation between the neighborhoods in which people use private vehicles for transportation and the number of positive cases is of 0.39, considerably lower than in neighborhoods where the main form of commuting to work is public transportation (0.80) or on foot (0.78).[19] This partly explains why Brazil had about 13 percent of those infected with Covid-19 in the world (as of October 15, 2020), while Brazilians are 2.5 percent of the world population.

(Un)governance

Emergency aid (or 'Corona-Voucher' as intended by the Ministry of the Economy), combined with the Employment and Income Maintenance Emergency Program provided income for about 43 percent of the Brazilian households.[20] This relatively high percentage compared to other South American countries contrasts with the reality of 46 million Brazilians 'invisible' to the programs. The criteria for obtaining the aid required documents and registration via a mobile application that the extremely vulnerable population just did not have. Millions of Brazilians do not have a bank account, leading the population to gather in kilometer-long lines in the vicinity of banks and public agencies to withdraw the benefit – exposing a population that already lives under the precariousness/vulnerability dyad to virus infection.

The measures to alleviate the consequences of the pandemic in the formal and informal economies, albeit much stronger than those of most South American countries, reduced income from 40 percent to 90 percent of the original figures (Cardoso, 2020b), making it impossible for the informal workers to stay home. A myopic comprehension of the country's economy led the minister of the Economy to save big business instead of small and medium ones, which create 66 percent of jobs and are going bankrupt by the hundreds of thousands, because the promised subsidized loans never reached them. This will have a huge negative impact in the post pandemic recovery, for unemployment rates will be sky-high for a long period.

These are symptoms of a serious crisis of governance. There was no central coordination or guidelines to combat the pandemic. President Bolsonaro denied the seriousness of the disease and has insisted, from the beginning, that it was no more than a light cold, prompting Brazilians to return to work to save the economy.

He also neglects the deaths, stating that everybody will die some day and that this is a small price to pay for the sake of the economy. When the dead reached 100,000 he just said that 'life must go on. We must find our way out of this problem'.[21]

As a matter of fact, the federal government considered following WHO guidelines when it counted only a few positive cases. However, the signs that a pandemic would inevitably impact the country's (meager) economic results reoriented the federal government's strategies and speeches. Obsessed with his own reelection, Bolsonaro started to use his constitutional prerogatives to hinder social isolation. In the first few weeks, when governors took the first steps to establish social isolation for the entire population, the federal government proposed 'vertical isolation', or quarantine restricted to the elderly and people with pre-existing illnesses. Experts immediately showed that this would not contain the outbreak, for it disregarded the precariousness and high population density of most Brazilian homes, especially in the favelas and poorer neighborhoods.

A month after the first death in the country, the Supreme Court was provoked to decide on the constitutionality of a Provisional Bill against social isolation issued by the federal government. The decision established that states and municipalities could impose restrictions on circulation and define which activities would or would not be suspended. However, the absence of joint institutional strategies coordinated by the federal government had consequences. At that point, the country had surpassed 1,000 deaths and, as it should be expected in regard to a disease that spreads exponentially, in a short time the hospital system of the state of Amazonas collapsed and its government had to hire refrigeration containers to temporarily allocate dead bodies. The same happened in Belém (capital of Pará) and Fortaleza (capital of Ceará).

The Ministry of Health had a third incumbent named after the refusal, by the two previous ones, both physicians, to implement the president's order to impose chloroquine and hydroxychloroquine as the standard SUS treatment protocol. The Ministry was handed to a military that populated the office with 1.2 thousand militaries, and the first measure was to impose chloroquine to the SUS, because Bolsonaro believes the medicine is an effective treatment.[22] The army's pharmaceutical laboratories directed loads of money and energy to the production of chloroquine and hydroxychloroquine instead of antibiotics and vaccines, their original duty. The Ministry also changed the methodology of counting those contaminated and dead, strongly underestimating the actual figures, and stopped publicizing the data in its website. After protests by the WHO and the constitution of a consortium of major news media companies that started collecting and publishing statistics on the evolution of the disease in a daily basis, the Ministry of Health resumed the official statistical records.

As of October 15, only 9 percent of the population had been tested for Covid-19, in spite of promises of massive testing, which was opposed by president Bolsonaro, and the import of tests was halted. Misinformation, fake news, denial and necropolitics guide the federal government's actions.

Alternative institutional initiatives

In the absence of the federal government, many interesting initiatives came to the fore. The states of the Northeast Region (NE) made of the recently created Consortium of the Northeast a means to coordinate the sanitary actions of the region's nine states, the home of almost 60 million Brazilians (28 percent of the total population).[23] A Scientific Committee to Combat Coronavirus was created, putting together distinguished NE scientists, physicians and epidemiologists to gather, systematize and analyze data on the evolution of the disease in the region, to guide the governors' public policies in a way that no other region did, not to mention the federal government.[24]

The incidence of the Covid-19 was actually contained on the eve of the disease, while the NE Consortium negotiated ventilators directly with China, constructed field hospitals and increased the number of ICU beds, preparing for a stronger outburst. By the end of August, however, five out of nine North-Eastern states were above (sometimes 50 percent above) the national mean in terms of deaths per million inhabitants, and in some states, like Ceará (1,039 dead per million as of October 2020), the health system collapsed in April as the disease hit the hinterland where public hospital beds were scarce, bringing hundreds of people to the capital Fortaleza. The same happened in Sergipe (954 dead per million by October 2020).

The combination of high levels of informality and poverty in the larger cities with poor SUS resources in the hinterland seems to account for most of the incapacity of these states to follow successful containment policies or to treat part of the affected population, in spite of their collective responsibility approach to the disease.

The opposite happened in Bahia (473 dead per million by October 2020), the most populated state of the region. Informality is high there as well, but in the capital, Salvador, a systematic testing policy helped to detect and isolate the most vulnerable, while social distancing seems to have been more effective even in the poorer areas. The SUS did respond to the actual demand, and the coordination of the actions of the center-right mayor of Salvador with the left-wing governor of Bahia was crucial to the state's relative success.[25] Most of the measures were suggested or designed by the NE Scientific Committee. However, this did not prevent most of the NE states reaching a 'saturation phase' in August.[26]

In other regions, many states could not reach agreements with their neighbors, and this led social movements, NGOs and other civil society associations in favelas and poorer areas to take measures to protect their neighborhoods. The Central Única das Favelas (Unified Coordination of Favelas – CUFA), for example, mobilized workers' unions, firms, NGOs and individual donors, and managed to provide basic food baskets and income for more than 900,000 families distributed in almost 5,000 favelas in Brazil. Associations, social movements, public and private institutions and universities have also joined efforts in building solidarity networks to contain the advance of the pandemic among Traditional Peoples and Communities such as indigenous, quilombolas, caiçaras, fishermen, riverside populations, among other communities, many of them in the Amazon Region.

Conclusion

Decentralized initiatives, important as they may be (for they show that some responsive public authorities are acting to protect people in the territory they rule, and also show that part of the most vulnerable population is not apathetic and has decided to take their lives in their hands, against all odds), have proved to be insufficient to contain the disease. It may be the case that many lives have been spared because of them, that is, the disaster could have been much worse. But we actually do not know the real extension of the infection (tests are scarce) or even the number of deaths.

In fact, between March 1 and October 5, the number of dead by SARS not classified as Covid-19 (57.8 thousand) was 13.4 times that of the same period of 2019 (4.3 thousand).[27] This is a clear indication that the death figures are underestimated by at least 50,000 cases. Besides, thousands of people are dying at home, without ever reaching the SUS, and they are buried as 'dead by natural causes'. A study by the National Council of Health Secretaries (CONASS) estimated that these deaths are 22 percent higher in 2020 than in the 2015–19 period.[28] Thus Brazilians do not know the actual incidence of the disease. Renowned worldwide for its statistical expertise in health matters, Brazil is now facing the consequences of the systematic boycott by the federal government of official information.

The federal government spent nearly 12 percent of GDP in aid to firms (the vast majority of which large companies, including multinationals and banks), formal employees and also to the most vulnerable population: but it failed to save small and medium firms. The subsidy program designed for them was wrongly implemented.[29] Instead of using the public banks for subsidized loans, backed by the Federal Treasury, the money was handed to private banks that imposed many barriers to loans due to the forecast of default during the crisis. As of June 2020, some 700,000 small and medium firms had shut for good,[30] destroying 1.5 million formal jobs.[31] A self-fulfilling prophecy, of course. Banks did not save them because of fear of default, and their disappearance proved the banks 'right'.

Finally, probably thousands of lives could have been saved if the public authorities had forced private hospitals to harbor SUS patients when local SUS facilities collapsed. Nothing prevented them from acting like the city of Bogotá, in Colombia, which took over the administration of private hospital beds and made them available, according to a proximity criterion, for the most serious cases of Covid-19. On the contrary, the federal government acted *against* the other two executive powers' (state and municipal) intentions to do so, which in turn led them to raise field hospitals overnight, many of which did not meet minimum safety criteria or had basic health equipment,[32] with poor working and hygiene conditions, as well as delayed salaries for doctors and nurses. By the end of August the governor of Rio de Janeiro was removed from office due to corruption charges involving the subcontracting of field hospitals, ventilators and protection equipment.[33]

The consequence of this conflictual, sometimes corrupt, irresponsible governance? For more than three months, beginning in mid-May, Brazil has registered more than 1,000 deaths per day. The rate began to decrease slightly (to more than 900) only by the end of August and to 600 by the end of October, accumulating nearly 160,000 (or 762 per million Brazilians). And counting.

Notes

1 Source: World Development Indicators.
2 https://noticias.uol.com.br/saude/ultimas-noticias/redacao/2020/03/19/primeira-vitima-do-rj-era-domestica-e-pegou-coronavirus-da-patroa.htm (accessed September 2020).
3 https://veja.abril.com.br/mundo/america-latina-e-caribe-e-regiao-do-mundo-com-mais-mortes-pela-covid-19/#:~:text=A%20Am%C3%A9rica%20Latina%20se%20tornou,AFP%20baseada%20em%20dados%20oficiais (accessed October 2020).
4 *Plan Ceibal* available at www.siteal.iiep.unesco.org/sites/default/files/sit_accion_files/siteal_uruguay_5043.pdf (accessed October 2020).
5 www.elpais.com.uy/informacion/educacion/mil-anotaron-comer-escuela.html (accessed August 2020).
6 www.chileatiende.gob.cl/fichas/77255-bono-de-emergencia-covid-19 (accessed October 2020).
7 www1.folha.uol.com.br/mundo/2020/04/medidas-duras-contra-covid-19-no-peru-esbarram-em-problemas-sociais.shtml (accessed October 2020).
8 https://bono2.yomequedoencasa.pe/#!/ (accessed October 2020).
9 https://g1.globo.com/bemestar/coronavirus/noticia/2020/04/05/com-corpos-de-mortos-por-coronavirus-nas-ruas-cidade-do-equador-recebe-doacao-de-mil-caixoes-de-papelao.ghtml (accessed October 2020).
10 Almost 120 state-owned companies were privatized during the 1990s, including energy production, telecommunications, roads, railways, ports, mining, steel industry, petrochemicals, airplane (Embraer), most of the public banks of the federal states and many more. See https://oglobo.globo.com/economia/confira-as-principais-privatizacoes-no-brasil-desde-os-anos-90-21732658 (accessed August 2020).
11 IBGE data, in www.ibge.gov.br/explica/pib.php (accessed August 2020).
12 Bolsonaro's campaign was restricted to the social media and WhatsApp, and was quite obscure vis-à-vis the public debate.
13 www.diap.org.br/index.php/governo-bolsonaro/89892-13-mps-perdem-validade-nos-6-meses-do-segundo-ano-do-governo-bolsonaro-2 (accessed August 2020).
14 A Provisional Bill (Medida Provisória) is a prerogative of the president created by the 1988 Constitution. Once enacted, it has immediate force of law. However, if the Congress does not appreciate it in 120 days it loses validity. If approved with amendments, the president can veto them. And the Congress can either approve them as is or reject them.
15 www.brasildefato.com.br/2018/05/31/governo-corta-verbas-da-educacao-e-da-saude-para-bancar-diesel-mais-barato (accessed August 2020).
16 https://economia.ig.com.br/2020-03-21/cortes-no-sus-e-teto-de-gastos-sao-desafios-no-combate-ao-coronavirus.html (accessed August 2020).
17 https://valor.globo.com/brasil/noticia/2020/05/08/menos-de-10-dos-municipios-do-pais-tem-leito-de-uti-aponta-ibge.ghtml (accessed August 2020).
18 https://noticias.uol.com.br/saude/ultimas-noticias/redacao/2020/03/19/nove-em-cada-10-cidades-do-pais-nao-tem-leito-de-uti-e-exportam-pacientes.htm (accessed August 2020).

19 www1.folha.uol.com.br/equilibrioesaude/2020/08/mortes-por-covid-19-tem-mais-relacao-com-autonomos-donas-de-casa-e-transporte-publico.shtml?utm_source=newsletter&utm_medium=email&utm_campaign=newsfolha (accessed August 2020).
20 https://biblioteca.ibge.gov.br/visualizacao/livros/liv101737.pdf (accessed July 2020).
21 www1.folha.uol.com.br/equilibrioesaude/2020/08/vamos-tocar-a-vida-diz-bolsonaro-sobre-iminencia-de-100-mil-mortes-por-covid-19.shtml (accessed August 2020).
22 Followers of the president started a social media movement saying 'We don't need vaccine, we have Chloroquine'.
23 The Interstate Consortium for Sustainable Development was created in February 2020 to coordinate regional investments and public policies. All governors belong to parties of opposition to Bolsonaro. See https://jc.ne10.uol.com.br/canal/politica/nacional/noticia/2020/02/11/governadores-inauguram-sede-do-consorcio-nordeste-em-brasilia-399586.php (accessed August 2020).
24 www.comitecientifico-ne.com.br/ (accessed August 2020).
25 https://bahiaeconomica.com.br/wp/2020/03/30/rui-costa-e-acm-neto-estao-no-caminho-certo-mas-precisam-dar-inicio-a-testagem-massiva-da-populacao/ (accessed August 2020).
26 https://preprints.scielo.org/index.php/scielo/preprint/view/1136/1703 (accessed August 2020).
27 Source: SIVEP-gripe microdata tabulated for this chapter.
28 www.conass.org.br/indicadores-de-obitos-por-causas-naturais/ (accessed October 2020).
29 https://recontaai.com.br/atualiza-ai/o-erro-e-prometer-e-nao-cumprir-diz-sindicato-sobre-falta-de-credito-a-empresas/ (accessed August 2020).
30 https://oglobo.globo.com/economia/mais-de-700-mil-empresas-que-fecharam-as-portas-nao-vao-reabrir-apos-fim-da-pandemia-24535458 (accessed July 2020).
31 www1.folha.uol.com.br/mercado/2020/07/fechamento-de-empregos-formais-desacelera-mas-atinge-15-milhao-na-pandemia.shtml (accessed July 2020).
32 https://exame.com/brasil/enfermeiros-dormem-no-chao-em-hospital-de-campanha-do-maracana-no-rio/ (accessed August 2020).
33 https://g1.globo.com/rj/rio-de-janeiro/noticia/2020/08/28/afastamento-de-wilson-witzel-entenda.ghtml (accessed September 2020) The governor is a political enemy of president Bolsonaro and contends that the removal, an act of the Federal Public Attorney totally dominated by the president, was arbitrary and persecutory.

References

Avritzer, Leonardo. (2018). 'Operação Lava Jato, judiciário e degradação institucional', *in* Fábio Kerche and João Feres Júnior (eds.), *Operação Lava Jato e a democracia brasileira*. São Paulo: Contracorrente, pp. 37–52.

Bacigalupe, Gonzalo, Gonzales, Rafael, Cuadrado, Cristóbal, Sandoval, Vicente and Farias, Cristian. (2020). O desastre chegou ao Chile: A falida estratégia de combate à pandemia de Covid-19. *Blog DADOS*, available at: http://dados.iesp.uerj.br/chile-pandemia (accessed July 2020).

Cardoso, Adalberto. (2020). *À beira do abismo. Uma sociologia política do bolsonarismo*. Rio de Janeiro: Amazon.

Cardoso, Adalberto. (2020b). Crises, reformas e quarentena: consequências no mundo do trabalho. Paper presented at the *Seminários de Quarentena*. Rio de Janeiro, IESP-UERJ. Available at www.youtube.com/watch?v=fMni0d_mEQ0 (accessed August 2020).

Cardoso, Adalberto and Préteceille, Edmond. (2020). *Classes médias no Brasil. Estrutura, perfil, condições de vida, mobilidade social e participação política*. Rio de Janeiro: UFRJ (forthcoming).

Croda, Julio, de Oliveira, Wanderson Kleber, Frutuoso, Rodrigo Lins, Mandetta, Luiz Henrique, Baia-Da-silva, Djane Clarys, Brito-Sousa, José Diego, Monteiro, Wuelton Marcelo, Lacerda, Marcus Vinícius Guimarães (2020). Covid-19 in Brazil: advantages of a socialized unified health system and preparation to contain cases. *Revista da Sociedade Brasileira de Medicina Tropical*, Vol. 53, https://doi.org/10.1590/0037-8682-0167-2020.

De Paula, Luiz Fernando and Moura, Rafael. (2019). A Lava Jato e a crise econômica brasileira. *Jornal dos Economistas*, No. 360, Aug. Available at www.corecon-rj.org.br/anexos/C1D017FCEE732F4E1B9B4E13C46AD36E.pdf (accessed August 2020).

Fraschina, Santiago. (2020). Con 2 de cada 3 hogares cubiertos por el IFE, Argentina tiene la política de transferencias directas más importante de la región. Universidad Nacional de Avellaneda. www.undav.edu.ar/index.php?idcateg=198 (accessed July 2020).

Gentilini, Ugo, Almenfi, Mohamed, Orton, Ian and Dale, Pamela. (2020). Social protection and jobs responses to Covid-19. *World Bank Group*. https://openknowledge.worldbank.org/handle/10986/33635 (accessed August 2020).

ILO. (2018). *Women and men in the informal economy: A statistical picture*. Geneva: International Labour Office. Available at www.ilo.org/wcmsp5/groups/public/---dgreports/---dcomm/documents/publication/wcms_626831.pdf (accessed August 2020).

Peci, Alketa. (2020). A resposta da administração pública brasileira aos desafios da pandemia. *Revista de Administração Pública*, Vol. 54, No. 4, http://dx.doi.org/10.1590/0034-761242020.

Santos, Wanderley G. (2017). *A democracia impedida. O Brasil no século XXI*. Rio de Janeiro: FGV.

Singer, André (2012). Os sentidos do lulismo. Companhia das Letras. ISBN 978-85-8086-358-1. Retrieved 12 August 2015.

17

CUBA DANCING WITH COVID-19

Citizenship and resilience

Roberto Zurbano Torres

Cuba is, perhaps, the only country where the Cold War has not yet ended: a war sustained by political and economic harassment from the United States that has lasted 60 years. The island created a popular-democratic Revolution in 1959 that impacted the continent. Millions of people supported measures such as the nationalization of foreign companies, and agrarian and urban reforms which gave land and houses to thousands of families. The Literacy Campaign taught 90 percent of the population to read and write and created the basis for its current scientific development. Despite popular support and international recognition of the Revolution, the US government was hostile. Cuba responded by declaring itself socialist and aligning itself to the rhythm of other communist countries. These countries provided military and economic aid to support Cuba in the development of its social programs.

It is difficult to talk about Cuba without referring to the dispute with the United States. It marks its history, its present and, perhaps, the future of the island: two countries that dance to conflicting geopolitical rhythms. Cuba developed its political and economic life facing the greatest world power but unable to take advantage of US economic and scientific development. The island adopted a public health model in the face of ideological conflicts and diplomatic and commercial isolation promoted by the United States in retaliation for its socialist status. Twelve governments dedicated substantial resources to break the island's resistance: economic sabotage, biological wars and the prohibition of obtaining financial credits, industrial parts, food and patented medicines in the United States.

From tradition to the public health model

The beginning of the 19th century witnessed the initiation of a medical tradition in Cuba led by doctors trained in Europe. This coincided with French professionals who arrived on the island after the Haitian Revolution. They returned to specialize in emerging specialisms, making the island a point of world medical reference. In Cuba, a 'successful' Spanish colony, an enslaved mass of blacks formed part of the capital of the sugar oligarchy. There was particular concern for the health of black people: they were work machines and also used for experiments by European doctors. After the end of the war (1898) the US Army introduced an epidemiological plan for the devastated island. Many Cuban doctors were trained in hospitals and laboratories in the United States and, together with colleagues trained in Europe, developed Cuban medicine and its infrastructure.

The 1959 Revolution produced an exodus of doctors and scientists which, in turn, impacted and reduced the health service. The new government championed medicine as a political task and built medical schools throughout the country. In the midst of Cuba-US hostility and in the face of such an influential enemy Cuba looked for survival formulas. Faced with these difficulties their strategy consisted of elegantly dancing among them, avoiding them and thinking beyond the recovery of a sanitary structure depressed by the exodus and shortage of instruments and medicines. The ideas, like dancers themselves, leaped over the restrictions. The government celebrated the professionals who remained in the country and, together with the study of medicine, promoted exchanges with countries of the socialist bloc and other nations.

The key to its current scientific development stems from a quasi-prophetic speech that Fidel Castro Ruz, leader of the Revolution, delivered in 1960, when he announced: 'The future of Cuba must necessarily be a future of men of science'. This was the starting point of a social model where science became the basis of the country's socioeconomic development. This model was achieved gradually through new curricula, by annually recruiting tens of thousands of medical students and by graduating specialists who made up research teams and academic exchanges.

Overcoming the crisis

Before the fall of the Berlin Wall 80 percent of Cuba's trade was with socialist countries. When it fell, the island lost its main suppliers and suffered severe economic crisis. Socialist Cuba and its emancipatory project were devastated; its health structure suffered equally. The state made tourism its economic priority, began stimulating foreign investment and redirected the labor market towards fast-growing sectors. Science, once privileged, was not included in the new plans. But far from damaging the sector it forced scientists to rethink their mission in the face of the new crisis. Despite rigid internal bureaucracy the scientific sector survived: it was jealously protected by Fidel Castro himself and, in addition, initiated a bio-political strategy that allowed groups of scientists and health managers to create the current model that inserted the science sector, and its institutions, into the global economy.

Research centers and institutes respond vigorously to Covid-19, in particular those belonging to the 'Scientific Pole', where 'innovative drugs and vaccines are produced, which are exported to more than forty countries' (Lage 2018: 71). This scientific enclave, which lies to the west of the capital, is home to several advanced technology research and development centers that produce hundreds of patents, drugs, technologies and medical supplies of international standard. In 2012 Scientific Pole institutions and pharmaceutical industry companies joined together to form BioCubaFarma, consisting of 38 companies and 22,000 workers.

The preparation

The epidemic arrived in the middle of the process of economic transformation, following the Communist Party Congress and the recently approved Constitution. The first established the Guidelines for Economic and Social Policy. The second restructured laws and jurisdictions, and the economic opening that renews society. Article 21 of the Constitution reads:

> The State promotes the advancement of science, technology and innovation as essential elements for economic and social development. It also implements forms of organization, financing and management of scientific activity; it encourages the systematic and accelerated introduction of its results in the production and service processes, through the corresponding institutional and regulatory framework.
>
> *(Official Gazette: 915)*

The pandemic halted this process of social transformation. A centralized economy, burdened between the US economic blockade and an inefficient local bureaucracy, did not seem capable of overcoming the tragedy. Even so, health indices remain among the best in the region, thanks to a policy of free universal access to healthcare. There is no private medicine nor health insurance companies. The strength of Cuba's health structure lies in its preventive system supported by a network of primary care clinics of family doctors (with nine doctors per 1,000 inhabitants). Added to this are specialized clinics, hospitals, laboratories, drug factories, high-level research centers, nurtured by universities and by a business structure that inserts them in the market of knowledge and human capital available to international organizations. Along with a competitive practice in dealing with disasters and epidemiological risks, especially in underdeveloped countries. When Covid-19 reached the island, Cuba was prepared to face its lethal pace.

Upon learning of the epidemic in Wuhan, Cuba issued an early warning. It was picked up by the press but without alarm. On January 29, a month after China's notification of the disease, the Council of Ministers approved a Plan for the Prevention and Control of the new coronavirus, a day before the Emergency Committee of the WHO International Health Regulations declared the International Health Emergency. The Pedro Kouri Institute of Tropical Medicine (IPK) in Havana briefed Cuban epidemiologists and experts; some traveled to Mexico for a Pan

American Health Organization training course. In the third week of February, the IPK began the first PCR tests of people suspected of contagion from abroad.

Meanwhile, social networks demanded the closure of airports to international tourism. Being a country where tourism is its main economic lifeline, the government tried not to affect it until the last minute. Cubans, inside and outside the island, pushed hard, without immediate result. The President of the Republic, Miguel Díaz-Canel Bermúdez and the Prime Minister, Manuel Marrero Cruz, held meetings where they announced measures to face the threat, which had not yet been declared a pandemic. On March 3, the Political Bureau of the Communist Party launched an emergency plan with 497 measures, later approved by the Council of Ministers. On March 9, the Prime Minister and the Minister of Public Health reported on national television on the situation and the measures taken. The government centralizing information is usual in socialist states. In Cuba, all health statistics and other sectors are handled with state discretion and it is difficult to elaborate, find or question the data offered by state organisms.

The dance begins

On March 11, the WHO declared the pandemic. Coincidentally, on the same date, the first cases of Covid-19 were detected in Cuba: three Italian tourists who had arrived via Havana's main airport and stayed in the tourist town Trinidad. Social media picked up the information with alarm. There was an immediate deployment of already prepared health and scientific sectors: the first medical protocols, screening in communities, PCR tests of infected personnel and 100 percent contact tracing. A preventive campaign was launched with thousands of people mobilized for health work and specialized medical teams being formed in each province. The vast experience gained from dealing with cyclones and hurricanes along with such epidemics as hemorrhagic conjunctivitis, swine fever, dengue, along with various acts of US biological warfare, were all incorporated. There was experience and organizational capacity from the authorities and appropriate perception of risk by the population.

On the second day the Cuban press announced that the President and Prime Minister would lead meetings of a working group to follow up on the Plan for the Prevention and Control of Covid-19. This group met daily, until October 10. They launched preventive campaigns in official media and social networks. In addition, each morning a particularly charismatic Ministry of Public Health official appeared on national TV to present and comment on the day's epidemiological situation. Hospitals and intensive care units did not collapse, nor were the medicines approved in national and international protocols for the disease lacking. Several medicines that have facilitated the recovery of 93 percent of infected Cubans are produced nationally and applied successfully inside and outside of Cuba. Suspected cases were each held for two weeks in isolation centers where they received free treatment. At this point the government offered wage guarantees to vulnerable workers and others affected by the closure of their work centers.

Sanitary restrictions were increased in work and study centers, public transport, gastronomic centers, markets and especially in hospitals. The pandemic was handled as a matter of national security. On March 23 the Political Bureau of the Communist Party met, chaired by First Secretary, Army General Raúl Castro Ruz. They approved over 100 measures intended to break the chain of transmission: physical and social distancing, closures of work centers and schools, travel restrictions, prohibitions of mass gatherings (religious, sports, cultural, etc.), quarantine, isolation of suspected or confirmed cases, recommendations to stay at home and even mandatory quarantine in some cities and residential areas.

On March 24 further measures were announced including—much called-for on social media—the closure of borders. The country's 14 provincial Defense Councils were activated, also visually: from then on these authorities would wear military rank uniforms. This detail clearly expresses the verticality in the social treatment of the pandemic. At the beginning of the HIV epidemic patients were confined to a kind of hospital camp called Villa Los Cocos; for many it functioned as a sanitary prison: they were not allowed to go outside but if that was necessary they were accompanied by a guard, who would return them hours later to confinement. This practice was criticized because of the rights of patients and later changed to outpatient treatment of the disease.

The socialist state assumes public health as state policy with decisions executed vertically in vaccination campaigns, epidemics and pandemics. It is a health service that has responded to previous campaigns of US biological warfare such as the 1981 dengue hemorrhagic fever which killed one hundred children. The Cuba-US dispute has generated this kind of war mentality, incorporating military terminology and rigid schemes that prevent citizen participation and contributions. Without competition from a non-existent private sector the public infrastructure capitalizes on the country's health work. This explains the resistance suffered by traditional or alternative medicine.

The dysfunctional relationship between Cuba and the US has caused anthropological damage to political thought of the island, creating a mentality that is called 'of a besieged plaza' (a military phrase, as if surrounded inside a square): defensive, with a sense of victimization and distrust towards the outside, or to reprisal and immobility from the inside. The social body also suffers from phobias and manias that could be alleviated with participatory therapies. It would be worth thinking of a strategy that, without ignoring the ideological beliefs that sustain Cuban public health, makes for more flexibility regarding other social participation practices. I offer dance as an example when thinking about transforming such rigid institutions. Dancing is a de-automatizing act of the body (physical, political, social): it moves horizontally and dialogically, broadens the visual field and seeks sociability on equitable terms. From this perspective, I interpret the Cuban experience with Covid-19, from the tactical vision of the dancer facing a partner, in a ballroom with land mines.

On March 27, the first local transmission of the virus was announced in the city of Cárdenas, in the tourist hub of Varadero. Stringent controls increased but despite a persistent health campaign, people were slow to adapt to restrictions. Within a month following the local transmission, symptoms that we now recognize as part of the emotional scenario of Covid began to emerge: uncertainty, depression, anxiety and so on. Professionals and psychology students organized phone and online counseling to alleviate family and other tensions. This type of counseling had previously only been used for drug addiction but was now extended in the face of increased domestic violence during the pandemic. According to Cuban experts, 'Covid-19 not only affects the biological component of health, it can also have a far-reaching psychological impact. The pandemic has already been related to emotional tensions such as fear of infection, fear of others and fear of family and social stigmatization'.

New media stars

The response of Cuba's public health system to the pandemic was excellent and included young medical students supporting the work of medical personnel in cities and in the countryside. One of the new and notable things that resulted from Covid-19 was the legitimization of the country's greatest asset, its scientific heritage. Thanks to Covid-19 the work of a large and hard-working scientific community, previously invisible to wider society, was made public. On April 2, the President of the Republic brought together for the first time a group of expert scientists from medical, biotechnological and pharmaceutical fields directly involved in confronting the pandemic. It exposed the country's scientific strategy to the media and erased the aura of secrecy that had previously surrounded its institutions. From that day on, such meetings were held weekly.

The press celebrated these specialists, institutions, research teams and their international awards. They published results from the Finlay Vaccine Institute, the Center for Genetic Engineering and Biotechnology, the Center for Molecular Immunology, the Center for Biomedical Research, the Institute of Hematology and Immunology, the Center for Neurosciences of Cuba, the Center for Immunoassay, the Institute of Pedro Kouri Tropical Medicine, the Center for Drug Research and Development and so on. The media coverage created much empathy for doctors and scientists; it reinforced their social recognition and the need to dedicate more funds for research, repair of medical institutions and improving salaries, living and working conditions of those so essential to society. Since March 29 each night at 9 pm Cuban medical personnel have been applauded by a public that recognizes their extraordinary work in the face of the epidemic.

This applause is also in honor of the 3,000 members of the 'Henry Reeve' International Specialist Medical Brigade who are supporting Covid work in 39 countries, including First World countries such as Italy and Monaco. The Brigade—there are 52 brigades who, over 15 years, have worked in areas affected by hurricane, earthquakes and epidemics (cholera in Haiti, Ebola in Africa)—have recently been nominated for the Nobel Peace Prize. The US government has tried to sabotage and discredit the Cuban medical system with diplomatic and economic pressures so governments in the region do not request or accept the Cuban Brigades in their countries.

During the pandemic Cuban solidarity has also been visible in other, extraordinary ways. On March 16 the government authorized the entry of a British cruise ship, MS Braemar—already refused entry to other requested ports in the Caribbean—which had reported an outbreak of Covid onboard. On March 28 Cuba authorized a German airline humanitarian flight—also refused by neighboring countries—to repatriate British passengers. These actions generated a robust for-and-against debate regarding the risk to the country both on social media, in the foreign press and on the street. The Cuban president explained their actions as acts of solidarity of the Revolution, insisting that Cuba had followed all national and international medical protocols and taken all necessary precautions to protect the population.

Good news broke on August 19. Specialists from the Finlay Institute announced the development of Soberana01, the first possible Cuban vaccine against Covid-19: an important moment for the science of the only Latin American country that faced the epidemic with its own resources. The name of the vaccine expressed the battle for the sovereignty of science in Cuba: a challenge for any developing country. The news brought relief to millions of Cubans and five days later the first phase of clinical tests began.

Towards a new model of governance

The emergency responses developed from being provisional to more permanent as scientific and political learning and achievements were established during exchanges, decision-making, down to the smallest details, in order to control the pandemic. From such dialogues, decisions, solutions and information management, a governance model emerged that incorporated the active role of science, listening to social networks and more flexible criteria when implementing laws and policies that facilitate new conditions of living and work during the pandemic.

One evident deficit, however, following the lockdown of cities, the reduction of public transport and the minimal mobility of people, was the appalling distribution of food, medicine and cleaning products. The shortages and poor organization of distribution created unrest. Added to this was the role of three currencies in domestic use and the inequality of provincial markets. The Revolutionary National Police and the Revolutionary Armed Forces were mobilized. Their mission impossible was to organize the long queues of people crowding in front of markets and pharmacies; students were called in to prevent some people from buying multiple times. These were deficiencies in the urban fabric that the pandemic exacerbated, that provoked thousands of complaints and resulted in social unrest. The official media blamed the population without denouncing the lack of administrative solutions or explaining the tensions that the shortage and immobility generate in the population.

The model of governance in the making attempted to profile the contribution of science in the production of food, energy, medicine and other deficiencies.

From the same perspective, and indirectly responding to demands made on social networks, technology was brought closer to people through innovations such as e-commerce, teleworking and e-government, which were implemented in a limited way already before the pandemic and which the pressure of these days turned into realities, not totally successful and still costly, but irreversible.

The actions, reactions and decisions experienced in these days demand a consensus difficult to achieve in a society as vertical as Cuba, with little citizen participation and the fragile work of civil organizations. The Internet was a battlefield between government lines, the proposals of civil society and the pressures of political opposition, inside and outside the island. High political tension turned the pandemic into a field of conflict between various positions that wielded criticism and demands on issues other than health. The necessary consensus was not achieved but many citizen demands were tactically accepted by politicians. Consensus is a process of recognition and disposition in the face of conflicts that requires conditions, but an extreme situation such as the pandemic seemed to activate this possibility in the face of concerns of people, institutions and organizations with different or opposite interests. Although the differences reached moments of great hostility, the confrontations did not have a social impact that put at risk the health of the population, the control measures or the established social order.

Various entrepreneurs respond with initiatives: Clandestina, a Cuban design store, offered masks for children and adults emblazoned with innovative phrases and tropical colors, private restaurants invented menus 'to go' and some donated meals to vulnerable people in their neighborhoods. A well-known taxi company (the Cuban version of Uber) offered lower prices to help people with hospital visits. Organic farms on the outskirts of the city offered fruits, vegetables and yogurt at reasonable prices. Neighbors organized WhatsApp groups to find out where certain products could be bought or to exchange food or medicine for more essential goods. The Yucabyte site discovered that the Porter @ app, which was created by the Informatics University for the use of shopkeepers, and linked to the Ministry of the Interior, features in addition to coleros (people queuing), other 'categories of interest' that have nothing to do with the purpose of the application (Yucabyte: 3). Faced with an increase in violence, and with the lukewarm response of the National Assembly to the Request for Comprehensive Law Against Gender Violence made by 40 Cuban women in November 2019, the Cuban feminist network YoSíTeCreo created a platform to support victims of gender violence which had increased during the pandemic.

Such initiatives were read and heard about in digital magazines and podcasts: comments, interviews and critics revealed collective actions and reactions with fresh and informative freedom, informing people what was happening in their neighborhoods. Artists, influencers and activists toured the provinces—both physically and digitally—with diverse offers: their reflections and creativity closely linked to positions of socially responsibility, including perspectives that contrasted with the inadequacy or partiality of the press and other official institutions.

Social activism, the great absence

Social activism needs to be thought of as a right and as something urgent for each citizen. It is an organized response that generates in individuals and communities a high capacity for empathy and creation, powerful vaccines against any epidemic. During Covid-19, government prejudices marginalized the activist a little more: aware of the visible and invisible deficiencies in the community they are part of. Activism takes place against the current, as the government considers it a political opposition. Perhaps they are right in defining as opponents those activist groups that do not consider themselves parties, even if they assume anti-systemic agendas. But, the accusation of opposition to activism is a strategic error that in such a complex context must be reconsidered.

Social activism does not withdraw from this governmental vision and it continues to empower communities lacking in equality and equity (which must be reinforced in times of crisis). Resilience does not occur by decree, but in daily dialogue, in the search for common understanding and open positions towards solutions. Thus, such citizen resilience generates greater self-esteem and collective responsibility in the face of difficulties. Contagion, confinement and distancing changed activism, relocating its role to those who require understanding and support: people who did not abide by the 'Stay at home', due to unhealthy or overcrowded homes, low wages or dependence on the informal market. The current health condition should not overshadow the socio-political health of the nation, to which environmentalism, feminism or anti-racism, to just give three examples, contribute greatly.

Racism is a psychosocial pandemic that nullifies memory, criticism and reparation efforts. Anti-racist activism contributes to healing a social disease that involves many people, aware of it or not. It is curious how the statistics distinguish Covid-19 patients by gender, age, nationality and so on, but not by skin color, a data historically haggled over. Anti-racist activism will investigate how the pandemic makes black lives more vulnerable in Cuba, where it is still difficult to understand that the legacy of slavery remains. The activists are archaeologists of intimate social truths, buried under layers of social violence, economic domination and political opportunism. They think of other difficult lives. Although they suffer ridicule, punishment and marginalization, they do not abandon their task. Without them, a healthier society will not be possible.

Conclusion

The health management of the pandemic has been efficient and has demonstrated the role of science in Cuba as part of socioeconomic development. The scientific journal *Nature* highlighted Cuban biotechnology as 'the most established biotechnology industry in the developing world, which has grown even in the absence of the venture capital model that rich countries consider a prerequisite' (Nature 2009: 130). This indicates that this is the path of other Cuban industries and that the health sector could find, in this path, a way to restore clinics and hospitals, optimize their technology and offer better national and international services than before the economic crisis.

However, the political handling of the crisis within Cuban society was not very confident. It involves a complex process not resolved with scientific formulas, but with political will, strategies and public policies in the short, medium and long term, in proactive and participatory terms, combining forces and social actors. If science managed to leap over the walls of North American blockade, bureaucracy and administrative inefficiency, creating scientific exchanges and competitive companies, we must seek a similar process in Cuban ideological life, economic restructuring and daily life. Despite the exodus of young people and the aging of the population, the 'besieged plaza' that restricts critical thinking continues to weigh on instead of opening new institutions and capacities for society to heal with Cubans' own management towards a new society.

The pandemic catalyzed old, unresolved conflicts in a country that forks, like Borges' garden paths, between a half-socialist and half-capitalist structure; between two currencies in circulation and between two ways of treating the intellectual capacity and human capital formed by the Revolution. One that instrumentalizes these forces to satisfy the interests of a dominant group, little interested in granting claimed citizen rights. And another path where responsible intellectuals do not postpone their civic proposals and repress their criticisms, for the sake of social improvement that generates economic development.

Lessons from the pandemic are clear: that new social practices and governance models must be incorporated as irreversible processes. But it is essential to find a model of public coexistence to recover from citizen deficiencies and structural limitations—not ignoring the complex international scenario, or the financial persecution of the United States, intensified during the pandemic, and its attempt to devalue Cuban health. Just as the 'new normal' is conceptualized, a new public coexistence could be conceptualized, establishing citizen pacts that will not be easy without deploying economic, social and political possibilities and the capacities of all generations and sectors (I include social activism, private sector, diaspora, religious institutions, etc.). The post-pandemic will bring greater challenges for both the biological and social body that, on this island of Sun, must dance together, for life.

References

Castro Ruz, Fidel, www.cuba.cu/gobierno/discursos/1960/esp/f150160e (accessed September 2020) Cuba's biotech boom, *Nature*, vol. 457, 2009, p. 130.

From Centro Habana, October 2020.

Giselle: This is the menu: (Dis)protection of personal data in Cuba, www.yucabyte.org (accessed September 2020).

Official Gazette of the Republic of Cuba, No. 37 Extraordinary of August 29, 2014.

Lage, Agustín 2018 Twelve essential and urgent truths about science in Cuba, *Issues Magazine*, 93–94, Cuba, January, June.

18

NICARAGUA AND COVID-19

Authoritarian indifference

Kai M. Thaler

In early 2020, the official stance of the Nicaraguan government was that the Covid-19 pandemic was a problem for other countries and Nicaragua had nothing to worry about. A few early cases were dismissed as results of patients' travel abroad. Even as cases mounted in bordering countries, local doctors and international health officials raised concerns about rising respiratory illness reports, and Cuban officials identified Covid-19 cases originating in Nicaragua, President Daniel Ortega's administration retained its unwavering optimism—or willful delusions. Nicaragua was alone in the Americas in the depth of official inaction, even once the government finally acknowledged Covid-19's foothold in the country (Thaler 2020; Salazar Mather et al. 2020). What laid the groundwork for this denialism? And what does the subsequent toll of the pandemic and the government's lax response tell us about the state of Nicaragua's political, social, and economic institutions?

I argue that the Covid-19 pandemic and the Nicaraguan government response reveal the depths of the authoritarian control held by Ortega, First Lady-turned-Vice President Rosario Murillo and their family: they possess institutional reach from the national to local level and throughout government and civil society, even if popular legitimacy has eroded. The crisis and response have also made lethally clear the ruling family's prioritization of self-interest over all else—even their most loyal supporters' health and lives. Since Ortega took office in 2007, his and Murillo's ruling *Frente Sandinista de Liberación Nacional* (FSLN) trumpeted poverty reduction and free healthcare for the Nicaraguan people as priorities, but the Covid-19 crisis has revealed the toxic mix of a low-income, largely informal economy and a still-weak, highly unequal healthcare system.

After two years of violent repression following 2018 mass protests and the internal collapse of Nicaragua's closest ally, Venezuela, international isolation has made it difficult for outside actors to pressure Ortega and Murillo, or to effectively aid the population from abroad. Meanwhile, despite over a decade of harassment and repression, civil society, has proven resilient, promoting and coordinating popular, autonomous responses to Covid-19. Ultimately, the pandemic has rendered more starkly the costs of the Ortega-Murillo family's continued control of Nicaragua, after years of suggestions Ortega was a guarantor of stability.

Nicaraguan government's lagging pandemic response

As Covid-19 began its march around the globe, most Central American governments scrambled to make sense of scientific information about the new coronavirus and shifting international health guidelines. The region's first known Covid-19 death occurred March 15 in Guatemala. Nicaragua's neighbors closed their borders, prepared quarantine facilities, and ramped up public health measures and restrictions on large gatherings, but the Nicaraguan government took the opposite approach. Borders remained open for travelers, the government denied quarantine facilities were necessary, and Murillo promoted large government-sponsored events and sports leagues (Robinson 2020; Thaler 2020). Most infamously, Ortega and Murillo organized the March 14 'Amor en Tiempos del Covid-19' (Love in the Time of Covid-19) rally and parade in Managua, which drew thousands of people—but not the ruling couple.

Despite doctors, businesspeople, foreign officials, and Catholic Church leaders raising alarms and organizing their own prevention measures, the government painted Covid-19 as no problem for the country, saying the health system was prepared and that God would protect Nicaragua. Beginning around March 10, doctors reported suspected Covid-19 cases, submitted samples for testing, but received no response from MINSA, the Ministry of Health (Miranda Aburto 2020a). Once Nicaragua's first official Covid-19 case was identified on March 18, the government continued denying the need for more preparation. This denial was maintained when community spread began and doctors reported rising cases of 'atypical pneumonia', the designation given to suspected Covid-19 patients, who went untested due to the government's failure to organize large-scale testing, and government efforts to obscure Covid-19 data. After April 2, Nicaragua was Latin America's only country with open borders (Bow 2020a).

This pattern continued for months, with the government downplaying the pandemic, lacking transparency around testing and distribution of international health aid, promoting public events and tourism, keeping schools open, and undermining civil society actors' and doctors' autonomous public health responses (Luna 2020a; Miranda Aburto 2020b; Romero 2020). Ortega himself was absent throughout much of the spring and summer—normal by his standards, but particularly jarring during a public health crisis (Thaler 2020).

Despite their public indifference to the pandemic, Ortega and Murillo acted to protect themselves, their family, and the backbone of the regime—the security forces. Reporters uncovered orders from mid-March for disinfectant and gloves for Ortega and Murillo's residence (Silva 2020) and police began wearing masks in late March (Baltodano 2020). That same month, the government dispatched public employees and FSLN cadres door-to-door to provide health information, but these 'brigades' were not given personal protective equipment, making them potential vectors (Miranda Aburto 2020c).

In mid-May, as cases mounted, the government quietly made some preparations, officially redirecting international loan funds toward the Covid-19 response, but still limiting testing and keeping data secret, releasing implausibly low case numbers, and promoting untested treatments (Navas 2020). The government also failed to secure missing components for 26,000 donated Covid-19 test kits, even as cases were growing, hospitals became overwhelmed, and nighttime 'express burials' became common (Bow 2020c; Miranda Aburto 2020d; López Ocampo and Sheridan 2020).

Officially, as of October 17, 2020, there have been 5,353 confirmed Covid-19 cases (805 per million people) and 154 deaths in Nicaragua (23 per million people), a country of about 6.6 million people, with case and death spikes in late May and late June. Testing data are unavailable, the only Central American country for which this is the case. Due to the government's lack of transparency and obscuring and undermining of accurate health data, civil society groups and dissident doctors in mid-March started the Observatorio Ciudadano (Citizens' Observatory) to collect data about confirmed and likely Covid-19 cases. As of October 17, the Observatorio identified 10,733 total Covid-19 cases (1,615 per million) and 2,780 deaths (418 per million).

These Observatorio data are still likely an undercount, but based on Worldometer data, they suggest Nicaragua's death rate is around the 20th worst in the world, only surpassed by Panama in Central America (see Table 18.1, data as of October 17, 2020), despite a case rate around 131st globally. Nicaragua has approximately the same population as El Salvador, but based on Observatorio data, Nicaragua has had one-third as many cases per million compared to its more densely populated neighbor (1,615 versus 4,842), but a per capita death rate three times higher (418 per million versus 141). Based on Observatorio data, Nicaragua's Covid-19 death rate has been more than twice that of Guatemala and over 1.5 times that of Honduras

TABLE 18.1 Covid-19 in Central America

Country	*Covid-19 cases*	*Deaths*	*Cases per million*	*Deaths per million*	*Population*
Belize	2,728	43	6825	108	399,714
Costa Rica	94,348	1,183	18472	229	5,107,745
El Salvador	31,456	917	4842	141	6,495,849
Guatemala	101,028	3,515	5,609	195	18,011,279
Honduras	86,691	2,556	8,712	257	9,950,286
Nicaragua (official)	5,353	154	805	23	6,647,548
Nicaragua (Observatorio)	10,733	2,780	1,615	418	6,647,548
Panama	123,498	2,557	28,492	587	4,334,467

and Costa Rica, despite far fewer cases per million. Ortega and Murillo's allies in Venezuela, amid state collapse but strong official lockdown and public health policies, had twice as many cases per million (3,018), but only 26 deaths per million (one-sixteenth Nicaragua's rate).

While underlying health system weakness is partially to blame, Nicaragua's lack of preparation and widespread testing led to underprepared hospitals, patients seeking care too late, and, ultimately more deaths. The government response and lethal Covid-19 outcomes are rooted in Nicaragua's institutional environment.

Authoritarian consolidation and Ortega-Murillo family dominance

Daniel Ortega was elected to the presidency 2006, returning to Nicaragua's highest office after being head of state in the FSLN's revolutionary government from 1979–1990. After the 1990 turn to full electoral democracy, Ortega consolidated control of the FSLN party apparatus, gradually purging rivals. The FSLN was previously a leftist party, ideologically rooted in Marxism-Leninism, Catholic liberation theology, and anti-imperialist nationalism. In the late 1990s and early 2000s, however, Ortega remade the FSLN along Christian democratic lines, allying with the Catholic Church hierarchy, capitalist business elites, and rightwing President Arnoldo Alemán (Close 2016; Peraza C. 2016; Spalding 2017; Thaler 2017). Parts of the FSLN's historic mass base remained behind Ortega, and once in office, he used targeted social programs, patronage jobs, and partisan distribution of public aid to shore up support among the poor, a crucial, but relatively inexpensive task in the second-poorest country in the Americas.

During his first decade in office, Ortega steadily centralized power, eroding state institutions' independence and giving them partisan branding (the FSLN won legislative control in 2011), cracking down on independent civil society organizations, and using redirected state money from Venezuelan oil deals to build business empires for the Ortega-Murillo family and their allies Close 2016; Jarquín 2016; (Thaler 2017; Martí i Puig and Serra 2020). Murillo grew in influence during this period, tightly controlling official government communications and viewed by many Nicaraguans as the 'power behind the throne'. Murillo ascended to the Vice Presidency in the blatantly fraudulent 2016 elections, making her power official and explicitly opening the possibility of a political dynasty—four decades after the FSLN-spearheaded 1979 revolution toppled the longstanding Somoza family dictatorship.

Ortega and Murillo's power seemed secure, bolstered by a growing economy, firm FSLN control of the state, new alliances with Nicaragua's growing Evangelical Christian population, and increasing family control of Nicaraguan media. Meanwhile civil society organizations were corporatized or persecuted and the opposition was divided (Jarquín 2016; Steigenga, Coleman, and Marenco 2017; Thaler 2017). In late 2017, according to Latinbarómetro (2017) surveys, Ortega was Latin America's most popular president, and despite democratic erosion, Nicaraguans reported optimism about the future.

This picture of stability shattered in April 2018. Elderly pensioners and student allies took to the streets in response to planned social security cuts for retirees and workers—and were beaten by pro-government thugs. The protests expanded, and after police and pro-government paramilitaries killed several young protesters, demonstrations grew into a nationwide civil uprising against Ortega and Murillo's regime. Ortega and Murillo's governing bargain crumbled, as the Catholic Church and business leaders joined protesters, calling for dialogue and new elections. Many longtime FSLN supporters turned on Ortega and Murillo.

It briefly looked like the ruling couple might fall, but in June and July 2018, they struck back with a vengeance, purging opposition supporters from public institutions and sending police and paramilitaries to violently reclaim the streets, while the military stayed in its barracks. Pro-government forces killed over 300 people, wounded and imprisoned thousands, and sent tens of thousands more into exile (Grupo Interdisciplinario de Expertos Independientes 2018; Inter-American Commision on Human Rights 2018). By mid-2018, Ortega and Murillo had lost most of their public support (Latinobarómetro 2018) and international legitimacy.

By early 2020 when the Covid-19 pandemic emerged, Ortega and Murillo faced even fewer accountability mechanisms than before April 2018. The FSLN and its paramilitaries, centered around the Sandinista Youth, have national reach, and there is no real political opposition in the government, down to the local level. Independent media outlets operate but face harassment and censorship, while Ortega-Murillo family-controlled outlets and social media let the government shape their supporters' media narrative.

Ortega and Murillo became even more insular and defensive after 2018, prioritizing officials' loyalty and willingness to tow the government line. In early April, for instance, mid-pandemic, Health Minister Carolina Dávila Murillo was replaced with Dr. Martha Reyes Álvarez, the latter having proved her loyalty by attacking Cuban reports of Covid-19 cases emerging from Nicaragua (Luna 2020b). Government officials have provided and parroted absurd justifications for the lack of early Covid-19 control measures. A white paper released in late May, two months into Nicaragua's outbreak, claimed the country was following the failed 'Swedish strategy' of avoiding lockdowns to protect the economy (Secretaría Privada para Políticas Nacionales 2020)—despite Nicaragua's far lower testing capacity, healthcare and economic resources, and data transparency.

This personalization and centralization of power meant Ortega and Murillo's inner circle lacked dissenting voices. Thorough political control foreclosed the possibility of regional or local leaders independently enacting public health measures, something that enabled more effective subnational pandemic responses in federalized Brazil, Mexico, and the US, despite national leaders' denialist stances.

The Covid-19 crisis revealed that Ortega and Murillo no longer have accountability mechanisms constraining their actions, or any remaining sense of obligation beyond their family. Already in 2016, Close (2016: 138) argued that Ortega had constructed a political system that was 'verticalist (power is structured and exercised hierarchically), hyperpresidential, personalist with a touch of … "amoral familism", and increasingly hegemonic'.[1] After April 2018, these features were heightened, but Ortega and Murillo still appeared to value and feel accountable to their supporters, organizing public events and giving resources and opportunities to loyalists.

The Covid-19 response demonstrated a complete transition to amoral familism: Ortega and Murillo showed no concern for the common good beyond their family's material interests. They remained indifferent to Covid-19's toll even as it hit their staunchest supporters hard, killing top FSLN officials, Evangelical ministers, and sports figures. Outcry from independent media, medical leaders, the opposition, the Catholic Church, and business associations all fell on deaf ears. Having weathered the 2018 protests, Ortega and Murillo feel free to pursue whatever policies they choose, and no one remains domestically to dissuade or stop them.

Economic precarity and an unequal, hollowed-out healthcare system

Beyond Ortega and Murillo's claims of divine protection, their stated reasoning for not implementing border closures, lockdowns, and other Covid-19 control measures was that it would be too harmful economically. In Ortega's (2020) first major speech after the pandemic hit Nicaragua in April, he stated lockdowns were not an option, because 'if this country stops working, it dies, and if the country dies, the people die'.

The Covid-19 crisis placed lower-income countries like Nicaragua in a tough spot: with the majority of workers in the informal sector and living on limited resources, not working could quickly mean starving. Yet this situation could have been avoided through government assistance for poor Nicaraguans, as other countries in Central America and around the world provided during the pandemic. Ortega and Murillo's failure to offer similar assistance and their claims the country would starve under a lockdown make clear the government's failures to sustainably reduce poverty and to create an economy benefiting all Nicaraguans.

Ortega and Murillo changed the FSLN's slogan to 'Christian, socialist, in solidarity', yet rather than developing a truly socialist coordinated market economy, once in office, Ortega chose extraction: he continued the neoliberal macroeconomic policies of his post-1990 predecessors and built up family members' and FSLN cronies' wealth. The economy grew from 2007–2017, continuing preexisting trends, but this was accompanied by rising inequality and stagnant real wages, with around three-quarters of the population still informally employed (Sáenz 2016; Thaler 2017; Banco Central de Nicaragua 2020). The 2018 protests and crackdown stopped growth, with prior declines in Venezuelan economic support combining with economic disruptions and plummeting tourism to push Nicaragua into recession. Coordination on labor policy between the government, business associations, and FSLN-linked labor unions also stopped in 2018, leaving Ortega, Murillo, and remaining allies in full control of economic policy.

The recession was projected to continue in 2020 even before the Covid-19 pandemic, but Ortega and Murillo managed to avoid the full economic collapse many predicted in 2018. Economic stability was clearly a priority in the Covid-19 response, though to protect Ortega-Murillo family wealth, not the public. The failure to provide increased economic aid to the population, like 2018's announcement of social security cuts, reveals Ortega and Murillo's unwillingness to sacrifice any of their own hundreds of millions, if not billions, of dollars in ill-gotten riches (Nicaragua Investiga 2019) to help out the Nicaraguan people. None of this wealth was put into action to dampen the recession's effects on the masses, or to make it feasible for Nicaragua's poor workers to stay home to slow Covid-19.

Half-filled economic promises were mirrored in the health sector. Nicaragua's government is constitutionally bound to meet citizens' healthcare needs, and there were hopes Ortega would fulfill this mandate, given his socialist rhetoric and the revolution's 1980s expansion and improvement of healthcare access. Funding remained limited, however, with highly unequal healthcare accessibility and quality. Areas outside major cities are underserved and undersupplied, with Nicaraguans who can going to private providers or abroad for care (Pizarro 2011; Sequeira et al. 2011; Sotelo Vargas and Vargas-Palacios 2020). The health sector also became increasingly politicized, with the FSLN seeking to control medical unions and pressing workers to publicly demonstrate support for the government. Politicization deepened in 2018–2019, as the government purged medical professionals who participated in protests or simply treated wounded protesters (Huete-Pérez 2018; Vargas-Palacios, Pineda, and Galán-Rodas 2018; Sotelo Vargas and Vargas-Palacios 2020).

When Covid-19 struck, Nicaragua's health system had already lost hundreds of workers to firings and emigration, while government policing of hospitals in 2018 diminished public trust. The government's promotion of mass events and rejection of pleas and aid from the Pan-American Health Organization (PAHO) showed political control, not public health, remained Ortega and Murillo's primary concern, alarming doctors and experts (M. C. Jarquín, Prado, and Gallo Marin 2020; Huete-Pérez and Hildebrand 2020; Salazar Mather et al. 2020). In May, over 700 Nicaraguan doctors warnedthe health system might collapse without preventive action, due to limited resources and supply shortages (Luna 2020e). The government ignored this advice, instead seeking to silence healthcare workers, firing those who challenged policies or leaked accurate information (Amnesty International 2020; De Cordoba 2020; Kincaid 2020). Even public health centers have high charges for Covid-19 tests, US$150 or about half the average monthly income of formal sector workers, and the government has continued taxing essential medical equipment (Luna 2020f; Today Nicaragua 2020).

Ortega and Murillo continue prioritizing personal power and wealth over public welfare, even when their own supporters are suffering. The government's willful disregard for and insulation from pleas and warnings by Nicaraguan experts has been mirrored internationally.

The Ortega-Murillo regime's international isolation

A strength of Ortega and Murillo's government before 2018 was balancing stable relations with both the US, the regional hegemon, and Latin America's Venezuelan-led leftist bloc. Rhetorically, Ortega embraced anti-imperialism and adopted late Venezuelan President Hugo Chávez's internationalist language of 'Bolivarianism', joining his Bolivarian Alliance for the Americas (ALBA). Yet Nicaragua retained good US relations, remaining a Central American Free Trade Agreement member, pursuing neoliberal macroeconomic policies, and cooperating on anti-narcotrafficking efforts and restricting migration (Martí i Puig 2016; Thaler 2017). The US and European Union gave weak rebukes for election fraud in 2016, but Ortega and Murillo weathered them without any trouble.

Ortega and Murillo's foreign standing quickly eroded once the government began massacring protesters in 2018. Other Latin American leaders condemned the government crackdown, calling for dialogue. The long-dormant Nicaragua Investment Conditionality Act (NICA Act) finally passed the US Congress, restricting international financial institutions' loans to Nicaragua, and the US, EU, Canada, and Switzerland sanctioned top government officials, updating sanctions into 2020. International human rights organizations and UN High Commissioner for Human Rights Michelle Bachelet have consistently condemned the Ortega-Murillo regime's abuses, continuing during the Covid-19 pandemic.

The Covid-19 crisis has deepened Ortega and Murillo's isolation. Latin America's leftist bloc has disintegrated following electoral losses, leaders' contentious removal from office in Brazil and Bolivia, and Venezuela's political and economic collapse. Ortega and Murillo managed to alienate their closest remaining stable ally, Cuba, with their Covid-19 denialism, while their failure to cooperate with PAHO and to take reasonable Covid-19 prevention measures created new feuds with Nicaragua's neighbors. PAHO officials repeatedly offered assistance and called on the Nicaraguan government to let their advisers visit and to openly provide Covid-19 data, only to be rebuffed (Cruz 2020; Luna 2020c; Lister 2020; Munguía 2020a; 2020b). The leaders of Costa Rica, El Salvador, and Honduras all decried Nicaragua's lax official Covid-19 response, and a serious dispute erupted with Costa Rica, which unilaterally closed its border with Nicaragua and filed complaints with PAHO (Álvarez 2020b; Leiva 2020; 100% Noticias 2020).

The Nicaraguan government's Covid-19 response has undone any efforts to stabilize the country's reputation after the 2018 political crisis. This global pariah status may make it difficult to attract foreign investment to reboot the economy after Covid-19, especially if there are (reasonable) doubts about the government implementing an effective vaccination program. At a time when global cooperation is key to combating Covid-19 and avoid economic disaster, the Ortega-Murillo regime has chosen isolationism and antagonism, harming the Nicaraguan public.

Civil society's resilience in the face of repression

Even before 2018, independent civil society groups, media outlets, and opposition political parties were restricted and repressed, but continued organizing and speaking out against erosion of democracy, corruption, and human rights violations (Jarquín 2016; Cortés Ramos, López Baltodano, and Moncada Bellorin 2020). One ray of hope in Nicaragua's Covid-19 crisis has been civil society groups promoting responsible public health practices, countering government disinformation with independent data, and drawing global attention to government malfeasance.

Beginning in March 2020, civil society groups promoted self-isolation (#QuedateEnCasa, 'stay home', trended on social media), business restrictions, and mask-wearing, despite harassment from the government and its supporters. The Catholic Church restricted services and sought to provide medical advice and care, despite harassment and even terrorist attacks from government supporters. Journalists and independent citizens worked to counter false information spread by government supporters on social media. These efforts sought to mobilize a communal spirit of responsibility, recalling the collective public health campaigns of the revolution.

Doctors organized calls to follow scientific guidelines and the advice of the World Health Organization and PAHO, growing frustrated as the government continued to ignore their pleas (Álvarez 2020a; Bow 2020b; Delgado 2020; Medrano 2020). Doctors registered their concerns with Nicaragua's remaining independent media organizations, leaking information from hospitals, while journalists sought to provide scientific guidance from abroad (Confidencial 2020). Most vitally, beginning March 14, the Observatorio Ciudadano collected data on suspected and confirmed Covid-19 cases and deaths, providing independent, reliable information, while the health ministry obscured the truth.

These civil society efforts may not have been able to shift government policy, which only changed when Covid-19 cases grew too prevalent to ignore, but they have offered vital independent voices in the face of government inaction and disinformation and helped mobilize a spirit of communal responsibility. Civil society action also helped spark decentralized personal and community measures to slow the pandemic, easing the potential burden on the health system and likely reducing the overall toll of Covid-19. Nicaraguan civil society's resilience provides a source of optimism for the post-pandemic future and the difficult task of rebuilding the stressed economy, health system, and social fabric.

Conclusion

Have other factors been at play in the Nicaraguan government's Covid-19 response? Ortega argued international sanctions hamstrung the government's response, but, as mentioned above, sanctions have been targeted, not general, and Ortega and Murillo have vast resources they could use for public interests. Sanctions also did not prevent Nicaragua from receiving international donations to aid the Covid-19 response (Luna 2020d; Romero and Munguía 2020).

Given Nicaragua's lower-income status, labor informality, and weak healthcare system, was the country destined to face a high Covid-19 toll, and thus better off minimizing the short-term economic costs? Nicaragua's death rate suggests otherwise, and a July 2020 survey found over 50 percent of Nicaraguans saying Covid-19 was the country's most urgent problem, compared to 15 percent prioritizing the economy (Orozco 2020). Restrictions and public health measures early on help slow epidemics, reduce the likelihood of health system collapse, and can protect the economy in the long term (Correia, Luck, and Verner 2020). Further, the Ortega-Murillo government's denigration of preventive measures, promotion of mass events, and hiding data did not help 'manage' the pandemic's impacts—they actively worsened them.

The rate of increase in Covid-19 cases and deaths has slowed from July to the time of writing in October 2020. The virus may have hit the most vulnerable populations first, with individuals' health precautions and the Nicaraguan population's relative youth reducing impacts going forward (young populations have been suggested as key in low Covid-19 death tolls in sub-Saharan Africa). As rising case numbers Europe in September and October 2020 show, however, Covid-19 can return with a vengeance.

From 2007–2018, Ortega and Murillo's political bargain with the Nicaraguan people was premised on providing stability and economic growth, even if political and social freedoms were narrowing. The 2018 protests and repression broke this bargain, but Covid-19 deepened the degree to which Ortega and Murillo's rule has become destabilizing and detrimental to Nicaragua. The ruling couple have proven unwilling to sacrifice any of their power and family riches, even if it means thousands more Nicaraguans will die from Covid-19 than if economic aid and effective public health measures were implemented.

Opposition disorganization and fragmentation make political challenges to Ortega and Murillo difficult, even if the scheduled 2021 elections are already unlikely to be free and fair. Ortega and Murillo's personalization of state institutions was complete after 2018, and the Covid-19 crisis reinforced that a post-Ortega-Murillo Nicaragua needs a wholesale reconstruction of political and economic institutions (Cortés Ramos, López Baltodano, and Moncada Bellorin 2020), on a scale unseen since the 1979–1990 revolutionary period. This project will require vision, commitment, and leadership from Nicaraguans from across the political spectrum; the strength and resilience Nicaraguan civil society has displayed throughout the Covid-19 crisis; and continuing support from international institutions.

Note

1 Close (2016) adapts the concept of amoral familism from Banfield (1958), whose original work on rural Italy has been rightly criticized for its biases.

References

100% Noticias. 2020. 'Nayib Bukele Preocupado Por Negligencia de La Dictadura de Daniel Ortega Ante Coronavirus.' *100% Noticias*, March 21.

Álvarez, Leonor. 2020a. 'Orteguismo Inunda Redes Sociales Con Noticias Falsas Cuando Crecen Reportes de Casos de Covid-19.' *La Prensa*, May 8.

———. 2020b. 'Rosario Murillo Enfila Sus Dardos Contra Costa Rica: "Países Que Se Dicen Europeos."' *La Prensa*, May 19.

Amnesty International. 2020. 'Open Letter to Daniel Ortega, President of Nicaragua, Sent by International Organizations.' London.

Baltodano, Isela. 2020. 'Régimen Orteguista Manda a Los Policías Protegidos Con Mascarillas a Las Calles.' *La Prensa*, March 25.

Banco Central de Nicaragua. 2020. 'Salario Nominal y Real.' Managua: BCN.

Banfield, Edward C. 1958. *The Moral Basis of a Backward Society*. Glencoe, IL: The Free Press.

Bow, Juan Carlos. 2020a. 'Nicaragua, El Único País Latinoamericano Con Las Fronteras Abiertas.' *Confidencial*, April 2.

———. 2020b. 'El Ataque de Ortega Al #QuedateEnCasa y Otros Tres Errores Contra La Covid-19.' *Confidencial*, May 1.

———. 2020c. 'Dos Meses Después, Donación de 26,000 Pruebas Covid-19 No Se Ha Usado.' *Confidencial*, June 7.

Close, David. 2016. *Nicaragua: Navigating the Politics of Democracy*. Boulder: Lynne Rienner.

Confidencial. 2020. 'Médicos Denuncian 'inseguridad' En Hospitales Frente Al Covid-19.' *Confidencial*, March 25.

Cordoba, Jose De. 2020. 'Nicaraguan Doctors Who Spoke Up Are Fired.' *Wall Street Journal*, July 28.

Correia, Sergio, Stephan Luck, and Emil Verner. 2020. 'Pandemics Depress the Economy, Public Health Interventions Do Not: Evidence from the 1918 Flu.' https://doi.org/10.2139/ssrn.3561560.

Cortés Ramos, Alberto, Umanzor López Baltodano, and Ludwing Moncada Bellorin, (eds.) 2020. *Anhelos de Un Nuevo Horizonte: Aportes Para Una Nicaragua Democrática*. San José, CR: FLACSO.

Cruz, Ana Lucía. 2020. 'PAHO: Nicaragua Is the Only C.A. Country with No Covid-19 Test Reports.' *Confidencial*, June 28.

Delgado, Antonio Maria. 2020. 'Defying Pandemic Fears, the Nicaraguan Government Shuns Social Distancing.' *Miami Herald*, April 2.

Grupo Interdisciplinario de Expertos Independientes. 2018. 'Nicaragua: Informe Sobre Los Hechos de Violencia Ocurridos Entre El 18 de Abril y El 30 de Mayo de 2018.' Washington, DC: GIEI.

Huete-Pérez, Jorge. 2018. 'Nicaragua's Human Rights Crisis Requires International Response.' *PLoS Neglected Tropical Diseases* 13 (3): 1–4.

Huete-Pérez, Jorge, and John Hildebrand. 2020. 'Nicaragua's Covid-19 Crisis Demands a Response.' *Science* 369 (6502): 385.

Inter-American Commission on Human Rights. 2018. 'Gross Human Rights Violations in the Context of Social Protests in Nicaragua.' Washington, DC.

Jarquîn, Edmundo, ed. 2016. *El Régimen de Ortega: ¿una Nueva Dictadura Familiar En El Continente?* Managua: PAVSA.

Jarquín, Mateo C., Andrea M. Prado, and Benjamin Gallo Marin. 2020. 'Nicaragua's Response to Covid-19—Authors' Reply.' *The Lancet Global Health*, no. 20: 30220.

Kincaid, Jake. 2020. 'Nicaraguan Doctors Say Population Now Fighting Two Enemies: The Government and Covid-19.' *Miami Herald*, July 15.

Latinobarómetro. 2017. *Informe 2017*. Santiago: Corporación Latinobarómetro.

———. 2018. *Informe 2018*. Santiago: Corporación Latinobarómetro.

Leiva, Noe. 2020. 'Honduras and Costa Rica Take Measures to Stop the Entry of Nicaraguans.' *Tico Times*, May 16.

Lister, Tim. 2020. 'Nicaragua's Ortega Says Covid-19 Is under Control, Unlike in 'capitalist' Countries. Local Epidemiologists Disagree.' *CNN*, July 22.

López Ocampo, Ismael and Mary Beth Sheridan. 2020. '"Express Burials" Raise Fears That Nicaragua Is Hiding a Coronavirus Tragedy.' *Washington Post*, May 17.

Luna, Yader. 2020a. 'Negocios, Iglesias y Universidades Toman Sus Propias Medidas Ante Covid-19.' *Confidencial*, March 17.

———. 2020b. 'Daniel Ortega Replaces Health Minister in Nicaragua amid Coronavirus Pandemic.' *Confidencial*, April 3.

———. 2020c. 'OPS: "Situación de Covid-19 En Nicaragua Es Indeterminada."' *Confidencial*, April 24.

———. 2020d. 'Ortega Reitera Queja Contra Sanciones, Para Asumir "retos" Como Covid-19.' *Confidencial*, May 4.

———. 2020e. '"Elevado Riesgo de Muerte Por Falta de Recursos Sanitarios", Alertan Más de 700 Médicos.' *Confidencial* , May 28.

———. 2020f. 'Ortega Impone Impuestos "ilegales e Inmorales" a Ventiladores, y Mascarillas Para Prevenir Covid-19.' *Confidencial*, July 3.

Martí i Puig, Salvador. 2016. 'Nicaragua: País Bolivariano, Pero No Del Todo.' *Política Exterior*, no. November/December: 28–34.

Martí i Puig, Salvador and Macià Serra. 2020. 'Nicaragua: De-Democratization and Regime Crisis.' *Latin American Politics and Society* 62 (2): 117–36.

Medrano, Mario. 2020. 'Más de 500 Médicos En Nicaragua Piden Al Gobierno Estrategia Frente Al Covid-19 y Protección Del Personal Sanitario.' *CNN Español*, May 7.

Miranda Aburto, Wilfredo. 2020a. 'Gobierno Centraliza y Calla Sobre Pruebas de Coronavirus.' *Confidencial*, March 19.

———. 2020b. 'Rosario Murillo Orders Recreational Activities in Nicaragua Despite the Coronavirus.' *Confidencial*, March 19.

———. 2020c. 'Visitas Casa a Casa: Bajo Indiferencia de La Población y Reticencia de Empleados Públicos.' *Confidencial*, March 21.

———. 2020d. 'Nicaragua's "Express Burials" Raise Fears Ortega Is Hiding True Scale of Pandemic.' *The Guardian*, May 19.

Munguía, Ivette. 2020a. 'PAHO "Concerned" About the Nicaraguan Government's Response to Covid-19.' *Confidencial*, April 8.

———. 2020b. 'PAHO: "In Nicaragua Covid-19 Spread Is Already at Community Level."' *Confidencial*, May 28.

Navas, Lucía. 2020. 'Régimen Modifica Acuerdo Con BCIE Para Usar US$11 Millones Para Enfrentar Emergencia Por Covid-19.' *La Prensa*, May 8.

Nicaragua Investiga. 2019. '¿Cuánto Dinero Tiene Daniel Ortega? La Incalculable Fortuna Del Presidente.' YouTube. 2019. https://youtu.be/46Kyx2cjWuo.

Orozco, Manuel. 2020. '5ta. Encuesta de Opinión Publica de Nicaraga.' Washington, DC: Inter-American Dialogue.

Ortega, Daniel. 2020. 'Discurso Del Presidente de Nicaragua, Comandante Daniel Ortega.' *El 19 Digital*, April 15.

Peraza C., José Antonio. 2016. 'Colapso Del Sistema Electoral.' In *El Régimen de Ortega: ¿una Nueva Dictadura Familiar En El Continente?*, edited by Edmundo Jarquín, 116–40. Managua: PAVSA.

Pizarro, Ana María. 2011. 'The Health System's Many Pending Issues.' *Envio*, no. 363.

Robinson, Circles. 2020. 'Nicaragua Abre Sus Puertas a Turistas Que Llegan En Cruceros.' *Confidencial*, March 17.

Romero, Keyling T. 2020. 'Minsa Prohíbe Solidaridad de Monseñor Álvarez Para Prevenir Coronavirus.' *Confidencial*, April 6.

Romero, Keyling T. and Ivette Munguía. 2020. 'Régimen Ha Recibido Más de US$15 Millones de Ayuda Por Covid-19.' *Confidencial*, May 10.

Sáenz, Enrique. 2016. 'La Gestión Económica: ¿Despilfarro de Oportunidades?' In *El Régimen de Ortega: ¿una Nueva Dictadura Familiar En El Continente?*, edited by Edmundo Jarquín, 209–65. Managua: PAVSA.

Salazar Mather, Thais P., Benjamin Gallo Marin, Giancarlo Medina Perez, Briana Christophers, Marcelo L. Paiva, Rocío Oliva, Baraa A. Hijaz, et al. 2020. 'Love in the Time of Covid-19: Negligence in the Nicaraguan Response.' *The Lancet. Global Health* 8 (6): e773.

Secretaría Privada para Políticas Nacionales. 2020. 'Informe Sobre El Covid-19 y Una Estrategia Singular.' Managua.

Sequeira, Magda, Henry Espinoza, Juan Jose Amador, Gonzalo Domingo, Margarita Quintanilla, and Tala de los Santos. 2011. 'The Nicaraguan Health System: An Overview of Critical Challenges and Opportunities.' Seattle: PATH.

Silva, Diego. 2020. 'Ortega Ordena Compra Urgente de Alcohol En Gel y Guantes Para Evitar Coronavirus En El Carmen.' *Despacho 505*, April 8.

Sotelo Vargas, Gender and Elena Vargas-Palacios. 2020. 'Políticas de Salud En Nicaragua.' In *Anhelos de Un Nuevo Horizonte: Aportes Para Una Nicaragua Democrática*, edited by Alberto Cortés Ramos, Umanzor López Baltodano, and Ludwing Moncada Bellorin. San José: FLACSO.

Spalding, Rose J. 2017. 'Los Empresarios y El Estado Posrevolucionario: El Reordenamiento de Las Élites y La Nueva Estrategia de Colaboración En Nicaragua.' *Anuario de Estudios Centroamericanos* 43: 149–88.

Steigenga, Timothy, Kenneth M. Coleman, and Eduardo Marenco. 2017. '"En Dios Confiamos": Politics, Populism, and Protestantism in Daniel Ortega's Nicaragua.' *International Journal of Latin American Religions* 1 (1): 116–33.

Thaler, Kai M. 2017. 'Nicaragua: A Return to Caudillismo.' *Journal of Democracy* 28 (2): 157–69.

———. 2020. 'Nicaragua Is Stumbling into Coronavirus Disaster.' *Foreign Policy*, April 17.

Today Nicaragua. 2020. 'Nicaragua Is the Only Country in the Region That Charges for Covid-19 Tests.' *Today Nicaragua*, July 19.

Vargas-Palacios, Elena, Ricardo Pineda, and Edén Galán-Rodas. 2018. 'The Politicised and Crumbling Nicaraguan Health System.' *The Lancet* 392 (10165): 2694–95.

Africa

19

RWANDA AND COVID-19

Leadership and resilient health system

Jeanine Condo and Edson Rwagasore

Rwanda, a country of 13 million, is among the countries in Africa with a growing economy. Its innovative reputation and its use of 'country proof of concept' have benefitted the country over the last two decades. Today, Rwanda uses drones to deliver blood and other essential medical drugs and consumables to overcome the geographic complexities that limit rural access to medical services. In agriculture, drones are used to estimate crops' surfaces, and in transport, the nationwide use of electronic cards to pay bus fares, known as 'tap and go', has reduced unnecessary transactions. With telephone penetration at more than 80 percent of the population, the use of mobile-money, known as 'MOMO', is another nationwide electronic transaction system to pay retailers from small supermarkets to pharmacies, shops and so on.

As soon as Covid-19 was declared, Rwanda adopted a national rapid response team, coordinated at a centralized level with local administrative bodies to implement measures at the district—sectoral—and village levels. The rapid response team, formed at the prime minister's office, was in charge of delivering clear messages to the community, developing measures to protect the population and mobilizing human resources and funds to fight Covid-19 as well as its economic consequences. Rwanda used robots to conduct basic clinical checks among patients with Covid-19, and also set up these robots at Kigali International Airport (KIA). The country's response has been informed from its past experience combating other communicable and non-communicable diseases, including Ebola, Zika, Chikungunya and others viruses that are observed in the region.

After the declaration of a new outbreak of coronavirus disease-19 (Covid-19) by the National Health Commission of China on December 31, 2019 and the March 11, 2020 WHO declaration of a Public Health Emergency of International Concern (PHEIC), Rwanda developed a Covid-19 preparedness and response plan based on the following key guiding principles: (1) strong political and financial commitments within the country and across the region; (2) utilization of existing institutions and scientific evidence; (3) a multidisciplinary approach that integrates aspects beyond clinical management including technical, social, political and regulatory aspects; (4) protection of Rwandans and people living in Rwanda through prevention and control mechanisms and; (5) continual strengthening of national disease prevention and emergency response.

In the wake of the country's first Covid-19 case in March 2020, Rwanda followed a complete lockdown strategy, closing schools, public transport, shops and interprovincial movements, while allowing only basic services that provide access to food and health services. The Ministry of Health, Ministry of Local Government and other institutions concerned with the pandemic outbreak quickly created a structured and coordinated incident management system to fight against Covid-19. Different groups were developed to handle: (1) management and operations, including multi-sectoral and multi-partner coordination mechanisms to facilitate implementation of the action plan; (2) workforce capacity development and analysis of human resource needs (clinicians, media, mapping of vulnerable populations, etc.); (3) logistics, stakeholder engagement and mobilization of financial resources from within the country and across the region (printing of SOPs, data collection and reporting tools, etc.); and (4) monitoring and evaluation (development of M&E frameworks). The rapid implementation of nationwide interventions following lockdown is a reflection of a responsive and responsible government to fight against Covid-19 while minimizing the risk of new infection and number of deaths among its population. (Condo et al., 2020; Lazarus et al., 2020).

National capabilities for testing, surveillance and response were also assessed and strengthened by adopting new tools and a platform that allowed for the digitalization of health data and geo-mapping of cases across countries. Protocols for testing and referral systems were implemented to avoid or minimize any risk of contamination from sample collection, sample packaging, sample transportation and sample analysis. Within 6–24 hours, results are shared via text message to individuals tested for Covid-19. When results come back positive, a contact tracing process begins, using recall history and prompt retrieval of all persons in contact with the active case within the 2–14 days preceding the laboratory test result.

Community awareness and engagement strategies were immediately put in place with the involvement of the top leadership of the country. Clear messages were communicated to raise awareness of Covid-19, including common symptoms, where to seek help and how to prevent its spread. For example, the President of the Republic of Rwanda, Paul Kagame, shared appropriate hand-washing techniques on Twitter and through different communication channels as well as other steps that communities should take. The government sought to ensure that all Rwandans and people living in Rwanda understood the steps undertaken by its institutions, and debates and talk shows on TV and radio were coordinated to maximize engagement in the community. During these talk shows and news, ministers were invited to explain what the government was doing to curb Covid-19, using local language to allow individuals across all socio-economic layers to expresses his/her own opinion, question, concern and so on.

Partial release of lockdown after reduction of reported cases

During complete lockdown all points of entry to the country were closed. After the partial release of stringent lockdown measures, points of entry staff began systematic screening. Measures for the early detection of potential cases, identification of appropriate isolation rooms and timely containment practices were put in place. For example, crossborder truck drivers were tested systematically and a system of driver exchanges was put into place by Eastern African Countries (EAC) to minimize contamination from drivers to general population. Each truck coming from outside Rwanda was assigned to another Rwandan driver to drive the truck from the border to within the country. The relaxation of lockdown measures also included measures that certain workers in both the private and public sectors should work from home. Working hours and curfew hours were communicated through the office of the prime minister to the community using local newsletters, radio, TV and Twitter messages.

All public and open spaces, including markets, shops, offices and bus stations, were instructed to implement the following mandatory measures:

(1) All individuals were instructed to use water and soap systematically before entering compounds/buildings.
(2) A system of temperature recording was immediately initiated across all spaces across the country. Individuals with high fever were not permitted to enter buildings and were requested to consult their nearest clinic. Direct communication with the Ministry of Health was established for follow-up with individuals with a fever or any other signs leading to Covid-19.
(3) Use of individual containers alcohol was encouraged and reinforced during working hours so no sharing occurred.
(4) Individuals were instructed to not leave their house without wearing a facial mask, even those driving in private cars.
(5) Social distancing measures were systematically implemented with signs on floors indicating where each individual queuing should stand.
(6) Youth volunteers were deployed at transportation hubs to reinforce social distancing and wearing facial masks.

The graph below summarizes key steps taken by the government to curb the coronavirus pandemic in Rwanda.

The health sector and Covid-19

Rwanda, like many countries across the world, implemented preventive measures to protect its population and people living in Rwanda. Leadership and strong governance were key for reducing new cases. As of October 22, 2020, there are 5,017

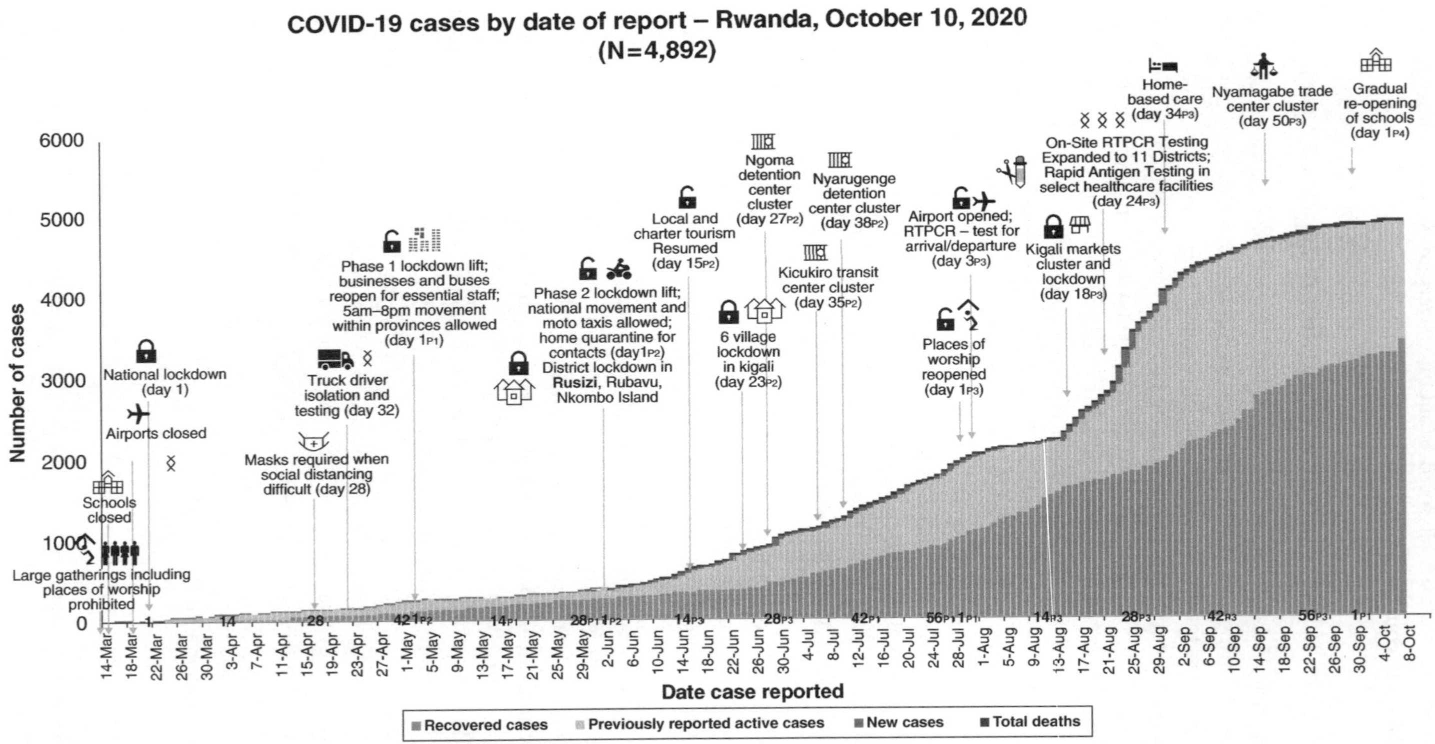

Cases per million population (Case fatality rate) = 378 (0.6%); Global=4,671 (3%); Africa=1,271 (2%); South Africa=11,571 (2%); Ethiopia=701 (2%); Surrounding Countries: Kenya=744 (2%); Uganda=203 (1%); DRC=121 (3%): Data unreliable; Tanzania, Burundi.

FIGURE 19.1 Government steps to curb the coronavirus pandemic in Rwanda

positive tests out of 540,136 tests performed, which reflects a positivity rate of 0.93 percent. The total number of deaths is 34.

Due to the stringent measures implemented during lockdown, other health services such as immunization, nutrition growth monitoring program (GMP) and family planning may have been affected by the lockdown measures put in place between March and May 2020. An analysis conducted by the National Early Childhood Development Program (NECD) shows a decline in the number of children under five who have reported for monthly GMP. Likewise, people who are exposed to non-communicable diseases (high or low blood pressure, diabetes, cardiovascular diseases, etc.) or chronic diseases (HIV/AIDS, Hepatitis, etc.) that require continuous pickup of medication may have faced difficulties related to transport from home to health facilities, reducing their level of adherence to treatment. Although the government of Rwanda mobilized funds to support existing health activities, most human resources have been involved with the fight against Covid-19. This shift has placed a substantial burden on the delivery of other routine services.

Rwanda's approach to managing Covid-19 and its consequences

Rwanda's complete lockdown was implemented from the second week of March to May 4, 2020, following Rwanda's first confirmed positive case. During the first week of lockdown, a command post was set up along with an extensive contact tracing program. The command center first carried out a complete screening of workers at ports of entry, including flight attendants. The command center is mainly managed by the Ministry of Health, and employs health providers and local government employees to support the existing health workforce. Since its onset, Rwanda has communicated its Covid data on a daily basis both internationally and locally. This has also been done using local languages, thus reinforcing the population's understanding and awareness for the measures put in place. So far, Rwanda has placed emphasis on testing high risk groups, such as Rwandans returning from abroad or foreigners in transit to Rwanda. Testing was made available at all points of entry, including airports and all borders with all neighboring countries. This strategy minimized spread of the disease into the general population.

Access to essential services, such as medical services, markets and food shops, was not affected by the lockdown, but transport from home to health facilities was often hard to find. At a decentralized level, provincial and districts authorities enforced social distancing measures of 1–2 meters, mandated use of handwashing stations and implemented programs to provide mass access to masks and to teach their appropriate use. Many of the country's lockdown measures were difficult for portions of the population that live on a daily income that depends on the availability of daily work, thus affecting their overall purchasing power for foods and other basic needs. To partially remedy these difficulties, the government of Rwanda implemented fixed price tariffs on food goods to avoid price increases during lockdown.

Rwanda's approach to individual and community Covid-19 screening

More than 400 individuals from the government and private sectors were mobilized to support the country's command posts, which focused on the following tasks: (1) overseeing the command post activities; (2) strengthening Covid-19 surveillance in health facilities across all districts; (3) activation of district response team across all districts; (4) enhancement of temperature recording processes and systematic screening of all individuals working at points of entries, anyone who crossed the borders and who worked in crowded places such as banks, clubs or bars; (5) strengthening risk communication and community engagement.

Rwanda's community screening strategy focused first on hotspots, followed by systematic screening of all individuals, starting in the capital city and then moving to districts and provinces bordering Rwanda and neighboring countries. Covid-19 screening processes were carried out mainly by robots, doctors and medical students who just finished their last year of medical school. The use of robots facilitates social distancing between health providers and patients as well as avoidance of unnecessary contact (Musanabaganwa et al., 2020). Efforts were taken to train the country's health workforce on how to correctly conduct throat swab collection, and laboratory technicians were equipped to transport samples for analysis at the national reference laboratory under Rwanda Biomedical Center (RBC).

Individual and community Covid-19 contact tracing

Rwanda has identified contact tracing as a critical step to reduce contamination within its communities. Once a Covid-19 case is suspected, a sample is collected at an identified satellite sample collection site, and the result becomes available within six hours using PCR (Nachega et al., 2020). If the result comes back positive, the infected individual is placed into isolation and a contact tracing procedure is initiated using the following steps: (1) open an investigation using trained Covid-19 case investigators; (2) conduct memory history to recall all possible contacts (within one meter) during the contagion window, from two days to 14 days before the onset of symptoms; (3) follow-up with all contacts to monitor any signs pointing to possible Covid-19 infection, including but not limited to cough, fever and sore throat. This step also includes communicating with household members and examining travel histories.

Mitigation strategies to cope with the economic consequences of lockdown

Rwanda's full lockdown was accompanied by measures to help support populations in the poor and very poor categories. This was possible due to consistent community censuses of population structures by local governments who estimate their population characteristics as part of a universal health insurance process to provide subsidies for vulnerable populations. This process classifies the Rwandan population into four groups based on wealth assets called *ubudehe*, namely rich, middle, poor and very poor. Lists of vulnerable populations were made available, and soon after, all government staff and most private sector employees volunteered to donate one month's salary as a mitigation strategy to supplement the gap in feeding those in the last two categories of *ubudehe*. Soon after, Rwandans were motivated to complement government efforts to continue supporting vulnerable populations through *isibo*, well-organized neighbors or individuals living together. This rapid response to mitigate economic challenges faced by vulnerable groups was facilitated by the existing strong health system and strong local government systems and structures in place.

Strong, resilient leadership and management skills constitute a prerequisite for overcoming the burdens of the pandemic. For the last two decades, a culture of accountability, including proper asset management, has been instilled in all government officials to achieve Rwanda's 'Vision 2020' and now 'Vision 2050' targets. Prior to Covid-19, the government was able to implement preventive measures following the International Health Security regulations, and as a result, Rwanda never recorded any cases of Ebola. Likewise, strong collaboration across borders made the implementation of preventive measures possible to minimize importation of case across borders. During Covid-19, consistent support from leadership in addition to teamwork across government and non-governmental organizations has resulted in a more coordinated effort.

Strong, resilient health system to supplement measures to curb Covid-19 cases in country

Over the last decade, Rwanda's health system has delivered a number of significant health outcomes (WHO, 2020). These include an 80 percent reduction in maternal mortality from 2005 to 2015 and a 70 percent reduction in infant mortality during the same period. Life expectancy has increased from 49 years in 2000 to 67 years in 2018. Primary health care is now universal due to government efforts, and over 90 percent of all Rwandans are enrolled into a health insurance plan. Access and use of maternal and child health services (MCH) have improved significantly over decades. Women of childbearing age enjoy full antenatal care, and universal coverage of first antenatal care is estimated at 99 percent in 2014/15, up from 8 percent in 2000. Over 90 percent of women now have skilled assistance during delivery, and child immunization coverage has improved over the last 10 years with over 93 percent of children aged 12–23 months receiving all basic vaccines, with no significant variation between boys and girls or between rural and urban locations (Gurusamy and Janagaraj, 2018).

Facing future pandemic outbreak

The development of private sector health services and manufacturing of pharmaceutical products and equipment are expected to drive employment and growth.

Rwanda has set out a range of incentives to attract investment into the health sector. These include (1) a corporate income tax holiday of up to seven years when investing an amount equivalent to USD 50 million; (2) an accelerated depreciation rate of 50 percent for the first year; (3) foreign companies investing at least USD 250,000 are allowed to recruit three foreigners without a labor test; (4) exemption of VAT on imported medical equipment. These incentives are targeted at attracting investment in the following areas: (1) production of pharmaceutical products and medical equipment; (2) medical supply distribution companies to ensure that medical products are accessible; (3) health facilities such as clinics, specialized hospitals, and diagnostic centers; (4) medical tourism in the niche subsectors of oncology, cardiology and nephrology; (5) medical education and training institutes such as medical schools, nursing paramedical schools, medical engineering schools, and eLearning platforms.

Rwanda's experience with Covid-19 revealed the importance of having a comprehensive and integrated health surveillance system, of which the digitalization of Community-based Health Insurance (CBHI) and health services are key components. Other important systems identified during Covid-19 include a resource tracking tool as well as community outbreak surveillance and reporting instruments. So far, the Ministry of Health and Ministry of ICT are working together to implement a system that is user-friendly but also comprehensive and integrated to respond to future health crises.

East Africa Regional response to Covid-19 and missed opportunities

Rwanda, like many countries in the continent, is facing limited capacity in testing and laboratory platforms to satisfy the growing demand for rapid Covid-19 testing results. Countries in the EAC have implemented different strategies during the Covid-19 crisis resulting in different mitigations strategies. For example, while Rwanda implemented its nationwide lockdown strategy, Tanzania focused on economic growth as a national priority. The progress of number of cases and therefore its management differed across countries. Figure 19.2 shows the number of cases in

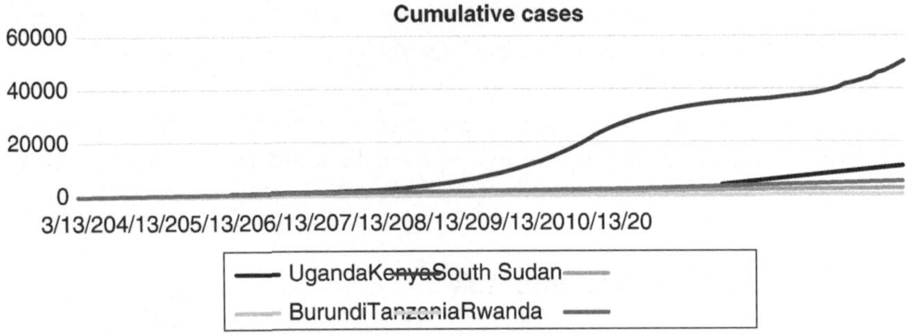

FIGURE 19.2 Distribution of cases in East Africa region

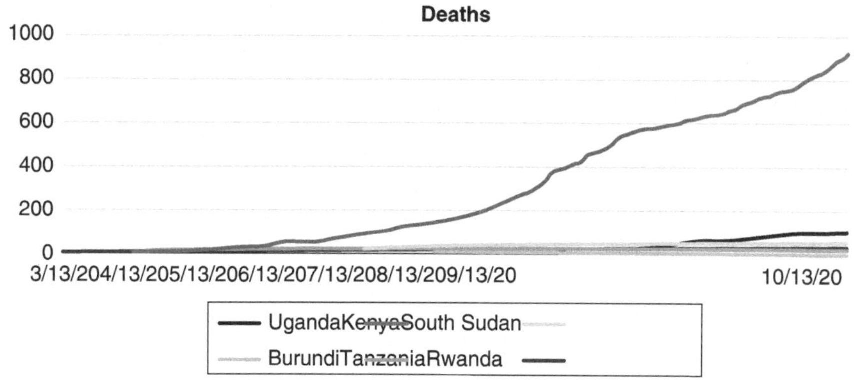

FIGURE 19.3 Distribution of number of deaths due to Covid-19 in East Africa region

EAC and the number of deaths from each country from the declaration of Covid-19 cases up to date.

In view of the above and in order to sustain the gains from the measures put in place so far, a lockdown guideline across countries in the region should be harmonized to minimize spread or importation of cases across borders, thus limiting the vicious circle of contamination and re-contamination within the same population within and across the region. An analysis conducted by David E Phillips et al. stresses the need for implementing strategies and using success stories to better plan health interventions. Non-harmonization has negative impacts on health indicators and outcomes. The same author suggests that Covid-19 could lead to a 45 percent increase in child deaths and a 39 percent increase in maternal deaths across low- and middle-income countries (Phillips et al. published in Johns Hopkins Coronavirus Resource Center, 2020).

The pandemic has left us with key lesson learnt, namely the urgent need for harmonization of governance systems in general and health systems in particular, with strong monitoring and surveillance systems from local to regional levels. These systems should be strong, transparent, supported and resilient to reflect population health across and within countries. Rwanda reveals that good governance, a solid healthcare system and coordination between local and national governments headed by capable leaders paid off in terms of an efficient and well-coordinated response to the Covid-19 pandemic.

References

Condo, J., Uwizihiwe, J. P. and Nsanzimana, S. (2020). Learn from Rwanda's success in tackling Covid-19. *Nature, 581*(7809): 384–384.

Gurusamy, P. S. R. and Janagaraj, P. D. (2018). A success story: the burden of maternal, neonatal and childhood mortality in Rwanda-critical appraisal of interventions and recommendations for the future. *African Journal of Reproductive Health, 22*(2): 9–16.

Johns Hopkins Coronavirus Resource Center. (2020). Covid-19 Dashboard by the Center for Systems Science and Engineering (CSSE). https://coronavirus.jhu.edu/map.html, accessed September 2020.

Lazarus, J.V., Ratzan, S., Palayew, A., Billari, F. C., Binagwaho, A., Kimball, S. and l-Mohandes, A. (2020). Covid-SCORE: A global survey to assess public perceptions of government responses to Covid-19, *PloS one*, *15*(10), e0240011.

Musanabaganwa, C., Semakula, M., Mazarati, J. B., Nyamusore, J., Uwimana, A., Kayumba, M., Umutesi, F., Uwizihiwe, J. P., Muhire, A., Nyatanyi, T., Harvey, T., Hitimana, N., Byiringiro, F., Mutesa, L., Nsanzimana, S. (2020). Use of technologies in Covid-19 containment in Rwanda. *Review of Public Health Bul. Vol. 2*(2): 7–12.

Nachega, J. B., Grimwood, A., Mahomed, H., Fatti, G., Preiser, W., Kallay, O. and Ngamije, D. (2020). From easing lockdowns to scaling-up community-based Covid-19 screening, testing, and contact tracing in Africa: shared approaches, innovations, and challenges to minimize morbidity and mortality. *Clinical Infectious Diseases*, ciaa695, https://doi.org/10.1093/cid/ciaa695.

World Health Organization (2020) Achieving quality health services for all, through better water, sanitation and hygiene - Lessons from three African countries. www.who.int/publications/i/item/9789240009493, accessed September 2020.

20

KENYA AND COVID-19

Ahmed Kalebi

When the first Covid-19 case was suspected in the country, Kenya lacked the capacity to carry out any testing. The Ministry of Health's (MOH) designated reference laboratories were not prepared to conduct Polymerase Chain Reaction (PCR) tests, forcing the patient's sample to be referred to South Africa for confirmation. It took the assistance of the World Health Organization to prepare reference laboratories, as the MOH lacked the reagents necessary to conduct tests. At this time, many low and middle-income countries (LMIC) were caught flat-footed, unable to produce their own reagents for PCR tests. These countries were entirely dependent on importation from developed countries, who were in the throes of the pandemic and thus unable to export. The situation was compounded by a stoppage of global flights, further affecting the shipment of samples. The result was a lack of capacity to undertake testing to make a timely diagnosis. From this precarious starting point, this chapter examines the response of the Kenyan government to the Covid-19 pandemic, outlining how the county's institutions have fared, focusing in particular on healthcare, public health administration, social security and economic support.

Patient zero

In Kenya, the first confirmed case of Covid-19, the 'Patient zero', was a young woman who had returned to the country from the USA through London and traveled home having passed through screening at the airport without being flagged; later she presented herself to a designated center for isolation in Nairobi after developing mild symptoms. The sequence of events thereafter raised concerns and public suspicion that the case was stage-managed. Although it was a genuine case, it was wrongly handled; the situation was unnecessarily dramatized and sensationalized to instill fear among citizens, which made it look like a militaristic affair instead of a health issue, and the government used the opportunity to put in place guidelines to curb community spreading (Human Rights Watch, 2020). Before patient zero was isolated, the systems in place and measures enacted were clearly inadequate to ensure the disease was not imported into the country; rather there was a lot of confusion on who was responsible to prevent any infection getting into the country and how the situation should be managed.

Just like many other countries that were still grappling with the sudden spread of the virus, the MOH's Port Health Services introduced questionnaires to be filled by travelers who were expected to self-declare their symptoms if they had any, as well as people they had come into contact with and the countries they had visited (Kenya Airports Authority, 2020a). However, due to lack of proper supervision, the questionnaires were often not properly filled out. This was quite a shambolic system in comparison with countries like Rwanda, which had implemented more stringent screening procedures. In Kenya's case, the government-issued measures and guidelines were not properly observed as passengers' temperatures would be taken in some flights, while in others, passengers simply walked through immigration without any temperature screenings or questionnaires. There was no systematic approach to the Covid-19 pandemic considering one could have traveled to Kenya from a relatively safe country via countries that were hotspots for infection rates, for example, China and Italy (The Print, 2020).

Thus, although the government put in efforts to implement enhanced surveillance at Jomo Kenyatta International Airport (JKIA) against Covid-19 (Kenya Airports Authority, 2020b), it focused on screening travelers coming from China and European countries while ignoring flights from other countries. For example, travelers from the UAE were not screened. The process was not rigorously implemented, there was no robust debate and discussion on how the pandemic could be handled better, and without proper records and verification of where somebody was staying and very minimal contact tracing, the response was superficial and inadequate. Across the globe, governments picked up suspected Covid-19 patients and isolated them. However, Kenya's patient zero, having arrived from US, traveled home using a taxi and stayed for couple of days, mingling with other people. When she did not feel well, she presented herself to Mbagathi Hospital to seek medical attention; there was no self-quarantine as advocated by the government.

Patient Zero was confirmed on Friday, March 13, 2020, however there was another patient whose case was never confirmed to the public due to circumstances under which the patient was identified. This author's laboratory organized for samples to be collected from another patient who did not travel outside the country, but reported sick on March 16. When her test results came back positive from South Africa, the case was reported to relevant health institutions in the region. The revelation was met with bureaucratic wrangling. The laboratory had to defend itself, noting that it was the private sector and could not turn down a patient's requests to have a test done. Instead of interrogating the patient and doing contact tracing, the response from concerned authorities was drastic, threatening to reprimand the doctor who ordered the test and shut down the laboratory.

Concerns about community transmission in Mombasa were raised to top officials in the Ministry of Health, but it was never discussed in public or in any other forums. As the coastal city experienced intense community transmission early in April and May unlike any seen elsewhere in the country, leading to total lockdown of parts of the city, it revealed the institutional failures for a more robust and transparent assessment of the actual situation.

Responding to an international crisis

When the first case of Covid-19 was announced in China on January 9, 2020 (ECDC, 2020), there were a few calls to stop inbound flights from China. However, the government failed to act, allowing flights from both China and Europe, despite reports showing the first imported case was from Europe. This represents a failure of institutions, allowing flight operations to continue, despite the common knowledge that flights were coming from places with reported cases of Covid-19. The hue and cry from the public was ignored, and it became clear that a number of imported cases were getting into the country. Infected persons failed to self-report to relevant authorities, and therefore potential for seeding the infection in the community was raised.

Due to backlash from the public and apparent lack of self-quarantine, the MOH eventually directed that all incoming passengers must be placed under mandatory quarantine, while international flights remained. The initial move to enforce compulsory quarantine for inbound travelers, however, was ineffective, as passengers were held in airport hallways where they mingled without masks. Eventually, designated centers were identified and passengers were moved there for two weeks of quarantine, but these facilities were mainly hostels in colleges and were not suitable for quarantine. Amidst glaring deficiencies, the government decided to appoint the KMPDC (Kenya Medical Practitioners and Dentist Council) to coordinate the centers for quarantine and isolation; yet the KMPDC is primarily a regulatory body, and is not an operational arm of the MOH.

The systems that were in place were both weak and woefully inadequate. Rather than presenting a clear plan, what emerged was more of a show than a carefully thought-out strategy. The handling of patient zero revealed that there was no advanced crisis preparedness. What followed was the formation of a National Covid-19 task force, as well as steering committees and interministerial teams in an attempt to address the growing concern from the public about the country's preparedness. Before the government suspended all international flights on March 25, Kenya Airways offered a one-way complimentary ticket to Kenyans stranded in New York who wished to return home. Captain Daudi Kimuyu Kibati was the second patient to die in Kenya of Covid-19 complications due to inadequate medical attention. Captain Kibati was in charge of the last flight from New York to Nairobi, which evacuated Kenyans stranded in the United States before the government's ban on international flights took effect (Daily Nation, 2020).

Corruption and complications

As the government began to implement public health measures, the word 'quarantine' became associated with punitive measures by government security agencies against the public, as anyone found to have flouted curfew and cessation of movement got placed under mandatory quarantine, and some of the centers were quite filthy. In addition, anyone who was in contact with those who had tested positive was also taken into mandatory quarantine, while the ones who tested positive were pushed into mandatory isolation in designated hospitals, even if they were asymptomatic. These actions generated a lot of stigma, and many started refusing to go for testing, even when offered for free.

Confusion also arose in terms of who was in charge of managing the pandemic, the central government of the county governments. Though some element of coordination was portrayed between the two arms of government, it became clear that there was a disconnect as county governments protested attempts by the central government to take over some of their mandates under the Constitution, including the power to employ medical staff in their counties and the handling of funds channeled for this effort. There were also numerous *faux pas* by both the central and county governments related to delays in implementing vital restrictions, including bans on religious congregations and restrictions on public transport.

Corruption also played a role in Kenya's botched response. Many donations, World Bank resources and funds from the exchequer are alleged to have been misappropriated. Leakage of public funds has been the subject of investigation by anticorruption agencies, criminal investigation authorities, the Parliament and donors. Checks and balances in institutions charged with procurement, such as the Kenya Medical Supplies Agency (KEMSA) and others charged with expenditure through Treasury, were disregarded.

Controversies about procurement at KEMSA and the scandal surrounding the so-called 'Covid Millionaires' also affected confidence in the health system. The KEMSA exposé (NTV, 2020) disrupted the government's talking points and messaging, causing people to lose trust and confidence in the government. Many Kenyans felt the government had betrayed them and that it was not doing anything serious. Further, senior officials from the Ministry of Health got involved in clearing their names from the scandal, which meant their focus shifted from fighting Covid-19 to defending their names. In addition, law enforcement agencies took the fight against Covid-19 less seriously following the exposé and people stopped wearing masks on public transportation, while no longer following the directive of a reduced number of people in Public Service Vehicles (PSV).

That was a pivotal moment for the country because of the corruption that was exposed and saw the public throw caution to the wind because nobody could speak authoritatively about the epidemic anymore. There was a lot of hype and scaremongering at the beginning of the crisis. Then, there were conspiracy theories that maybe the Covid-19 pandemic was not real. People cried wolf so much, that when the worst did not happen, they questioned why people from the slums were not dying as expected, but nobody explained to the general public why that was happening – they later felt the whole process was a sham.

Testing and tracing

At the beginning of the pandemic, the poor preparedness of the country's health institutions in terms of diagnostic capacity was revealed, as the country was almost entirely dependent on donors (World Bank, UNICEF, CHAI, and Jack Ma Foundation) to undertake testing, lagging behind countries like Rwanda, Uganda and even Djibouti in numbers of tests. Further doubts were raised about the validity and usefulness of the test data that did emerge. A number of companies had introduced the use of rapid tests (antibody and antigen tests) as early as May 2020, and the Health Ministry said that it would advance their use. These rapid tests had some limitations compared to PCR in terms of sensitivity and specificity but could be used on an emergency basis to substantially increase the total number of tests. Further, these tests were much cheaper and could actually inform public health decisions. Unfortunately the country lost the opportunity to use these tests as the MOH failed to approve their use. The Ministry claimed it did not want to confuse the public by telling people there was a test that could be used as an alternative to PCR, thereby causing people to run away from PCR testing. In reality, however, the country did not have the capacity to do enough PCR testing and the cost was high.

From many perspectives, the country performed poorly on testing, contact tracing, treating and surveillance of patients. In a number of counties, the testing for Covid-19 was not optimal. Statistics showed that whereas the country had hit almost 8,000 tests a day between June and July, in September it went below 3,000 tests a day, on average. The Ministry of Health acknowledged the drop in testing, saying there were supply chain issues with unavailability of reagents for the Roche and Abbot automated platforms, further denting the testing efforts. Further, mass testing across the country never happened. The MOH was not doing Point Prevalence Testing (PPT), such that there was a lack of good representation of how the trend of infection was developing in the country. The data from the tests done represented mainly hospitalized patients, truck drivers and travelers at the border, with no representative community-level testing. There has been virtually no testing in rural and low-income areas, including slums.

Six months down the line—in September—the MOH acknowledged the positivity rate was going down and that the infection rate seemed to be decreasing. Statistics released by the MOH as of September 23, 2020 showed that the country had a positivity rate of less than 5 percent, with the weekly positivity rate ranging between 4 percent and 5 percent, indicating a continuous decrease in positivity rate. Data at the Lancet Group of Labs showed that Kenya hit the peak of infection in July 2020, which was corroborated by Kenya Medical Research Institute (KEMRI). However, as per the Ministry's data, the country saw its peak in August 2020. MOH data are often characterized by a delayed turnaround time, as samples are often collected two weeks or more prior to being tested, resulting in time lags of up to four weeks. Indeed, one of the problems the country has faced is that decisions made by the government are informed by old, and not real-time data. Additionally, because of a prolonged turn-around-time, results are sent to contact tracing teams on the ground often more than ten days after sample collection, rendering the results meaningless to contact tracing effort, as the patients would usually be beyond the isolation period. This caused frustration for frontline workers and demoralized them to the point of not actively doing surveillance and contact tracing, as acknowledged by the Ministry of Health—a sign of structural and operational institutional failure.

Low mortality and luck

Fortunately the pandemic has had a mild impact on morbidity and mortality among the Kenyan people, despite possible infection rates of 34–41 percent, as estimated by the KEMRI, which worked out that the peak of the first wave of the epidemic in Kenya occurred in late July and early August. The fatality rate has been low, sparing Kenya the ravaging deaths seen in Europe, South America, the USA and some parts of Asia. Epidemiologically, Kenya has done much better compared to Europe and other continents where case fatality rates and positivity rates have been high. Local data show a case fatality rate of less than 1.5 percent, while the positivity rate overall has not exceeded 15 percent and the number of asymptomatic individuals has been 93 percent, meaning the disease hasn't been severe as experienced in other countries where a huge number of deaths were evident. In Kenya, no mass graves or increased burials were seen. This is a trend that has been seen across Africa, giving the impression the virus is not affecting African people as badly as it has in other places. The same trend was seen in in Tanzania, where the country was not doing much in terms of social distancing, wearing masks and testing, yet the virus did not ravage the population.

The fact that mortality rates have been low is not an indication of better management of the epidemic; data analytics were not informing decision making. There were discussions about reopening schools, restaurants, places of worship and even the airspace; however, the decisions were not made on the basis of epidemiological data. When the president opened both international and domestic flights, the country was at the height of infections as per data released by the Ministry of Health in late July and early August 2020. Debate about the reopening of schools centered on the country's low positivity rate, however it did not consider the fact that when other countries tried reopening schools, many ended up having a second wave of infection. These debates were further confounded by the fact that most data released by health officials were two weeks old or more; this meant the country might have been approaching a second wave of infections while people were still looking at numbers which were lower than reality.

Overall, Kenya and Africa have been very lucky, considering that many people did not wear masks, especially in the rural areas, and as time flew by, most people stopped wearing masks completely, except for a few cautious ones. People disregarding Covid-19 safety measures quickly became the norm with the general public, and politicians could be seen going about their day and holding rallies. At the community level, for example in Kibra slum, people mingle and children play while disregarding all Covid-19 safety precautions. The largest slum in Africa saw intense community transmission with a very high positivity rate. There was a likelihood that the positivity rate for the slum could have been as high as 60 percent. Urban slums were hit with high positivity rates, high rates of infection and community transmission, however, a lot of these infections were missed because testing was not being done intensively or they were misdiagnosed as other infections. Many people were actually diagnosed with malaria, yet there was no malaria in places like Nairobi, so it is more likely that their illness was actually Covid-19. Fortunately the pandemic has not been lethal. Various theories, such as the BCG vaccination, background immunity due to high burden of other infections and warm weather are possible contributors to better outcomes despite a low level of precaution. Slums fared very well in terms of numbers, despite little to no actual actions to handle the infections.

Infrastructure

In preparation for the pandemic, most counties were required to have at least 300 isolation beds, however, an audit by the Kenya Medical Practitioners and Dentists Council (KMPDC) showed that few actually met this criterion. Less than half of the counties met the criterion and for many who did, inspectors were hoodwinked by hiring beds and putting them in their facilities, while they did not actually purchase the beds. The majority of counties completely lacked any ICU facilities, while those with ICU facilities either lacked equipment or personnel, or both. The number of ICU beds were paltry across the country, even in private hospitals. The country was lucky the situation did not unravel as it did in Europe, because if it had needed ICU and isolation beds, the health sector would have been quickly overwhelmed due to lack of capacity. At the height of the epidemic, most of the private facilities in Nairobi were at capacity in July, however, by September 2020 occupancy rates had gone down. Facilities that had the capacity to handle the disease included Kenyatta University Teaching, Referral & Research Hospital (KUTRRH), Mbagathi Hospital and Mombasa Hospital, however the country in general had inadequate capacity.

While the country gradually improved in terms of installing isolation beds and creating health facilities for quarantine and isolation, decisions were made to shift towards home-based care. The home-based care initiative is seen as a success, since most patients were asymptomatic, hence there was no need to put every patient into institutional quarantine while they could be managed from home. Home-based care also helped in destigmatizing Covid-19. The Ministry of Health issued points about home-based care, but the reality of the matter was nobody was following the home-based care protocols and nobody was monitoring the patients. It was more on paper than it was practical. People who were to follow up on these patients often did not have the capacity to do so. Therefore, home-based care was a success in the sense that it decongested the isolation and quarantine centers, but on the other hand it does not exactly reflect a successful management practice.

Kenya's healthcare situation was further complicated by multiple strikes of healthcare workers. Despite money being allocated to fight Covid-19, there has been mismanagement on many fronts, and many personnel have complained about not receiving their salaries and their allowances. Workers' grievances were also centered on a lack of uniformity in terms of how counties were managing their health care workers. Some counties like Homa Bay and Kisumu had prolonged strikes, leaving the facilities unmanned. In this situation, the country was extremely lucky there was no explosion of cases during these times. Even Kenyatta National Hospital (KNH) threatened to go on strike, as the return-to-work formulae they had agreed on was not being honored.

Conclusion

Kenya's handling of the epidemic was not robust and decision-making processes were haphazard. This is perhaps best demonstrated by the lack of seriousness demonstrated by the country's leaders who were tasked with handling the pandemic. Nairobi Senator Johnson Sakaja, for example, chair of Senate Ad-hoc committee on Covid-19 Response, was arrested at the 'Ladies Lounge Club' for flaunting curfew regulations. Many politicians, including the president, spent time traveling the country, visiting churches and engaging with unmasked crowds in campaign rallies. This trend became the norm and by October there were no longer any meaningful measures being implemented by the populace. As a result, the present situation is worse than it was at the beginning. As of October 2020, the country was facing its second wave with a surge in hospital admissions, positivity rate and daily increase in numbers as well as fatalities. This became evident and the Ministry of Health acknowledged it in the third week of October, though many health experts had warned about the rising numbers as early as September.

Kenya has been extremely lucky to have survived Covid-19 without a high mortality rate. The case fatality rate has been 1.2 percent, which is pretty low compared to the global case fatality rate. When the first case was recorded, there was a lot of goodwill and attention from the public, but the government squandered the opportunity and unfortunately 'tenderpreneurs' have prevailed and won the day. The national government has not improved and counties simply pretend to be doing well. The Covid-19 pandemic has in many ways unraveled a rickety governance structure in Kenya, laying threadbare the inadequacies of the devolved governance system and public institutions in general.

References

Daily Nation (2020): *Covid-19: KQ Pilot Daudi Kibati Pays Ultimate Price.* May 13 (www.nation.co.ke/kenya/news/Covid-19-kq-pilot-daudi-kibati-pays-ultimate-price-284356). Retrieved on August 20, 2020.

ECDC (2020): *Event Background Covid-19.* July 2 (www.ecdc.europa.eu/en/novel-coronavirus/event-background-2019). Retrieved on August 20, 2020.

Human Rights Watch (2020): *Kenya: Quarantine Conditions Undermine Rights.* May 28 (www.hrw.org/news/2020/05/28/kenya-quarantine-conditions-undermine-rights). Retrieved on August 20, 2020.

Kenya Airports Authority (2020a): *The Covid-19 Travel Requirements Update 3: Travelers Health Surveillance Form.* March 27 (www.kaa.go.ke/press_release/). Retrieved on August 20, 2020.

Kenya Airports Authority (2020b): *Government Implements Enhanced Surveillance at JKIA Against Coronavirus.* January 23 (www.kaa.go.ke/corporate/careers/life-at-kaa/coronavirus-Covid-19-need-know-kaa-staff/).Retrieved on August 20, 2020.

NTV Kenya (2020): *Covid-19 Millionaires – NTV Investigates by Dennis Okari.* August 17 (www.youtube.com/watch?v=YC1pC6vZtW4). Retrieved on October 3, 2020. As lockdown eases, Kenyan doctors warn Covid still lurking www.news24.com/news24/africa/news/as-lockdown-eases-kenyan-doctors-warn-Covid-still-lurking-20201002.

The Print (2020): *Italy overtakes China, becomes world's deadliest Covid-19 hotspot.* March 20 (https://theprint.in/world/italy-overtakes-china-becomes-worlds-deadliest-Covid-19-hotspot/384287/). Retrieved on August 20, 2020.

21

AFRICA AND COVID-19

Ways forward

Nina Callaghan, Mark Swilling and Merin Jacob

The first coronavirus case in Africa was reported on February 14, 2020 (Travaley, 2020). Learning from the Ebola experience, as far back as January 2020 Liberia was one of the first countries in the world to start testing new arrivals in the country for the Covid-19 virus. The world was poised for a Covid-19 specter of death and sickness on the continent acknowledging poor health systems, a high disease burden including HIV, tuberculosis, malaria and fragile economies on the continent. News headlines in March 2020 warned of a 'ticking time bomb' with fears that overcrowded townships and slums would prevent effective social distancing. As of August 24, 2020, Africa has reported just over 1.1 million Covid-19 cases (0.08 percent of the African population) and 27,856 deaths (approximately 2.5 percent of the total infected population), a much lower number than had been anticipated. While Africa accounts for 16.72 percent of the global population (Worldometer, 2020), confirmed cases in Africa only account for 5 percent of the global total, with South Africa carrying the most confirmed cases and deaths of all African countries (Mwai, 2020).

Most African leaders have used a combination of what is referred to in the Introduction as 'hammer' and 'dance' measures. However, there is a third set of measures that the 'hammer and dance' couplet does not capture, namely the social protection measures needed to mitigate the devastating consequences of economic collapse for the most vulnerable in fragile highly unequal economies. The hammer and dance were evident across the continent: severe restrictions along with innovative responses around screening, testing and direct community health interventions (especially in West Africa with its Ebola experience still fresh in people's minds). But so too were social protection responses. While the continent has not been ravaged by Covid-19 to the degree expected, considering the stage the pandemic is in, economies are taking a beating. Africa is poised to lose 20 million jobs while a third of the continent's countries are at risk of debt distress (Ikouria, 2020). The United

Nations Economic Commission for Africa (UNECA) estimates the continent could lose half of its GDP growth, down to 1.8 percent from an estimated 3.2 percent as a consequence of disrupted value chains, stagnant exports and shrinking investment. The World Bank has gone further to model two scenarios of economic decline in Africa for 2020. Figure 21.1 below plots a severe crisis (dark grey) and a catastrophic crisis (light grey), while the off-white bar is a reference value for growth modeled before Covid-19 (Zeufack et al., 2020).

Aggressive 'hammer' measures to slow and prevent the spread of the pandemic have included lockdowns, curfews and travel bans, adopted by many African nations as infection rates steadily rose on the continent. The response has come at great cost with African leaders requesting debt relief, emergency funds and high levels of cooperation with international finance agencies. Embedded in these requests is the appeal to break with orthodox, punitive lending policies in the hope of getting through the worst of the pandemic on the continent and emerging with resources enough to cope with the aftermath.

This chapter will provide a comparative perspective on the impact of Covid-19 on African political economies. To contextualize these responses to the pandemic, a typology of varieties of African political economies may be useful. Unfortunately, according to two recent reviews (Nölke and Claar, 2013; Fainshmidt et al., 2018), the two dominant methods for assessing these varieties of political economies have thus far largely neglected the African context. Both the Varieties of Capitalism (VoC) and National Business Systems (NBS) approaches have been extended in recent years to take into account the new 'emerging' economic regions, but not the African region. Nölke and Claar's VoC-type application to the South African context is a notable exception (2013).

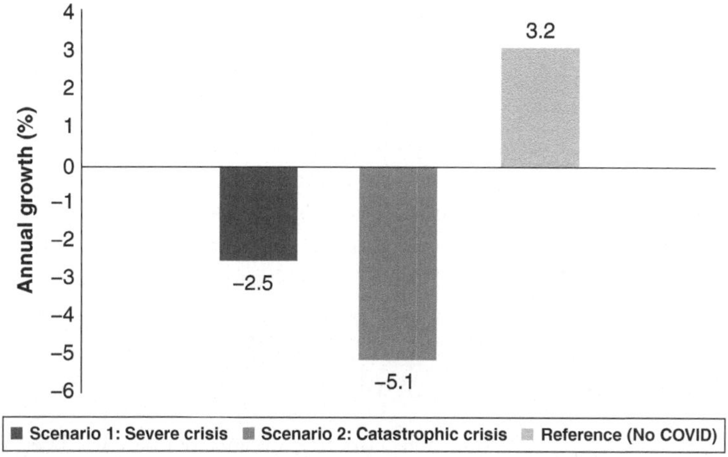

FIGURE 21.1 Effect of Covid-19 on Sub-Saharan Africa's growth rate (real GDP annual growth rate, %), 2020

By contrast, the Varieties of Institutional Systems (VIS) approach does include the African region within a wider global analysis. Compared to the VoC and NBS approaches, the VIS approach 'more comprehensively captures the institutional context provided by the state, financial markets, human capital, social capital and corporate governance institutions' (Fainshmidt et al., 2018, p. 2). Using the VIS analysis, tempered by the suggestive VoC approach to 'state-permeated market economies' proposed by Nölke and Claar, a slightly modified typology of African countries will be extracted from the global profile of countries developed by Fainshmidt et al. (2018). These institutional patterns help contextualize African responses to the Covid-19 pandemic in 2020.

General trends

Economic vulnerability indicators

Using the Supporting Economic Transformation (2020) index, several measurable indicators help to evaluate the impact of the pandemic on African countries (Raga and te Velde, 2020). The ten most significant indicators are as follows:

- Confirmed Covid-19 cases
- Reduction and cancellation of key airlines
- Travel restrictions
- Total trade with China as percentage of GDP (both exports to and imports from China)
- Inbound Chinese tourism
- Foreign direct investment (as net inflows in % of GDP, as well as China's outward FDI)
- External debt in % of GDP
- Current health expenditure as % of GDP
- Healthcare access and quality
- Migrants as % of population.

Drawing from the SET methodology, Ethiopia, Ghana, Sudan, Zambia and Burundi are the five African countries least resilient to the economic impacts of Covid-19 as Figure 21.2 illustrates. These countries top the list because they have less fiscal capacity to buffer the impacts along with poor quality health systems and poor access to them (Raga and te Velde, 2020). Out of the 50 least resilient countries across the world listed on the graph, half are in Africa.

Social protection

The effects of stringent aversion behaviors to contain Covid-19 has been devastating for loss of income and the collapse of the informal sector where 66 percent of working Africans are employed, most of them women (Makhubela, 2018).

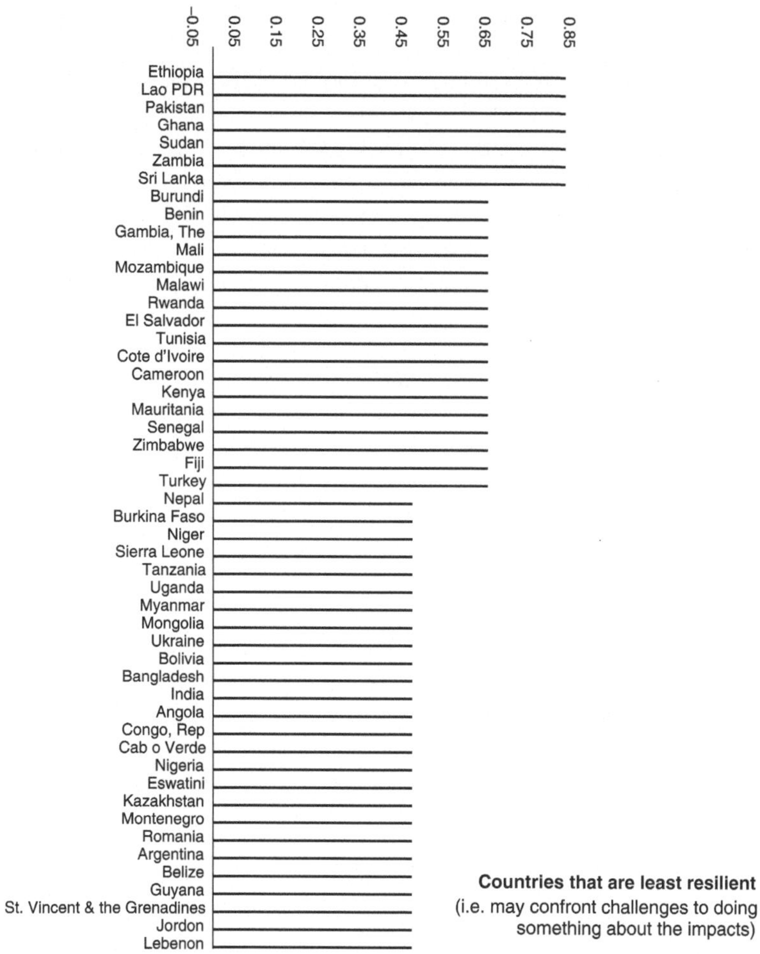

FIGURE 21.2 Economic vulnerability scale due to Covid-19 pandemic

Source: Raga and te Velde (2020).

South Africa, Ghana, Rwanda and Kenya have acted decisively but the suitability and effectiveness of those decisions are being criticized for not being contextual enough. Researchers, some health workers and economists say the measures are commensurate with international experience but are not sensitive to the structural features of African economies (Mahdi et al., 2020).

The suggestion is to relax the hammer measures and protect the most vulnerable via dance measures until 60 percent of the population achieves community immunity (Mahdi et al., 2020). Researchers have in general argued for less hammer and more dance – a phased approach to lockdown regulations to achieve majority community immunity while increasing testing is better than a generalized lockdown as it protects healthcare professionals and reduces stress on the healthcare system. It also allows space for other healthcare services like maternity, vaccinations, HIV and AIDS and other potentially neglected comorbid diseases. Increased livelihood opportunities, access to food and education are also more possible while the economic costs are less (Mahdi et al., 2020).

What is becoming abundantly clear during Covid-19 is that robust business and a healthy economy depends on a healthy society that is not subject to the brutality of inequality and poverty, compounded by social aversion regulations. The most resounding cry by social justice activists across many African states has been for more social protection from economic devastation: this is reflected in the demand for a universal basic income grant (UBI) and increases to existing social protection schemes in the face of the coronavirus crisis to support social distancing measures and help families to emerge and recover from the Covid-19 crisis. Social protection measures include conditional and unconditional cash transfers, school feeding schemes, public works programs, subsidized micro-finance, fee waivers, market price controls and policy changes (Omilola and Kaniki, 2014). Shoring up household poverty and food security is the primary driver behind these calls, acknowledging that most households across Africa are supported by the informal sector that have few to no protection measures.

Traditional development theories suggest that the informal sector is a buffer for the formal economy, and with fewer conditions for employment, the unemployed or former formal economy worker will take up informal employment. Researchers suggest this is not the case in South Africa where there is a high level of unemployment (29 percent) as well as relatively low informal employment (34 percent of workers) (Francis and Valodia, 2020). It is believed the coronavirus pandemic has caused the informal sector to shed more jobs, as a result of enforcing stringent lockdown regulations. Further support for this argument is evidence from the fallout of the 2008 global economic crisis that saw the informal sector contract by 7 percent while the formal sector recorded a 4 percent contraction for many middle-income countries (Rogan, 2016). The informal economy can therefore not be counted on as an absorptive sector.

Food prices have also climbed during this period due to unscrupulous retailers as well as higher value chain costs. Researchers in South Africa estimate that food poverty rates could more than double during strict lockdowns for households dependent on informal labor markets that are prevented from operating (C19 People's Coalition, 2020).

As economies contract, the need to ensure income rises and the argument around a UBI becomes stronger (Gentilini et al., 2020). Income is crucial when we acknowledge consumer spending is a central determinant to a country's gross domestic product and keeping companies profitable by creating demand, even if just for essential goods and services.

UBI is part of fiscal policy, a permanent welfare intervention that is financed through a host of sources – which means it is going to cost the fiscus. This kind of social protection is very different to helicopter money which is part of monetary policy designed to inject a cash supply into the economy, a temporary stimulus.

One such example is a one-off income payment that Namibia has implemented. It is intended to support households that have lost income due to Covid-19. As of June 2020, 173 countries across the world have introduced or adapted their social protection programs in response to Covid-19, including both helicopter money and extended benefits to existing grants. In sub-Saharan Africa, 22 countries have made changes to their welfare programs, largely driven by fee waivers for utilities, in-kind transfers and cash transfers.

Ethiopia, Rwanda, South Africa, Kenya, Lesotho, Namibia, Malawi, Mozambique and Mauritius all have strong social protection infrastructures (Mahdi et al., 2020). South Africa has substantially increased the child support grant and added a marginal top-up on all other grants for six months in an attempt to address hunger and financial distress for at least 18 million citizens dependent on social protection (Web and Vally 2020).

African countries who depend on commodity exports for national revenue have limited cash transfer programs like Chad, Central African Republic, Niger, Gabon, Equatorial Guinea and Cameroon. They will be the hardest hit by the Covid-19 economic downturn and would most likely be the first candidates for international funding and aid (Blin, 2020).

Nigeria is one resource-dependent country that has improved social protection substantially from poor initial coverage. Data from the World Bank show that in 2015 Nigeria supported an estimated 885,000 individuals with cash transfer programs increasing that number to over 9.3 million people during the Covid-19 pandemic. That is a staggering 1054 percent scale-up in social protection measures from pre-Covid-19 levels (Gentilini et al., 2020). Myanmar is the only other country in the world that has shown greater coverage improvement than Nigeria, recording a change of 8684 percent, considering that the global average of improving social coverage hovers at around 233 percent (Gentilini et al., 2020). The Democratic Republic of Congo has also made significant increases, with its change of 990 percent.

Many of these changes still need to be evaluated to understand how these social response measures will work out, going forward, and if they will become an institutional feature of each country's social assistance program. This will impact implementation, considering how long they have been planned and budgeted for and from which sources they will be funded.

Health as social protection

Many African countries have tended to invest more in innovative dance responses than in harsh hammer responses. South Africa is a good example of an extreme hammer response in the early phase of the pandemic that has worked quite well because space was created to prepare for a range of dance and social protection responses and the psychological shock put in place behavioral responses that have helped keep infection and death rates low relative to Europe, USA, Brazil and Russia (albeit high compared to other African countries). Mauritius and Senegal, on the other hand, have emphasized dance responses and ambitious social protection measures.

Mauritius is a sub-Saharan country with a high investment in social protection, allocating 9.3 percent of GDP, compared to the region's 4.5 percent average (Blin, 2020). Only Lesotho, Djibouti, Botswana and South Africa spend more than 6 percent of GDP on social protection (Blin, 2020). Mauritius looks to be one of the African countries that could weather the coronavirus crisis more successfully than others thanks to its broad social coverage and timely policy responses that have included an enforced lockdown and mass testing. The island nation also has one of the most robust health systems on the continent, providing free healthcare to all citizens while it's impressive 3.4 hospital beds per 1,000 population contrasts sharply to the rest of sub-Saharan Africa with just 1.2 beds per 1,000 population. It is noteworthy that Mauritius fares better than many Western countries like the United Kingdom, United States and Canada that have around 2.8 beds per 1,000 (Okereke and Nielson, 2020).

Senegal currently has the highest recovery rates of coronavirus infections on the African continent and the third highest in the world. The West African country is managing this on a comparatively small health budget, of around 6 percent of GDP, smaller than South Africa and up to three times smaller than the US (World Bank, 2016). Senegal is able to test everyone that walks into a health care clinic or hospital. The country's tiered health insurance schemes ensure everyone has access to affordable or free services. Senegal also has expert knowledge, organization and strategies in dealing with disease outbreaks like malaria, HIV/AIDS, Ebola and pneumonia and has put that wealth of experience to work against the coronavirus. Their medical laboratories have put together a Covid-19 test that produces a result within 10 minutes and it only costs USD 1. The test is now undergoing validation trials and production facilities in Dakar and the UK are readying to manufacture millions under a subsidiary of the Pasteur Institute, a specialist in infectious disease testing.

Activists and academics argue Africa's healthcare strengths lie in community healthcare workers and informal systems that have been used extensively in the continent's response to HIV and AIDS, tuberculosis and Ebola (Gichaga et al., 2020). Senegal and Liberia are good examples. Like elsewhere in some other African regions, these countries clearly display a strong institutional memory in dealing with large-scale health emergencies and epidemics. Community healthcare capacity should be built to help in the prevention, monitoring and response to Covid-19 infections as has happened in South Africa and Rwanda. In South Africa, 28,000 community healthcare workers have gone door to door to screen and test, focusing efforts in high density areas. When trained, community health workers can be trusted and this creates accessible sources in helping to dispel misinformation and promote hygiene practices. When enabled to screen and test, they can identify positive infections, link patients to healthcare facilities or advise families on isolation and quarantine. Currently Rwanda is directing its citizens to community health workers as the first referral when they suspect illness or have concerns.

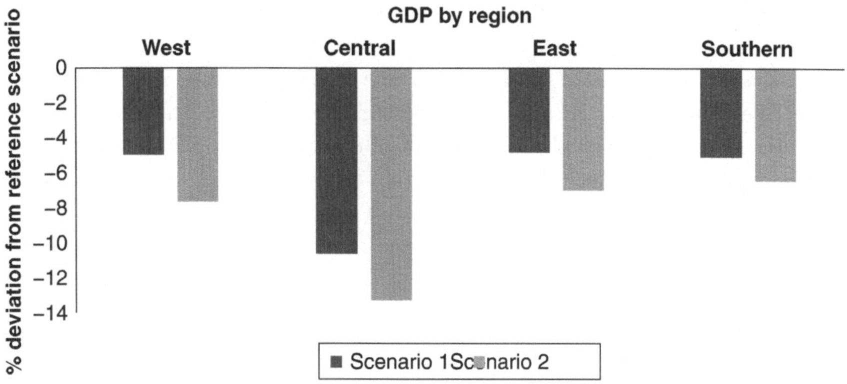

FIGURE 21.3 Impact of Covid-19 on Africa sub-regions, 2020

As technical strengths and resource endowments become clear across Africa's 54 countries, economic decline will not be even across the continent (Zeufack et al., 2020). Figure 21.3 shows how African regions are likely to be impacted by Covid-19 this year. The more optimistic scenarios indicated in dark grey are calculated according to a shorter active pandemic period, good country preparedness, a rapid and effective response to contain the virus and the reserve of government savings. In this scenario, the shocks to GDP are less severe than the second scenario, which is calculated on a longer pandemic period that sees a sustained decline in exports, private investment, private consumption and rising trade costs. Central Africa looks to be hardest hit, for its lack of social relief, quality of health services, state savings and peace and security. This region includes most of the continent's oil exporters, like Chad, Democratic Republic of Congo, Cameroon, Gabon and Equatorial Guinea, who are vulnerable to international shocks related to fluctuating oil prices. These countries also score in the lowest percentile when it comes to the environmental performance index which measures air quality, biodiversity and emissions. These indicators correlate with GDP and a country's preparedness to manage the pandemic (EPI, 2018). East Africa is the least affected sub-region thanks to more intra-regional trade, extensive social protection programs, being a net importer of oil and enjoying better peace and security (Calderon, 2020).

Social protection builds more resilience to weather the crisis and makes for a more enduring recovery. Studies by the Economic Policy Research Institute show that South Africa's social grants reinforce developmental impacts, improving household nutrition, education, health and access to vital services (Sampson, MacQuene and van Niekerk, 2006).

Flatten the debt curve

Scaling up welfare systems and Covid-19 health responses within a short timeframe is not what most African countries can afford. This is an acute reality as tax revenues fall during the pandemic along with national earnings from commodities like oil and minerals (Raga and te Velde, 2020). The continent currently has a total external and domestic debt stock of USD 500 billion. Debt was a problem across all middle- and low-income countries before Covid-19, the pandemic has just exacerbated the problem. The IMF is projecting that gross public debt for these countries (both domestic and external) would reach an average of 55.7 percent of GDP in 2020 (Gelpern, Hagan and Mazarei, 2020).

The G20 has agreed to freeze at least 76 poor countries' debt repayments while the IMF committed to a six-month standstill for 25 countries, most of them in Africa. The IMF has been approached by over 90 countries for emergency relief during the Covid-19 crisis, illustrating that this is not an African problem, but a much bigger debt crisis (Kharas, 2020). In March the IMF pegged the financial needs of developing countries at a conservative USD 2.5 trillion, a burden that will hamper the fight against the pandemic.

It is these very conditions around loan repayments that constrain a country's ability to make decisions in the interest of its development. While it remains beholden, the result is tighter austerity. It is these conditions that some economists blame for many African countries' socio-economic problems in the first place, pre-coronavirus (C19 People's Coalition, 2020). Repaying loans they can ill afford has led to cuts to social spending and health for many African countries that will prove disastrous in the face of the pandemic. Activists, economists and even some African leaders recognize that to acquiesce to IMF loan conditions will reinforce neoliberal policies and further entrench the export of austerity when African economies hard hit by Covid-19 would need to restart.

It is this fear that menaces South Africa, recipient of a USD 4.3 billion IMF loan towards its effort to raise USD 5.7 billion to fund Covid-19 responses. The loan is payable over a period of five years at an interest rate of 1.1 percent and comes with conditions to implement reforms to keep debt sustainable. The loan is not part of an IMF structural adjustment program but still implies conditions as a consequence of borrowing (Maeko, 2020). This would be consistent for all countries qualifying for loans from the IMF's rapid finance instrument, designed for Covid-19 relief specifically.

South Africa's state deficit is expected to rise to 81 percent of gross GDP in the period 2020–2021 and increased austerity is what opposition political parties, trade unions and ordinary citizens fear, along with the ever-present predation of corruption. Balancing the budget often means cuts to public spending, reduced social welfare and tax increases. South Africa has already seen the devastation of austerity measures, especially in the health and education sectors which undermines citizen rights and entrenches inequality. Spending on health for 83 percent of the population that is uninsured has only increased by 1.7 percent in real terms from 2014/15 to 2018/19 (Sibeko, 2019). This provides adequate context for the health crisis experienced in South Africa during the coronavirus pandemic, where state hospitals were found to be in varying conditions of disrepair and suffering a shortage of healthcare personnel. In these ways, austerity has not prioritized the constitutional rights of its citizens, and has decentered equality as a fiscal policy objective (Sibeko, 2019).

Varieties of Institutional Types and Covid-19 responses

The VIS approach integrates the variables that the VoC and NBS approaches take into account, but adds new ones, specifically the role of the state and the role played by financially powerful, politically connected extended families – both being particularly relevant to the African context where patrimonial forms of governance tend to be dominant (Booth and Golooba-Mutebi, 2011; Kelsall, 2013; Pitcher, Moran and Johnston, 2009). The VIS framework takes into account 'five dimensions of economic activity: (1) the role of the state in the economy, (2) the role of financial markets, (3) the role of human capital, (4) the role of social capital, and (5) the role of corporate governance institutions' (Fainshmidt et al., 2018, p. 4) Due to the space limitations of this chapter, it is not possible to describe the full theoretical and methodological approach adopted by Fainshmidt et al. (2018) other than brief descriptions of the five criteria and the key terms used to differentiate between varieties of institutional systems. They provide the following descriptions (Fainshmidt et al., 2018, pp. 4–7):

1. Role of the state: (a) *direct state dominance*: this refers to the way states direct their economies via a lesser or greater role in economic production via state-owned enterprises; (b) *state indirect intervention*: this refers to the variety of modes of intervention in the private sector via rents, patronage or active participation in corporate governance; (c) four *types of states*:
   - *Regulatory state* – rule setting, limited direct intervention;
   - *Welfare state* – protection of welfare and economic participation, including wealth redistribution;
   - *Developmental state* – accelerated industrialization, long-termist, rent-seeking present but not dominant, dense network formation between political and business elites;
   - *Predatory state* – extractive institutions, extensive rent-seeking, opaque decision-making, monopolization of power, patrimonial relations.
2. Role of financial markets: (a) *equity-based markets* (investment-led), and/or (b) *credit-based markets* (loan finance-driven), mixed with/substituted by (c) *family wealth* and (d) *state-provided capital.*
3. Role of human capital: (a) the degree to which *coordination with labor* occurs which, in turn, affects labor stability and wage levels, and (b) the extent and depth of *knowledge capital.*
4. Role of social capital: this refers primarily to the degree of *generalized trust* within society, which affects economic relationships and performance of firms/value chains.
5. Role of corporate governance: (a) degree of *ownership concentration* which affects how owners, management and labor interact – where public governance is

weaker, ownership concentration tends to be higher; (b) the extent of *family ownership* of a given country's economic assets – the norm is a few very wealthy families who own the large bulk of the key assets; and related to this (c) the extent of *family intervention in management* as opposed to reliance on professional managers to run the businesses.

Subject to slight modifications, this framework is useful. We would remove the category 'regulatory state' – all states set rules and regulations. Instead of referring to 'predatory states', we would prefer to refer to them as 'extractivist' states similar to the way this term is used in the Introduction. We also do not find it useful in the African context to distinguish between 'direct state dominance' and 'state indirect intervention'. Instead, the role of the state is, in general, interventionist, but more or less developmental. There are coordinated state-led economies that may not be particularly developmental (e.g. Senegal, South Africa), and developmental state-led market economies (e.g. Rwanda, Ethiopia).

Fainshmidt et al. (2018) build on the VoC and NBS literatures by reclustering their sample into seven configurations of institutional systems: State-led economies, Fragmented with Fragile State economies, Family-led economies, Centralized Tribe-led economies, Emergent Liberal Market economies (similar to VoC LME model), Collaborative Agglomerations and Hierarchically Coordinated economies (similar to the VoC CME model). Table 21.1 depicts the African countries from this survey, but with certain modifications based on our own understanding of these countries.

In our view, Rwanda, Nigeria, Ethiopia, Tunisia, Egypt and Uganda should be characterized as 'state-led' market economies (on Rwanda see Booth and Golooba-Mutebi, 2012), with Ethiopia, Rwanda and Uganda designated as more developmental (although there are, of course, extractive features). Uganda is included in this category, although in recent years the decades-long one-party rule is resulting in a weakening. South Africa is not an emergent LME despite trying to present itself that way. It should be characterized as 'centrally coordinated' (which is similar to Nölke and Claar's notion of 'state-permeated market economies' which they argue is more or less applicable to the South African context). However, the South African state has suffered the consequences of organized kleptocracy.

The obvious question is whether there is a distinctive pattern of responses to the pandemic according to type of state or cluster configuration. Many different types of states have imposed public health measures, including harsh hammer action in Senegal, Sierra Leone and Zimbabwe. Dance approaches (e.g. mandatory wearing of masks, etc.) have been applied in states as different as Botswana and Rwanda. As of August 2020, some African states have allowed a partial reopening of the economy and/or schools, including Benin, Botswana, Cameroon, Lesotho, Djibouti, Nigeria and Burkina Faso. However, precautionary measures remain in place in these countries such as wearing facemasks, using hand sanitizer and gloves and maintaining social distancing (Rutayisire et al., 2020). States as different as South Africa and Nigeria have scaled up social protection measures.

TABLE 21.1 Taxonomy of varieties of institutional systems in Africa

Configuration	*Configuration 1*	*Configuration 2*	*Configuration 3*	*Configuration 4*	*Configuration 5*
Type of institutional system	*State-Led*	*Fragmented with fragile state*	*Family-Led*	*Emergent LME*	*Centrally Coordinated*
The state					
Type of state	Developmental (D) and/or extractivist(E)	Developmental (D) *&/or* Extractivist (E)	Developmental (D) *&/ or* Extractivist (E)	growth-centred.,markets	Developmental
Financial markets					
Equity markets	Low	Low	Low	High	Low
Credit markets	High	Low	High	High	High
Family wealth	Mixed	High	High	Mixed	Low
State-provided capital	High	Low	Low	Low	high
Human capital					
Coordination with labour	Mixed	Low	Low	Low	Mixed
Knowledge capital	Low	Low	Mixed	High	High
Social capital					
Generalised trust	Low	Low	High	High	Low
Corporate governance					
Ownership concentration	High	High	High	High	High
Family ownership	Mixed	Mixed	High	High	Mixed
Family intervention	**High**	Low	High	Mixed	High

(*continued*)

TABLE 21.1 Cont.

Configuration	*Configuration 1*	*Configuration 2*	*Configuration 3*	*Configuration 4*	*Configuration 5*
Type of institutional system	*State-Led*	*Fragmented with fragile state*	*Family-Led*	*Emergent LME*	*Centrally Coordinated*
Countries in the configuration	Ethiopia (D)	Cameroon (E)	Algeria (E)	Botswana	South Africa (with extractive state characteristics)
	Nigeria (E) Rwanda (D) Tunisia (E)	DR Congo (E) Ghana (E), some (D)	Angola (E) Morocco (D)	Namibia	
	Egypt (E) Uganda (D) with fragile features	Kenya (E)			Senegal (D)
		Sudan Tanzania (D)			
Examples of Non-African States	Argentina China India Philippines Singapore Russia		Brazil Mexico Yemen	Hong Kong Singapore	Bulgaria South Korea Taiwan Ukraine

Source: based mostly on Fainshmidt et al. (2018).

Note: we have changed the far-right column from 'Hierarchically Coordinated' to 'Centrally Coordinated', and we have not allocated countries to the clusters in the same way that Fainshmidt et al. have done. We have also modified the meaning of state type.

TABLE 21.2 Measures African countries have taken in response to Covid-19

S/N	*Measures*	*African countries*
1	State loans or credit guarantees for companies	No African country
2	Income subsidies for affected workers	None, no African country
3	Tax deferrals	None, no African country
4	Regulatory forbearance to banks and corporate debtors	Nigeria
5	Social security deferrals or subsidies	None, no African country
6	Central bank grants debt repayment holidays such as loan moratoriums	Egypt, Nigeria
7	Salary donation or pay-cut by top public officials to contribute to coronavirus relief funding	Rwanda, Kenya, Malawi, Nigeria, South Africa
8	President takes a pay-cut, donates salary	Mali, Algeria, South Africa, Rwanda, Malawi
9	Provision of free water supply, food with government bearing the cost during the pandemic	Ghana, Rwanda
10	Tax holiday	Ghana
11	Countries that received support from foreign billionaires'	Nigeria, Zimbabwe, Ethiopia, Rwanda, Cameroun
12	Countries that sought and received support from local billionaires	Nigeria, South Africa[7]
13	Cash payments to all citizens to help them cope with financial difficulty during the pandemic	None, no African country
14	Corporate bailouts	None, no African country
15	Seeking debt forgiveness and other debt relief to reduce the economic impact of coronavirus	sub-Saharan Africa countries
16	Adopting accommodative monetary policies by central banks such as reducing interest rate	Congo, Nigeria, Egypt, Kenya
17	Good Samaritans and philanthropists donating food supplies	South Africa, Nigeria

Source: Ozili (2020).

In response to the Africa CDC recommendation to reduce the spread of Covid-19, 43 African countries have closed their borders, seven have closed international air traffic, two have imposed travel restrictions to and from specific countries, and three have imposed entry/exit restrictions (Rutayisire et al., 2020). In addition, some African countries have instituted mandatory quarantine for all travelers arriving into the country. For instance, people arriving in Rwanda since March 21, 2020 are subject to a mandatory 14-days of quarantine in selected health and testing facilities. Some African Union member states still allow citizens and residents to enter, conditional on 14-day self-quarantine requirements.

As is clear from the descriptions of responses by African Governments, many different types of states have responded in similar ways (Rwanda, Botswana, Nigeria), and similar types of states have responded in different ways (e.g. Rwanda, Ethiopia with respect to their President taking a pay cut).

As far as public perceptions of government responses are concerned, the Africa-wide survey conducted by the Partnership for Evidence-Based Response to Covid-19 (PERC, 2020) provides the most useful overview. In summary, 74 percent of Africans surveyed say their incomes have been reduced (in a range of 86 percent in Uganda to 38 percent in Sudan); 72 percent have experienced barriers to accessing food (in a range of 87 percent in Zimbabwe to 52 percent in Ethiopia), 38 percent said that the restrictions should remain in place (ranging from 52 percent in Mozambique to 26 percent in Nigeria), 60 percent believe restrictions should be eased to get the economy back on track (ranging from 75 percent in Sudan to 44 percent in Mozambique), 72 percent of the respondents are very or somewhat satisfied with the way their governments have responded (in a range of 86 percent in Ghana to 51 percent in Nigeria).

A fairly high average of 72 percent of respondents were satisfied with government responses to the pandemic, but the majority believe restrictions should be lifted to reboot the economy. This is clearly related to the fact that a high proportion experienced contraction in their incomes and restrictions on access to food.

The countries with the highest infection rates as a percent of the total population by October 2020 are South Africa (1.19 percent), Tunisia (0.39 percent), Egypt (0.1 percent) and Ghana (0.15 percent). The death toll as a percentage of infections is less meaningful, because if infections are low then deaths as a percentage of infections will be high. For example, Liberia only had 1,385 infections by October 2020 (0.03 percent of the population) and 82 deaths, which means the death toll as a percentage of infections is 5.92 percent.

It is also not possible to correlate a fragile state with a weak response because of the role international agencies play in these environments. Liberia is a good example. Liberia is often near the top of the list of fragile aid-dependent states. However, it was one of the first countries in the world to start testing for Covid-19 way back in January. This was because there were government and international agencies with extensive Ebola experience, and the population was used to responding to pandemic conditions. This, coupled with very early strict restrictions on who could enter the country, explains why the infection rate in Liberia is so low. It has nothing to do with lack of capacity for testing.

In conclusion, there is a wide variety of institutional systems in Africa which obviously affects responses to the Covid-19 pandemic. More importantly, how they are configured will affect their long-term economic responses in the post-Covid-19 environment. The analysis provided suggests that the forthcoming economic challenges will require the kind of developmental state-led economies that have started to emerge in Africa. With respect to the shorter-term pandemic responses,

Mauritius, Senegal and South Africa are examples of centrally coordinated market economies (with Mauritius probably more of an emerging LME) with well-developed health systems that were re-tooled for coping with the pandemic. However, conjunctural factors affected specific responses: high number of beds in Mauritius, Senegal's prior experience with pandemics and South Africa's 28,000 frontline community health workers. The experience of Liberia and Senegal suggests that a prior history of pandemics is what helps to equip authorities, aid agencies and the population for a rapid and effective response. Nigeria's fear of pandemic-induced social conflict catalyzed an extraordinary increase in social protection. The South African, Ethiopian and Rwandan experience suggests that coordinated hammer-type action at the start is key, but followed up thereafter by dance-type action, including engagements by frontline community workers to increase testing and other public health and social measures impacts.

Africa–China connections

In January 2020, in the early stages of coronavirus in China, low- and middle-income African countries dependent on trade and tourism felt the impact of China's lockdown long before infections even registered in African countries. Since 2009, China overtook the US as Africa's biggest trading partner, a relationship that includes direct foreign investment, trade in resources, manufactured goods and electronics.

China's record of favorable pricing and efficient logistics has made it a critical player in global demand and supply chains. Many African states have become dependent on Chinese imports like textiles, electronics and household goods. Kenya's port of Mombasa has become a regional transport and supply chain hub receiving goods bound for Uganda, Rwanda, Burundi, Democratic Republic of Congo and South Sudan (Okoth, 2020). Mombasa recorded its lowest arrivals of cargo ships from February 2020 to June 2020, most of the lost traffic from China. This has sent ripple effects across borders and down the supply chain, impacting the rail freight service that operates from the port (Kitimo, 2020).

Leaders in the East African region have come together to try and agree on crossborder trade regulations during Covid-19. They acknowledged the snarl up in freight and the impact on value chains due to each country having different regulatory responses to the virus, impacting the movement of cargo and people. Despite the efforts at collaboration, cargo has been stuck for months at Dar es Salaam and Mombasa ports, even as late as August 2020 (CNBC, 2020). Economic analysts in East Africa point to private sector interests that have begun to erode political agreements, where opportunities for selective movement of freight in an already constrained environment has offered narrow and concentrated profits for carrier businesses (CNBC, 2020). Sporadic unilateral decisions on the part of member states of the East African Community (EAC) have also thwarted the collective's intention for the free flow of goods. Kenya shut its borders with Tanzania and Somalia after spikes in Covid-19 infections at the respective border towns. The impact on ordinary people and small business owners has been devastating.

Thousands of small to medium-size enterprises on the continent have been forced to shut down after disruptions to supply chains and an inability to store large stocks. China is Kenya's biggest source market, accounting for up to 40 percent of all imports. Kenya Importers and Small Trader's Association say they've lost USD 300 million since the coronavirus outbreak (Kitimo, 2020). A fourth of all Ugandan imports come from China as well as 60 percent of all South Africa's clothing and textiles (Evans and Over, 2020).

The pandemic has revealed the complex nature of crossborder agreements, with African leaders having to consider their national interests with regional economic prosperity. It is a big test of political will and the skill of negotiation, with different modes of governance converging in the EAC, foreshadowing the kinds of real-time challenges Africa could face in enacting the much-lauded Africa Continental Free Trade Agreement (AfCFTA).

The flow of non-beneficiated natural resources out of Africa means that well-endowed countries do not benefit from their natural wealth, nor do they develop value chains and supportive industrial policies to harness their national and regional development (Massa, 2011).

Ethiopia, Kenya, Tanzania and Zambia have all benefited from Chinese rail projects thanks to the Belt and Road Initiative set up in 2013. Structured into most concessional infrastructure deals, however, is the agreement that public tenders for civil engineering and construction are awarded to bank pre-approved Chinese state-owned enterprises (McGregor and Havenga, 2019). This means that skills development, sector expertise and even opportunity for unskilled labor are lost to Africans.

Beneficiaries of Chinese loans are at further risk when national assets have been factored into state guarantees or public-private partnerships with Chinese contractors. With poor growth forecasts for the next few years, exacerbated by the Covid-19 crisis, over-indebted African countries are likely to default on loan agreements with China and other creditors (Kuo, 2020). Zambia is a good example (Servant, 2020). Kenya is in a similar debt bind with China and is potentially in danger of losing control of its port in Mombasa. The national asset is collateral in the USD 2.3 billion loan to Kenya Railways Corporation for a freight rail linking Mombasa and Nairobi. It is being built by the China Roads and Bridges Corporation (Kacungira, 2017).

Improved infrastructure not only serves nation states but also lays the foundation for intra-continental trade. The much-lauded Africa Continental Free Trade Area (ACFTA) will require this network of roads, rail, energy, water and communication technology that China is investing in (Hedenskog, 2018).

At the recent virtual gathering of African and Chinese leaders, the 'Extraordinary China-Africa Summit on Solidarity Against Covid-19', China made it clear that only non-concessionary loan repayments would be forgiven – a marginal sum as these types of loans make up only 9 percent of the total Chinese lending to the continent (van Staden, 2020). It is business as usual for repayments on interest-bearing loans, so none of the USD 150 billion owing has been forgiven (van Staden,

2020). However, China's President, Xi Jinping, did indicate that loan restructuring would be done on a case-by-case basis.

This overture is a significant indicator of how China plans to be part of Africa's Covid-19 economic recovery, considering Beijing is the continent's largest creditor. Debt relief efforts from larger institutions like the International Monetary Fund (IMF), World Bank and G20 are in danger of servicing Chinese creditors instead of bolstering national fisci. Besides a donation to the IMF relief fund, China has not yet responded commensurate with its role as a major development investor in Africa. And yet it is clear that an economic recovery would be difficult to imagine without them (Campbell, 2020).

Governance and corruption in Covid-19 South Africa

Governing the country during times of austerity and in the shadow of state capture during a pandemic has citizens on tenterhooks, and with good reason. Several government officials have been named in instances of corruption relating to Covid-19 tenders for personal protective equipment. Other irregularities center around tenders for quarantine camps, border security fencing, IT infrastructure, e-learning equipment as well as a host of service delivery complaints around failed food relief delivery, emergency water and sanitation and waste removal amounting to over USD 300 million (Mertens, 2020). These instances of misuse of scarce public funds are included in a litany of complaints received by the Public Protector. It is alleged that politically connected service providers won tenders at inflated prices and delivered poor quality equipment and services during the economic crisis for South Africa.

It appears that the legacy of state capture that resulted in hollowed-out institutions, decimated oversight bodies and manipulated processes have all converged on the Covid-19 crisis to help facilitate large-scale corruption across areas of need and response mechanisms. There are calls by civil society to review what they have identified as flawed procurement processes and diffuse governance (Omarjee, 2020). The national emergency conditions of the coronavirus lockdown allowed government to make extraordinary decisions, bypassing what would have been regular procurement protocol to enable a faster turnaround time. But a decade of state capture during former President Zuma's term 2009–2018 is evidence that massive loopholes exist in the procurement system pre-Covid-19 conditions. One of South Africa's largest unions, COSATU, has made the following recommendations to stem corruption (Omarjee, 2020):

- Centralize procurement under Treasury;
- Ring-fence contracts for local compliant manufacturers;
- Compel state entities to publish details of all contracts awarded;
- Ban politically exposed persons from doing business with the State;
- Finalize the Procurement Bill to be passed by Parliament;
- Investigate and prosecute tender corruption.

In a letter penned to fellow African National Congress (ANC) members, President Ramaphosa has called Covid-19 corruption 'an unforgiveable betrayal', acknowledging that the governing party is deeply implicated at all levels (Ramaphosa, 2020). He has reaffirmed his commitment to act against corruption to a promise-fatigued citizenry whose hope depends on stronger leadership.

A public administration lens is one way to try to understand what an uncaptured state looks like, better considering things like risk, monitoring and evaluation and an overhaul of procurement and oversight systems, but it is just one part of the story. Malfeasance surely has other roots, which asks deeper questions about inheriting colonial or Apartheid governance systems for modern democratic African countries, along with inherited ways of doing business. Economic growth paths that nurture black elites instead of redistributing wealth must be included in this line of questioning as the continent, and indeed the whole world, attempts to review its fragile arrangements exposed by the ravages of coronavirus.

Conclusion

The dire predictions of mass infections and deaths due to poor living conditions and healthcare in Africa did not materialize. Even in South Africa where the greatest number of infections were recorded for an African country (mainly because the capacity existed to do widespread testing), death rates as a percentage of infections (2.7 percent) turned out to be far lower than expected. As of November 11, 2020, hospital admissions of people infected with Covid-19 in South Africa had declined week-on-week for the fourteenth consecutive week.

African governments have deployed a wide range of methods to counter the Covid-19 pandemic. For many, such as Rwanda and South Africa, harsh hammer-like responses were evident at the start of the pandemic. However, in response to researchers and civil society pressure, this gave way to a range of dance-like responses. Senegal and Mauritius led the way in this regard. Nigeria and South Africa were examples of African countries that rapidly increased welfare benefit grants to support the poor. Liberia's and Senegal's advantage was extensive prior experience in dealing with pandemics, while Mauritius already had a well-funded health and welfare system in place. South Africa's formidable security force capabilities were immediately deployed to enforce extreme lockdown provisions that wrecked the economy, while the rapid escalation of testing was enabled by the existence of a vast cadre of frontline community health workers – the legacy of progressive health policies after democratization in 1994. Nigeria's dramatic increase in social grants can be interpreted as desperate action by a state that has hitherto cared little for the poor, but became worried about social conflict arising from predicted mass infections and deaths (which did not materialize).

There are a wide variety of institutional systems across the continent, from the centrally coordinated systems like South Africa and Senegal, to the state-led market economies (some developmental, some extractive), to the fragile states. Although hammer, dance and social protection responses are common across the continent, the degree and extent are determined more by conjunctural factors such as the prior existence of capacitated health systems, prior experience with pandemics, state capacity to act, economic resources and responsiveness to research and civil society. What really matters, however, is how African states respond to the deeper long-term challenges discussed in this chapter. Single resource-dependent fragile states are not well-equipped for tackling this challenge. State-led developmental states and developmentally oriented, centrally coordinated market economies will stand a better chance in the upcoming post-Covid-19 environment.

One thing is certain, the Covid-19 pandemic has had a profound impact on African economies. While the 2007/9 global financial crisis had a relatively limited impact on Africa's real commodity-based economies at a time of heightened demand for primary resources, the 2020 so-called 'pancession' has been a crisis of the 'real economy' and not just the financial economy. To this extent it has had a fundamental impact on African economies, bringing to an end a two-decade period of sustained economic growth for many leading economies.

As argued in the Introduction to the book, the pandemic has brought into relief deeper underlying contradictions that have hitherto been buried below various ideological narratives deployed by African political elites to mask the harsh realities of uneven African development. South Africa is a good case in point. The corruption scandals involving the politically well-connected in the looting of resources destined for poor and starving communities has caused so much anger, that finally for the first time the prosecuting authorities have started to take action against many of the looters-in-chief who have masked what they have done over the past decade behind populist rhetoric. If the pandemic has this effect, there may well be a silver lining around what has been a very dark cloud.

References

African Climate Reality Project (2018) *2018 EPI RESULTS*, *African Climate Reality Project*. Available at: https://climatereality.co.za/environmental-performance-index-releases-2018-results/ [Accessed August 26, 2020].

Blin, M. 2020. Mauritius heads into coronavirus storm with strong social welfare buffers. *The Conversation*, April 16.

Booth, D. and Golooba-Mutebi, F. (2012) Developmental patrimonialism? The case of Rwanda, *African Affairs* 111, 444: 379–403.

C19 People's Coalition. 2020. Help fight Covid-19 by rejecting International Monetary Fund (IMF) and World Bank Loans! *C19 People's Coalition*. Available at: https://c19peoplescoalition.org.za/reject-imf-world-bank/ [Accessed October 2020].

Campbell, J. 2020. Despite new China-Africa tension, Beijing has a pivotal role to play in Africa's Covid-19 Recovery. *Council on Foreign Relations*. Available: www.cfr.org/blog/despite-new-china-africa-tension-beijing-has-pivotal-role-play-africas-covid-19-recovery [Accessed October 2020].

CNBC, 2020. Covid-19: Rwandan bound containers held at Mo mbasa port. *CNBC*, July 8. Available: www.cnbcafrica.com/videos/2020/07/08/covid-19-rwandan-bound-containers-held-at-mombasa-port/ [Accessed July 15, 2020].

EPI, 2018. African Climate Reality Project (2018) *2018 EPI RESULTS, African Climate Reality Project*. Available at: https://climatereality.co.za/environmental-performance-index-releases-2018-results/ [Accessed August 26, 2020].

Evans, D. and Over, M. 2020. The economic impact of Covid-19 in low- and middle-income countries. *Centre for Global Development*, March 12. Available: www.cgdev.org/blog/economic-impact-covid-19-low-and-middle-income-countries [Accessed July 15, 2020].

Fainshmidt, S., Judge, W.Q., Aguilera, R.V. and Smith, A., 2018. Varieties of institutional systems: A contextual taxonomy of understudied countries. *Journal of World Business*, 53(3): 307–322.

Francis, D. and Valodia, I. 2020. Covid-19: The full economic impact will only be known later. *Covid-19 News, University of the Witwatersrand*, June 22. Available: www.wits.ac.za/covid19/covid19-news/latest/covid-19-the-full-economic-impact-will-only-be-known-later.html [Accessed July 5, 2020].

Gelpern, A., Hagan, S. and Mazarei, A. 2020. Debt standstills can help vulnerable governments manage the Covid-19 crisis. *Petersen Institute for International Economics*, April 7. Available: www.piie.com/blogs/realtime-economic-issues-watch/debt-standstills-can-help-vulnerable-governments-manage-covid [Accessed April 30, 2020].

Gentilini, U., Almenfi, M., Orton, I. and Dale, P. 2020. Social protection and job responses to Covid-19: A real-time review of country measures. *World Bank*, June 12.

Gichaga, A., Chandra, A., Wakaba, N., Qureshi, C. and Nepomnyashchiy, L. 2020. Covid-19 highlights the need for community health. *Think Global Health*, March 30. Available: www.thinkglobalhealth.org/article/covid-19-highlights-need-community-health [Accessed May 5, 2020].

Hedenskog, J., 2018. Russia is stepping up its military cooperation in Africa. *Swedish Defense Research Agency*.

Ikouria, E. 2020. Africa's top three asks to combat Covid-19 at the G20 meetings. Africa.com, April 9. Available: https://africa.com/africas-top-three-asks-to-combat-covid-19-at-the-g20-meetings/ [Accessed April 12, 2020].

Kelsall, D.T., 2013. *Business, Politics, and the State in Africa: Challenging the Orthodoxies on Growth and Transformation*. London: Zed Books.

Kacungira, N. 2017. Will Kenya get value for money from its new railway? *BBC*, June. 7 Available: www.bbc.com/news/world-africa-40171095 [accessed July 5, 2020].

Kharas, H. 2020. What to do about the coming debt crisis in developing countries. *Brookings*. Available: www.brookings.edu/blog/future-development/2020/04/13/what-to-do-about-the-coming-debt-crisis-in-developing-countries/ [Accessed August 2020].

Kitimo, A. 2020. Mombasa port, SGR reeling from no-show shipping lines. *The East African*, March 14, 2020. Available: www.theeastafrican.co.ke/news/ea/Mombasa-port-SGR-reeling-from-no-show-shipping-lines/4552908-5490992-e6s40h/index.html [Accessed April 12, 2020].

Kuo, M.A. 2020. Covid-19: The impact on China-Africa debt. *The Diplomat*. Available: https://thediplomat.com/2020/06/covid-19-the-impact-on-china-africa-debt/ [Accessed August 2020].

Maeko, T. 2020. South Africa gets $4.3bn IMF loan: In return, the country must reform. *The Mail & Guardian*. Available: https://mg.co.za/business/2020-07-29-south-africa-gets-4-3bn-imf-loan-in-return-the-country-must-reform/ [Accessed August 2020].

Mahdi, S., van den Heever, A., Francis, D., Valodia, I., Veller, M. and Sachs, M. 2020. South Africa needs to end the lockdown: Here's a blueprint for its replacement. *The Conversation*, April 9.

Makhubela, K. 2018. Africa's greatest economic opportunity: Trading with itself. *World Economic Forum*, January 16. Available: www.weforum.org/agenda/2018/01/why-africas-best-trading-partner-is-itself [Accessed July 5, 2020].

Massa, I. 2011. Export finance activities by the Chinese government. *Overseas Development Institute*, September. Available: www.odi.org/publications/6744-export-finance-activities-chinese-government [Accessed April 20, 2020].

Mazzucato, M. 2020. Capitalism's triple crisis. *Project Syndicate*. Available at: www.project-syndicate.org/commentary/covid19-crises-of-capitalism-new-state-role-by-mariana-mazzucato-2020-03?barrier=accesspaylog [Accessed August 2020].

McGregor, A. and Havenga, M. 2019. China's growing reach in Africa: Are we seeing a fair trade? *The Africa Report*. Available: www.theafricareport.com/17380/chinas-growing-reach-in-africa-are-we-seeing-a-fair-trade/ [Accessed August 2020].

Mwai, P. and Giles, C. 2020 Coronavirus: Is the rate of growth in Africa slowing down? *BBC*, September 1. Available: www.bbc.com/news/world-africa-53181555 [Accessed September 1, 2020].

Mertens, M. 2020. The looting starts deep in the bowels of government, that's where it must be stopped. *Daily Maverick*, August 21. Available: www.dailymaverick.co.za/article/2020-08-21-the-looting-starts-deep-in-the-bowels-of-government-thats-where-it-must-be-stopped/ [Accessed September 30, 2020].

Nölke, A. and Claar, S. 2013. Varieties of capitalism in emerging economies. *Transformation: Critical Perspectives on Southern Africa*, 81(1): 33–54.

Okereke, C. and Nielsen, K. 2020. The problem with predicting coronavirus apocalypse in Africa. *Aljazeera*. Available: www.aljazeera.com/opinions/2020/5/7/the-problem-with-predicting-coronavirus-apocalypse-in-africa/?fbclid=IwAR2tHsH-WXr8JH5n4zoIrW9mmZhJFHnS0mYb3mobXgpZ9G9gcxU1cqkVKww [Accessed August 2020].

Okoth, J. 2020. Kenya's economy has highest Covid-19 risk exposure in Africa. *The Kenyan Wall Street* 29 March. Available: https://kenyanwallstreet.com/kenyas-economy-tops-african-countries-with-the-highest-risk-exposure-to-the-deadly-corona-virus-ahead-of-other-destinations/ [Accessed March 30, 2020].

Omarjee, L. 2020. Covid-19 tender corruption a 'horror story' – Cosatu. *Fin24*. Available at: www.news24.com/fin24/economy/covid-19-tender-corruption-a-horror-story-cosatu-20200805 [Accessed August 2020].

Omilola, B. and Kaniki, S. 2014. Social protection in Africa: A review of potential contribution and impact on poverty reduction. New York: United Nations Development Programme (UNDP).

Ozili, P. K. 2020. Covid-19 in Africa: Socioeconomic impact, policy response and opportunities. *Policy Response and Opportunities (April 13, 2020)*.

Partnership for Evidence-Based Response to Covid-19 (PERC). 2020. Responding to Covid-19 in African Countries: Executive Summary of Polling Results: Cross National Findings. *Ipsos*. Available: www.ipsos.com/sites/default/files/ct/publication/documents/2020-09/executive-summary-cross-national-survey-31-august-2020.pdf [Accessed October 12, 2020].

Pitcher, A., Moran, M. H. and Johnston, M. 2009 Rethinking Patrimonialism and Neopatrimonialism in Africa, *African Studies Review*, 52(01):,125–156. doi: 10.1353/arw.0.0163.

Raga, M. and te Velde, D. 2020. Economic vulnerabilities to health pandemics: Which countries are most vulnerable to the impact of coronavirus? *Supporting Economic Transformation*. Available: https://set.odi.org/wp-content/uploads/2020/02/Economic-Vulnerability.pdf [Accessed May 5, 2020].

Ramaphosa, C. 2020. Let this be a turning point in our fight against corruption. Eyewitness News, August 23. Available: https://ewn.co.za/2020/08/23/read-the-full-letter-ramaphosa-sent-to-the-anc-on-corruption [Accessed September 15, 2020].

Rogan, M. 2016. Informal Employment and the Global Financial Crisis in a Middle-Income Country. *Women in Informal Employment: Globalising and Organising*, April 6. Available: www.wiego.org/blog/informal-employment-and-global-financial-crisis-middle-income-country [Accessed April 6, 2020].

Rutayisire, E., Nkundimana, G., Mitonga, H. K., Boye, A. and Nikwigize, S., 2020. What works and what does not work in response to Covid-19 prevention and control in Africa. *International Journal of Infectious Diseases*, 97: 267–269.

Sampson, M., MacQuene, K. and van Niekerk, I. 2006. Social Grants in South Africa. Policy Brief 1. *Overseas Development Institute.*

Servant, J. 2020. China steps in as Zambia runs out of loan options. *Guardian*, January 7. Available: www.theguardian.com/global-development/2019/dec/11/china-steps-in-as-zambia-runs-out-of-loan-options [accessed July 5, 2020].

Sibeko, B. 2019. The cost of austerity: Lessons for South Africa DRAFT. Available: https://iej.org.za/wp-content/uploads/2020/02/The-cost-austerity-lessons-for-South-Africa-IEJ-30-10-2019.pdf [Accessed July 2020].

Travaly, Y. and Mare, A. 2020. Learning from the best: Evaluating Africa's Covid-19 responses. Brookings, July 8. Available: www.brookings.edu/blog/africa-in-focus/2020/07/08/learning-from-the-best-evaluating-africas-covid-19-responses/ [Accessed August 10, 2020].

van Staden, C. 2020. Covid-19: Not much give from China in its relationship with Africa. *Africa Portal*, June 29. Available: www.africaportal.org/features/covid-19-not-much-give-china-its-relationship-africa/ [Accessed July 15, 2020].

Webb, C and Vally, N. 2020. South Africa has raised social grants: Why this shouldn't be a stop-gap measure. *The Conversation*, May 7. Available at: https://theconversation.com/south-africa-has-raised-social-grants-why-this-shouldnt-be-a-stop-gap-measure-138023 [Accessed August 10, 2020].

World Bank. 2016. Current health expenditure (% of GDP) – Senegal | Data. *data.worldbank.org*. Available: https://data.worldbank.org/indicator/SH.XPD.CHEX.GD.ZS?end=2016&locations=SN&start=2005 [Accessed October 28, 2020].

Worldometer. 2020. Population of Africa (2020) - Worldometer. *www.worldometers.info*. Available: www.worldometers.info/world-population/africa-population/#:~:text= The%20current%20population%20of%20Africa [Accessed November 13, 2020].

World Bank – PPIAF Chinese Projects Database, 2008.

Zeufack, A., Calderon, C., Kambou, G., Djofack, C., Kubota, M., Korman, V. and Cantu Canales, C. 2020. Assessing the economic impact of Covid-19 and policy responses in Sub-Saharan Africa. *Africa's Pulse* 21:1–124. Available: https://openknowledge.worldbank.org/bitstream/handle/10986/33541/9781464815683.pdf?sequence=18 [Accessed April 16, 2020].

Crosscutting themes

22

COVID-19 AND MIGRANT WORKERS[1]

The Gulf and Singapore

Habibul Khondker

The central argument of this chapter is that the impact of the pandemic on migrant workers may vary but not their shared experiences of vulnerability, uncertainty, and precarity. The vulnerability of migrant workers is rooted as much in the institutional and politico-economic framework of the countries of origin as in that of the countries of destination. In this chapter, we examine the impact of the Covid-19 pandemic on migrant workers in the Gulf Cooperation Council countries and Singapore who are faced with not only a life-threatening virus but also uncertainties about their jobs and income. Faced with a precarious situation in terms of both physical and mental health, with many migrant workers suffering job and income loss, the impact flows back to their countries of origin. The focus of the chapter is on the role of institutions in the home and host country for migrants to cope with the Covid-19 pandemic. In their countries of origin, migrant workers typically have a family, community, or local government to turn to; as foreign workers, they are dependent on the institutional support provided by host governments. Those who are undocumented remain at the mercy of host governments and the social network of their community. Foreign embassies may host labor attachés, responsible for looking after the welfare of the migrant worker citizens, but they are ill-equipped to deal with crises such as the pandemic. Migrant workers often fall through the cracks of institutional complexes of labor-sending and labor-receiving states. As migrant workers themselves have little bargaining power, they rely on their respective governments and their conditions depend on the bargaining power of their respective governments. For example, in the middle of the pandemic, Saudi Arabia put pressure on the Bangladesh Government to issue passports to 54,000 Rohingyas living in Saudi Arabia and threatened to send back Bangladeshi workers if the Bangladesh Government failed to comply (Dhaka Tribune, 2020b). Migrant workers remain victims of international migration diplomacy, which in turn is rooted in asymmetrical global power. The transnational dimension of power is often absent in the discussion of state-centered discourse of governance. Covid-19 responses allow for a cross-national examination of the political economy as well as relationships between states and their citizens.

The chapter is organized in the following manner. After a brief discussion of the plight of the migrant workers, we present an analytical framework to understand the impact of Covid-19 on the migrant workers highlighting two source countries – Bangladesh and India – and their respective institutional contexts. Following that, we examine the pandemic response *vis-a-vis* the migrant workers in the Gulf Cooperation Council (GCC) countries, Saudi Arabia, United Arab Emirates, Oman, Kuwait, Qatar, and Bahrain that make up the Gulf Cooperation Council, and finally Singapore. In the conclusion, we dwell on the lessons learned.

The plight of migrant workers and their vulnerability

International migrant workers (272 million in 2019) constitute 3.5 percent of the world population (World Migration Report, 2020). In 2018 (latest statistics available), migrants were responsible for global remittances of $USD689 billion. Millions of Global South migrants in the Gulf countries and other prosperous and labor-short countries play an important role in sustaining their families in their countries of origin, denting global poverty.

The virus has not been an 'equal opportunity' threat: poor and marginalized groups have been more adversely affected. That is, class remains central. In both liberal market economies (LME) and state-led market economies (SME) migrant workers and other marginalized groups faced the brunt of the crisis, facing factors rooted in pre-existing institutional arrangements or their lack thereof. If anything, Covid-19 magnified the disadvantage. In the absence of crisis-management institutional structures, short-term, make-shift arrangements were made by states and sometimes by formal and informal civil society organizations as well. (See Table 22.1.)

Drawing upon institutional analysis, this chapter takes into account the state's response to citizens *vis-à-vis* non-citizens, who lack rights and entitlements reserved for citizens in normal circumstances. We add the issue of governance to the varieties of capitalism thesis (Nederveen Pieterse, 2018) with additional focus on types of state and roles of civil society (state-society relations). The subjects of social protection, the rights of foreign workers and workers in the informal sector in general as outlined in the ILO and other international institutional arrangements deserve serious attention. In this chapter, we take a broader view of institutions to include political economy, state ideology, and normative structure guiding state-society relations as well as the larger global structures that influence state capacity. In the context of migrant-receiving countries, concerned international organizations as non-state actors may be included as civil society organizations. The conventional definition of governance, too, needs to be supplemented by the idea of metagovernance that includes the global context.

International organizations such as the International Organization for Migration (IOM) and ILO predicted that the pandemic would lead to dire consequences for

TABLE 22.1 Analytical framework

Country	*Governance type*	*State type*	*Civil society*	*Type of market economy*	*Public health institutions*
GCC	Traditional authority	Neo Developmental	Weak	Extractive/ Coordinated ME	Strong
Singapore	Republic	Strong Developmental	Moderate	State-led ME	Strong
India	Republic	Weak Developmental	Strong	Cronies-dominated ME	Weak
Bangladesh	Republic	Weak Developmental	Moderate	Cronies-dominated ME	Weak

Source: The table builds on Nederveen Pieterse (2018).

migrant workers, pointing to issues of exposure risk, access to health care, ability to cushion the economic impacts and social and cultural factors (IOM, 2020: 4). While global institutions such as the World Bank cheerleads the impacts of remittance in reducing the poverty level in the labor-sending countries (World Bank, 2018), they rarely focus attention on the risks and costs borne by migrant workers. The emergent migration diplomacy has failed to deliver because in a world dominated by neoliberalism, countries of origin see migrant workers as sources of foreign income, and host countries enjoy ready access to low-cost labor: a Faustian bargain. The Covid-19 pandemic gave rise to a multitude of tragedies worldwide; one poignant image was when several employers in Beirut, Lebanon dumped their Ethiopian domestic workers near the Ethiopian Consulate in Beirut (Reuters, 2020a; *The Economist*, 2020: 30) where they milled around, abandoned. Affected by economic free fall, many employers were unable to pay their domestic workers. The country's *kafala* system (not uncommon in the Middle East) linking their passports to their status as domestic service was abandoned only in September 2020 (*Arab News*, 2020).

Pandemic lockdowns forced the closure of business and construction sites. Tens of thousands of migrant workers were laid off or furloughed, and in some cases were forced to work for substantially reduced wages. As workers were often unable to maintain necessary social distance rules at worksites and typically lived in cramped housing conditions, exposure to the pathogen was much higher among migrants than among nationals in host countries (Guardian, 2020). Elsewhere, the virus also spread in densely populated commercial districts where many expatriates share housing to save on rent. Singapore's data showed a division between community-spread versus dormitory spread, the latter reflecting data for migrant or foreign workers. Many migrant workers without jobs and incomes remained stranded in their host countries. In both Singapore and the United Arab Emirates, governments provided free food assisted by local communities.

As the pandemic struck in the West, xenophobia shot up and migrants were often made scapegoats;

> Racial slander or outright violence against migrants or persons of perceived foreign nationality or origin. Such incidents of stigmatization and discrimination often happen against the backdrop of broader systemic inequalities that have serious impacts on public health, as well as in other domains, including education, employment, social services, and access to justice.
>
> (IOM Issue Brief, 14 July 2020)

The Covid-19 pandemic hit migrant workers around the world hard, exposing vulnerabilities and inequities in economic systems. Because of economic disruptions caused by the pandemic, there were massive job losses worldwide. For migrant workers, the loss of jobs has an accentuated effect, as many of them require earning to pay off debts incurred in the procurement of an overseas job, and having flow-on effects on their families in their countries of origin. Some essential jobs kept migrant workers employed, and living in dense housing, it also exposed them to a greater risk of contracting the disease. Losing jobs often detached migrant workers from associated health insurance and coverage.

A sample survey conducted on returnee migrants in Bangladesh in August 2020 revealed that they were not only suffering from unemployment (88 percent) and income loss, but 60 percent claimed they did not have enough food. Moreover, they complained that they were treated badly by the community and were stigmatized. The majority (86 percent) claimed that they did not receive any support from the government (Hasan, 2020). In addition to economic deprivations, migrant workers were also subjected to social stigma in both the host and the home countries. As migrant workers returned home, they were stigmatized as carriers of the virus. Their fortune changed overnight. Once referred to as heroes, remittance soldiers, and so on, migrants were instead viewed with suspicion as threats to their societies. They became strangers in their own countries, quarantined, socially distanced, and ostracized.

Stories about stigmatization dominated Bangladeshi media. Bangladeshi migrants in Italy, which is home to over 100,000 Bangladeshi migrants, were stigmatized in Italy following a Covid-19 test scandal in Bangladesh when one hospital issued a Covid-19 negative certificate fraudulently (Deutsche Welle 2020). Indian migrants faced a similar situation in India as they returned home from cities and other provinces of their own country (Kumar and Mohanty, 2020). In Nepal, returnee migrants from India were subjected to discrimination and oppression partly because of the bungled government policy and in a caste-dominated society they became a 'new low caste' (Chapter 5, this volume). Hate and discrimination against migrants has been exacerbated due to misinformation and fears associated with the Covid-19 pandemic. On May 8, 2020, the Secretary-General of the UN referred to 'a tsunami of hate and xenophobia' (UN News, 2020).

Worldwide, 2 billion or 61.2 percent of workers are in the informal sector. In India, 90 percent of workers are in the informal sector. In Bangladesh, the comparable figure is 85 percent. Many informal workers engaged in non-unionized employment in the cities of Bangladesh and India face the same vulnerabilities of migrant workers in the Middle East and parts of Southeast Asia. The common thread that links these two groups is their structural vulnerability due to the absence of social and legal protection.

Following the surprise lockdown in India in late March that closed down all transport, tens of thousands of migrant workers from the large cities began to return to their home villages, sometimes by foot and bicycle. Migrant workers trekked hundreds of kilometers to reach home and the support of their extended families, in the absence of social protections (Samaddar, 2020). According to the most recent census, in 2011, India had 456 million such migrants, amounting to roughly one-third of its population. Despite being Indian citizens, many find that crossing a state border puts them in a condition on par with international refugees since they often end up without a social protection net at their destination (Vijayaraghavan, 2020).

According to the Asian Development Bank, global remittances could drop by USD 108.6 billion in 2020 due to loss of employment of which Asia is likely to experience a slump of $54.3 billion. In 2019, remittances to the Asia-Pacific region amounted to $315 billion, but are disproportionately important in Pacific Island nations heavily reliant on remittance income per capita. Remittances to India are likely to drop by 23 percent from USD 83 billion last year to USD 64 billion this year due to the coronavirus pandemic, which has resulted in a global recession. Globally, remittances are projected to decline sharply by about 20 percent this year due to the economic crisis induced by the pandemic and shutdowns, according to a World Bank report on the impact of Covid-19 on migration and remittances (Mint, 2020). Remittance flows to Pakistan have dropped year on year by 32 percent from the UAE and 12 percent from Saudi Arabia. In the case of the Philippines, March saw a 39 percent decline in remittances from Kuwait, and a 20 percent decline from the UAE (Ghosh, 2020). Loss of income translates into a loss of remittances and the disappearance of economic support for households. Bangladesh received US$18.3 billion via remittances sent via formal channels in 2019, 73 percent of which came from the GCC countries. Remittances are the second-largest source of foreign earnings in Bangladesh following earnings from readymade garments. In 2019, remittances accounted for the equivalent of 30 percent of the national budget of US$62 billion, or 6 percent of the country's GDP (Sorkar, 2020). According to the Refugee and Migratory Movements Research Unit (RMMRU, nd), remittances account for 85 percent of daily expenditures for the families of overseas migrants. Sixty percent of these families are dependent on remittances for their daily expenses. Failure to secure an income means failure to recuperate the cost of migration, leading to an increase of debts in source countries.

Structurally, both India and Bangladesh are cronies-dominated market economies, where states are negligent in addressing social inequality and rely on migrant workers' remittance as a vital source of revenue. India and Bangladesh scored poorly in the Oxfam's Commitment to Reducing Inequality Index of 2020. The ranks of

India and Bangladesh were 129 and 113, respectively. In the ranking of workers' rights India's rank was 151 and Bangladesh's 109 (Oxfam, 2020).

Gulf countries

GCC countries are virtually dependent on migrant workers and other expatriate professionals for running their economies. Migrant workers range from 33 percent in Saudi Arabia to nearly 90 percent in Qatar and 85 percent in the UAE. According to the Population Division of the United Nations Department of Economic and Social Affairs (UNDESA), there were 35 million international migrants in the GCC countries and Jordan and Lebanon in 2019. Migrants in the six GCC states account for over 10 percent of all migrants globally, while Saudi Arabia and the United Arab Emirates host the third and fifth largest migrant populations in the world (ILO, 2019).

The Gulf countries fall in the category of state-led market economies of a conservative bent, where governments of the extractive state-led market economies protect the interests of the citizens (in some cases a small proportion of the total population) and a much smaller band of elites in the name of national interest. In pursuing these objectives, there are variations in the Gulf countries. The Covid-19 pandemic affected Gulf countries both directly and indirectly when petroleum prices collapsed. Even pre-pandemic, GCC countries experienced a fall in petroleum prices which sparked uncertainty about job prospects in the region. The global political economy of oil pricing impacted the fortunes of millions of migrant workers in the Gulf. (See Table 22.2.)

Although only 10 percent of the world's migrant population is hosted in the GCC, migrants make up a disproportionate share of their populations – 90 percent of the population of Qatar, upwards of 85 percent in the UAE, 70 percent in Kuwait, and 51 percent in Bahrain. Saudi Arabia and Oman are the only two states where migrants are a minority relative to citizens. As of late 2018, estimates of Oman's total population stood at 4,655,366, of whom 2,047,690 (44 percent) were foreign

TABLE 22.2 Covid-19 in GCC countries and Singapore (September 30, 2020)

Country	*Population (million)*	*Total cases*	*Deaths*	*Deaths per million*
Saudi Arabia	34.9	358,336	5,940	170
Qatar	2.8	139,783	239	85
Kuwait	4.2	143,917	886	206
Oman	5.1	124,329	1,435	278
UAE	9.9	174,062	586	59
Bahrain	1.7	87,600	341	198
Singapore	5.8	58,242	29	5

Source: Worldometer, www.worldometers.info/coronavirus/#countries (accessed on December 5, 2020).

nationals (Bel-Air, 2018: 7). In Saudi Arabia, foreign nationals make up 38.3 percent of the total population (Migration Policy Institute, 2020). The influx of South Asian workers began with the petroleum boom in the 1970s drawing chiefly from India, Pakistan, Bangladesh, Nepal, and Sri Lanka, as well the Philippines, Indonesia, Egypt, Ethiopia, and elsewhere in Africa. A large number of workers, especially the newly admitted, are heavily indebted. They often spend a fortune, drawing on high interest moneylenders, with the intent to repay using their expatriate wage. New workers were particularly vulnerable as Covid-19 hit the region, often the first to be laid off.

The employment of migrant workers in Gulf States is guided by a system of employer sponsorship known as the *kafala* system, which gives employers dual powers: over employment and right of residency. The term 'migrant workers' is generally limited to workers – male and female – who are hired under the *kafala* system. The term 'expatriates' refers to white-collar professionals who enjoy internationally competitive benefits and compensations. Apart from travel restrictions, expatriate professionals have mostly worked from home and remained unaffected by the pandemic. Many South Asian migrant workers in the Gulf are in extremely precarious circumstances brought on by global economic convulsions caused by the pandemic. Even at the early stage of the spread of the pandemic, migrant workers were fearful of job losses similar to those experienced in the crisis of 2008 (Wright, 2020). The challenge is not limited to the region's congested labor camps, where one room with bunk beds can sleep about a dozen workers. The virus has also spread in densely populated commercial districts where many expatriates share housing to save on rent. Many have lost jobs and are struggling. *The Guardian* reported: 'Crammed into work camps, stood down from their jobs, facing high rates of infection and with no way home, hundreds of thousands of migrant workers are bearing the brunt of the coronavirus pandemic in the Middle East' (Guardian, 2020). Overcrowding is one of the biggest factors for the surge in cases (Reuters, 2020b).

Gulf governments have spent hundreds of billions of dollars on stimulus packages to shore up the livelihoods of citizens but have offered no direct financial relief for migrants (Chulov and Safi, 2020). There were important variations in the response to the crisis in the Gulf countries. In the UAE, soon after the outbreak, the government issued welcoming messages stating that, regardless of documented or undocumented status, all were welcome at testing centers. The UAE launched a vigorous testing program, and by September 30, 2020, tested 9.7 million (UAE Government, 2020) of 9.9 million people (Worldometer, 2020). The mortality rate also remained very low by world standards at 0.5 percent (Gulf News, 2020). However, in Kuwait, which was probably the worst hit country in the Gulf, death rates have been high and migrant workers have made up the majority of the dead.

One of the strategies adopted in several Gulf countries was to repatriate migrant workers back to their countries of origin. From Qatar, Saudi Arabia, and Kuwait, planeloads of workers were sent back to India. Saudi Arabia was expected to expel 1.2 million of the 11 million foreign workers in the country by the end of 2020.

By the end of June 2020, 300,000 departed while another 180,000 were registered for departure (Ba'rel, 2020a). This was not purely a pandemic reaction. In Saudi Arabia, for example, a policy of reducing migrant workers was already in place. As petroleum prices fell internationally, many ostentatious projects were scaled back. By mid-May 2020, 900,000 South Asian migrants were stranded in the Middle East and as they began to be repatriated, they further added to already swelling unemployment in India. India's unemployment rate in April reached 23.5 percent, meaning 120 million people out of work (Sharma, Adhikari, and Anans, 2020).

With the ensuing economic downturn, many projects were either scaled down or closed. Many companies were forced to lay off foreign workers to cut their losses. In many cases, retirement or severance benefits were not paid as jobs were considered contract jobs. Even when clauses in employment contracts have stipulated the repatriation of workers at the expense of companies, firms have often not abided by these contractual obligations. Due to the conditions of lockdown, workers have been unable to go to the labor court or to find assistance from embassies to resolve their cases. The retrenchment and the pandemic have dealt a joint blow, further increasing their precarity. Some returnee migrants in Kerala from Doha reported in May that in addition to being laid off, those who were working were given fewer hours of work with reduced salaries (George, 2020).

Against this background of precarity, migrant workers 'ordinarily' live in a highly stratified social space, overlapping with national background and skill level. Supervisory roles often go to Indians while Bangladeshi and Nepalese workers are assigned to lower ranks. Domestic workers – mostly women – in the GCC make up 32.8 percent of the 38 million migrant workers in the Arab states. There are 3.77 million domestic workers in the Gulf countries (GCC) and domestic workers remain vulnerable and hostage to the whims of sponsors (due to the *kafala* system). Nurses are mostly from the Philippines, and contribute prominently to service sectors, especially health care services. Their role during the pandemic has been appreciated even from the highest levels of the government in the UAE.

In Gulf countries the process of nationalization of the workforce expedited the reversal of labor migration. Kuwait fired 400 professionals from the Ministry of Public Works abruptly in September 2020 (Serrieh, 2020). Many of the Gulf countries are reconsidering their continued dependence on foreign workers. Restriction on workers may affect the economic wellbeing of their families, risking food security. Continued restrictions on organized and orderly migration may give rise to increased irregular and shadowy border crossings (Yayboke, 2020). In all, the vulnerability of migrant workers is likely to increase. Despite border controls and increased securitization, irregular migration is common in all migrant-receiving countries in Asia. Irregular migration occurs in parallel with regular migration, though figures vary by countries and sub-regions, and data and sources on irregular flows are scarce.

Living arrangements of migrant workers in the Gulf countries have improved, yet the practice of room-sharing of six to eight people continues. Even prior to the pandemic, the UAE built an international image as a country that takes care of foreign workers. In the ensuing period, the government set up two dedicated websites, one for handling workers' claims against employers during the pandemic, and another for processing thousands of travel permits issued by citizens and foreigners alike (Bar'el, 2020b).

Singapore

Singapore is one of the state-led market economies of a developmental type where public interest ranks high as part of the overall priority of national development. Singapore has always relied on foreign workers for low-skilled employment, while nationals acquire more skill-oriented and supervisory roles. From the 1990s, Singapore began to focus on hiring high-end professionals in finance, IT, and biological sciences, offering permanent residency and citizenship. In Singapore, 36 percent of workers are migrant workers making up 1.42 million of Singapore's population of 5.6 million. As of December 2019, 1 million of the migrant workers held 'low skill' jobs in the construction, shipyard, and manufacturing sectors. Migrant workers generally come from low-income countries in search of better-paying opportunities to support their families (Iwamoto, 2020).

Singapore initially received accolades for its success in responding to the Covid-19 crisis, but as the number of affected cases began to swell amongst migrant workers in particular, the state took rapid action. The daily number of new Covid-19 cases escalated in early April 2020. The virus spread among 295,000 low-skilled migrant workers living in dormitories. As of May 6, there were 17,758 confirmed cases among dormitory residents. One dormitory housing approximately 13,000 workers saw 19.4 percent of residents infected (Koh, 2020). In Singapore, 200,000 foreign workers live in 43 dormitories that became the hotspots of the Covid-19 pandemic.

As of June 30, 2020, of the total infected in Singapore, migrant workers, euphemistically called 'dormitory residents', accounted for 94 percent of the cases. By September 16, 2020, the total infected tally was 57,514, of which migrant workers made up 54,271 or 94.36 percent (Ministry of Health, 2020). Singapore has been successful in lowering death rates, which stood at 27 as of mid-September. There were about 14,500 migrant workers in quarantine in Singapore as of August 21, 2020 (The Straits Times, 2020), some clearly infected *in situ*, in quarantine (Goh, 2020). The Singapore Government has planned to build new, improved housing for migrant workers (Phua, 2020).

Singapore mounted a successful and transparent program of testing workers, relocating cases to more hygienic conditions in hotels and docked cruise ships. Singapore was successful in taking timely actions to contain and isolate Covid-19 positive cases, taking aggressive action to contain, trace, and isolate close contacts. In carrying out the task, Singapore set up an inter-ministerial committee and mobilized volunteers.

Meritocratic Singapore has often prided itself in having a government of highly paid competent ministers and civil servants. Critics, mainly online, did not miss this opportunity to criticize their government and 'million-dollar ministers' for not doing as well as their counterparts did in Taiwan. 'Singapore was not so vigilant, and we are paying the price for such failures and missteps today', wrote one writer in an online magazine (Chopra, 2020). Even before the pandemic, unemployment in Singapore in the third quarter of 2019 reached a ten-year high (The Business Times, 2019).

Civil society organizations dedicated to the welfare of migrant workers such as Transient Workers Count Too (TWC2) along with religious organizations played an important role in publicizing the plight of foreign workers, coming to their assistance in the hour of need. This expanded the space of civil society and democracy in Singapore.

Conclusion

Covid-19 starkly exposed the condition of migrant workers, regular or irregular, worldwide. Migrant workers became poster children of marginalized groups, and the term precariat assumed new meaning. Migrants, whether international migrants, or local migrant laborers moving from village to cities for employment, share the common experience of deprivation and exploitation. In the Global South – whether in South Asia, South Africa or South America – migrant workers, disenfranchised and vulnerable, were burdened and impacted by the pandemic. The pandemic revealed both their vulnerabilities as well as their crucial role in the world economy.

The governance of migrant labor in times of crisis reveals more than just the immediacy of the crisis, but also a deep-seated, institutional, and structural relationship between the states and migrant workers. In normal circumstances, informal workers remain exceptionally vulnerable to economic and labor market shocks, being severely affected and unreachable. Many informal workers faced severe poverty and food insecurity. Their conditions were similar to those of undocumented workers in migrant destination countries. Prior to the Covid-19 pandemic-induced challenges, migrants endured multiple forms of employment exploitation and uncertainty in the GCC region because of their weak bargaining position. The situation has been mired by corruption and allegations of human trafficking by a class of exploiters in countries of origin.

According to official sources, between April 1 and September 6, 2020, a total of 111,111 migrant workers returned home, less than predicted, but the departure of migrant workers fell sharply: between January and August of 2019, around 460,000 Bangladeshi workers went abroad, compared with 176,000 workers in the same period the following year. This was at least in part due to the discontinuation of flights out of Bangladesh (Dhaka Tribune, 2020). Bangladesh's government has created a US$85 million fund to help returned migrants, offering them a soft loan without the need for collateral to train migrants so they can find better jobs abroad once the situation returns to normal, and also to provide them with seed money to jumpstart employment-generating activities (Sorkar, 2020).

What lessons can be learned? The pandemic revealed a fragmented healthcare system and low institutional capacity in migrant-sending countries, Bangladesh and India included, as well as a lack of political will to reduce dependence on foreign remittances regardless of the social cost. No matter the regime type, the presence of a strong public healthcare system is pivotal in tackling the pandemic crisis. The lesson is clear: so-called 'authoritarian regimes trample on individuals but can also be good for public health' (Pisani, 2020).

One of the lessons of the pandemic crisis is that it is not an equal opportunity calamity. Some classes, minority groups, and age-groups are more vulnerable than others. As far as foreign workers are concerned, vulnerability increases proportionate to the lack of formal contracts and other legal and social protections. It is time that labor-sending countries review the premises of some fundamental economic strategies. In the long run, they may need to create employment for a large number of potential migrants and restrict migration to a select few. Labor migration will not be halted but reduced: the reduced number of migrants should be better managed, with proper contracts, decent salaries, health insurance as well as basic rights.

Despite the initial shock, Singapore managed to handle the crisis effectively, showing that a disciplined and well-integrated citizenry who trust their government can play a key role in fighting the pandemic. Singapore also demonstrated that a well-run, state-led market economy can be more effective in a crisis than liberal market economies. In many countries, the presence of a responsible citizenry that can understand policies and the consequences of actions is a precondition for good governance. Social inequality is a barrier to the formation of responsible citizens.

Trust in public institutions is a precondition for success in handling crises. An honest and functioning government is a precondition for building a trusting relationship between citizens and the state. What matters most, according to Fukuyama (2020), are state capacity and trust in government, not regime type. That trust is earned over a period of time through tangible performance of the state, hence, the two variables are interdependent. Appropriate and functioning institutions and well-meaning, public-spirited, honest leaders can make a difference in leading a crisis-ridden country out of crisis. A bench line should be drawn for treating the vulnerable sections of people impacted most severely by crisis, whether in their home country or abroad. This group includes irregular or undocumented workers, who lack adequate housing, regular income, and access to healthcare. Actions are in order to prevent the roots of vulnerability.

While the pandemic sheds light on the global political economy, institutional structures of the extractive states, and unequal relations between the migrant-sending and migrant-receiving countries, it also points to possible avenues for progress. Governance matters, but metagovernance plays a key role for weak developmental states such as Bangladesh. While the literature on metagovernance (Jessop, 2011) pays heed to governance of governance and the overarching network of interactivity of the institutions, the discussion still remains state-centric. The concept should be broadened to include the global interstate system that often debilitates the state capacity of smaller, weak states. Reversing the idea, one can conclude that a global integrated response to the crisis would be effective for all the states despite their internal institutional weaknesses. A global rather than parochial nationalist response would help end the crisis.

Note

1 I want to thank Michaela Pelican, Ashiq, Aliya Khondker, and Olav Muurlink for their comments

References

Arab News (2020) 'Lebanon's New Domestic Worker Contract: End to "Kafala Slavery"?' September 13. www.arabnews.com/node/1733866/middle-east (accessed on December 12, 2020).

Bar'el, Zvi (2020a) 'Foreign Workers, Rich and Poor, Sent Packing from Gulf States Over Coronavirus Crisis,' *Haaretz*, June 30.

Bar'el, Zvi (2020b) 'UAE Can Afford to Pay for Coronavirus Fallout as Restrictions Bite,' *Haaretz*, April 16.

Bel-Air De, Francois (2018) Demography, Migration, and the Labor Market in the Gulf. Gulf Labor Markets, Migration, and Population (GLMM). *The Business Times*, Singapore (2019) Singapore Q3 unemployment hits 10-year high. (October 25).

Business Times, Singapore (2019) Singapore Q3 unemployment hits 10-year high. (October 25.) (accessed on July 21, 2020).

Chopra, Kush (2020) 'Where is the Often-Touted Exceptional Leadership of this Government in the COVID-19 Crisis?' *The Online Citizen*, www.onlinecitizenasia.com/2020/05/21/covid-19-and-the-quality-of-pap-leadership/ (accessed on July 12, 2020).

Chulov, M. and M. Safi (2020) 'We're poor people, Middle East Migrant Workers Look for Way Home amid Pandemic,' *The Guardian*, June 9.

Deutsche Welle (2020) 'Bangladeshi Migrants in Italy Stigmatized over Coronavirus Certificate Scam,' www.infomigrants.net/en/post/26190/bangladeshi-migrants-in-italy-stigmatized-over-coronavirus-certificate-scam (accessed on December 3, 2020).

Dhaka Tribune (2020) '70% Bangladeshi Returnee Migrants Struggle to Find Jobs,' August 12.

Dhaka Tribune (2020b) 'Dhaka Riyadh in Dispute over Issuing Passports,' September 23.

Economist (2020) 'Racism in the Middle East: Maids for Sale,' July 25.

Fukuyama, Francis (2020) 'The Thing that Determines a Country's Resistance to the Coronavirus,' *The Atlantic*, March 30.

Guardian (2020) 'Migrant Workers Bear Brunt of Coronavirus Pandemic in Gulf', April 19.

George, S. E. (2020) 'Forced to Return from the Gulf, Migrants in Kerala Are Wondering What Comes Next,' *The Wire*, May 7, https://thewire.in/labour/kerala-migrants-gulf-covid-19 (accessed on July 12, 2020).

Ghosh, Bobby (2020) 'Top World Bank Economist Explains the Impact of Coronavirus on Foreign Workers,' *The Economic Times*, July 7. https://economictimes.indiatimes.com/nri/working-abroad/top-world-bank-economist-explains-the-impact-of-coronavirus-on-foreign-workers/articleshow/76827158.cms (accessed on July 20, 2020).

Goh, Yan Han (2020) 'Recent Cases among Foreign Workers Involved Those Who Were in Quarantine Facilities,' *The Straits Times* (Singapore). August 22.

Gulf News (2020) https://gulfnews.com/uae/health/covid-19-uae-has-done-75-million-coronavirus-tests-low-mortality-rate-1.1599575980145 (accessed on December 30, 2020).

Hasan, Mehedi (2020) 'Returnee Bangladeshi Migrants Suffering Due to Stigma and Lack of Support,' *Dhaka Tribune*, August 19.

ILO (2019) 'Labor Migration,' www.ilo.org/beirut/areasofwork/labour-migration/lang--en/index.htm.

IOM (2020) Issue Brief, July 14.

Iwamoto, Kentaro (2020) 'Singapore Coronavirus Clusters Awaken Asia to Migrants' Plight,' Nikkei, June 9, https://asia.nikkei.com/Spotlight/Asia-Insight/Singapore-coronavirus-clusters-awaken-Asia-to-migrants-plight (accessed on July 12, 2020).

Jessop, Bob (2011) 'Metagovernance,' in *SAGE Handbook of Governance*, edited by M. Bevir, London: Sage, pp. 106–123.

Koh D. (2020) 'Workplace,' *Occup Environ Med* Epub ahead of print: June 8, 2020. doi:10.1136/oemed-2020-106626.

Kumar, C. and Mohanty, D. (2020) 'Migrant Workers Battle Stigma, Bias Back Home,' *Hindustan Times*, May 11.

Migration Policy Institute (2020) Saudi Arabia. www.migrationpolicy.org/country-resource/saudi-arabia.

Ministry of Health, Singapore (2020) Daily Report on COVID-19 www.moh.gov.sg/docs/librariesprovider5/local-situation-report/situation-report---16-sep-2020.pdf (accessed on October 12, 2020).

Mint (2020) 'Remittances to India Likely to Decline by 23% Due to Covid-19 According to the World Bank,' www.livemint.com/news/india/remittances-to-india-likely-to-decline-by-23-due-to-covid-19-world-bank-11587617295143.html.

Nederveen Pieterse, Jan (2018) 'Comparing Capitalisms, East and West,' in Lim, Hyun-Chin, Jan Nederveen Pieterse, and Suk-Man Hwang (eds) *Capitalism and Capitalisms in Asia*. Seoul: Seoul National University Press.

Oxfam (2020) The Commitment to Reducing Inequality Index. www.oxfam.org/en/research/fighting-inequality-time-covid-19-commitment-reducing-inequality-index-2020 (accessed on December 30, 2020).

Phua, Rachel (2020) 'COVID-19: Singapore to Build New Dormitories with Improved Living Standards for Migrant Workers,' CNA, June 1.

Pisani, Elizabeth (2020) 'The Unpalatable Lesson of Coronavirus: Dictatorships Can Be Effective,' *Prospect*, February 28.

Reuters (2020a) 'Ethiopian Maids "Dumped" in the Streets in Lebanon as COVID Hits,' July 17.

Reuters (2020b) 'Gulf Migrant Workers Left Stranded by Coronavirus Outbreak,' *Ha'aretz*, April 19, www.haaretz.com/middle-east-news/gulf-s-migrant-workers-left-stranded-by-coronavirus-outbreak-1.8780132.

Sammadar, Ranabir (2020) 'Burdens of an Epidemic: A Policy Perspective on Covid-19 and Migrant Laborers,' Kolkata: Calcutta Research Center.

Serrieh, Joanne (2020) 'Kuwait to Fire 400 Expat Employees at Ministry of Public Works: Al Arabiya, September 27.

Shaikh, Hina (2020) 'Responding to the Impacts of COVID-19 on Informal Workers in South Asia,' International Growth Center, May 13, www.theigc.org/blog/responding-to-the-impacts-of-covid-19-on-informal-workers-in-south-asia/ (accessed on July 12, 2020).

Sharma, K., Adhikari, D., and AZM. Anans (2020). 'Coronavirus Wrecks South Asian Migrants Livelihood in Middle East', *Nikkei Asian Review*, May 20.

Sorkar, M.N.I. (2020) 'Covid-19 Pandemic Profoundly Affects Bangladeshi Workers Abroad with Consequences for Origin Countries,' Migration Policy Institute, July 9. https://af.reuters.com/article/healthcareSector/idUSL8N2D23MQ (accessed on July 28, 2020).

Straits Times (2020) 'Coronavirus: 14,500 Foreign Workers in Singapore still Serving Quarantine,' www.straitstimes.com/singapore/coronavirus-14500-workers-still-serving-quarantine (accessed on December 10, 2020).

UAE Government (2020) https://covid19.ncema.gov.ae/en (accessed on December 12, 2020).

UN News (2020) 'UN Chief Appeals for Global Action Against Coronavirus-fueled Hate Speech,' https://news.un.org/en/story/2020/05/1063542 (accessed on July 12, 2020).

Vijayaraghavan, Hamsa (2020) 'Gaps in India's Treatment of Refugees and Vulnerable Internal Migrants as Exposed by the Pandemic,' Migration Policy Institute, September 10, www.migrationpolicy.org/article/gaps-india-refugees-vulnerable-internal-migrants-pandemic (accessed on July 12, 2020).

World Bank (2018) *Moving for Prosperity: Global Migration and Labor Markets.* Policy Research Paper.

Worldometer (2020) www.worldometers.info/coronavirus/#countries (accessed on December 5, 2020).

World Migration Report (2020) https://publications.iom.int/system/files/pdf/wmr_2020.pdf (accessed on July 10, 2020).

Wright, Andrea (2020) 'No Good Options for Migrant Workers in Gulf COVID-19 Lockdown,' https://merip.org/2020/04/no-good-options-for-migrant-workers-in-gulf-covid-19-lockdown/ (accessed on December 12, 2020).

Yayboke, Erol (2020) 'Five Ways COVID-19 is Changing Global Migration,' Center for Strategic and International Studies. www.csis.org/analysis/five-ways-covid-19-changing-global-migration (accessed on December 15, 2020).

23

COVID-19 AND SCIENCE

Italy and late modernity

Luciano d'Andrea and Andrea Declich

The Covid-19 outbreak acted at the same time as *a contrast liquid* to observe critical dynamics that have been neglected in the public debate and as an *accelerator* of social, political and cultural processes already in progress. As a contrast liquid, the crisis especially highlighted the vulnerability characterizing our societies, impacting hard on the weakest sections of the population (for example, on poorly housed people, or people in retirement homes or the impact of cuts in healthcare services of the last decades). The crisis also likely served as an accelerator of social and economic processes, although it is too early to understand which processes will be affected in the long run, such as economic and social polarization in society (OECD, 2020a), the shift to a green economy (Allan et al., 2020) or the digital transition (Euroactiv, 2020), for example in education (Tesar, 2020).

On a global scale, one of the major issues that the Covid-19 crisis revealed and perhaps accelerates is the fragility of governance systems. We are referring not only to the scarce capacity of governments to manage global crises, like a pandemic (Capano et al., 2020), but also their difficulties in governing increasingly fragmented, structurally weakening and rapidly evolving societies such as ours, also in normal conditions (Marsh, 2011).

Different approaches to this topic (ethical, political, cultural, psychological and even philosophical) have been proposed. Probably one of the most fruitful entry points is the relation between science and government. This relation is becoming more unstable, ambiguous and diversified than it was in the past, for at least two interconnected reasons: the growing relevance of scientific knowledge in the governance of societies (and therefore in political decisions) and the drastic transformations affecting science and its connections with the rest of society. Not surprisingly, then, the outbreak revealed how science-governance relationships are problematic in many European countries such as the UK (Freedman, 2020; Scally, Jacobson and Abbasi, 2020;), France (Moatti, 2020), the United States (Hamilton and Safford,

2020) and probably elsewhere. Italy is no exception and provides a good example to reflect on changes in science-government relations in a context of extreme emergency. The next section provides a brief outline of science-government relations in Italy. Then, a tentative phenomenology of how these relations developed in the Covid-19 crisis is presented. In the final section, some interpretive frames are proposed to analyze, from a broader perspective, the critical role played by science in the governance of contemporary societies.

Feeble science-government connections in Italy

In Italy, research institutions have long been undergoing a process of social and political marginalization. It could be sufficient to consider the amounts allocated for research and development in the period 2007–2018. Considering the amount of 2007 equal to 100 in PPP (Purchasing Power Parity) US dollars, in 2018 the index decreased in Italy to 79 and in France to 90, while in the UK it increased to 106, in Belgium to 108, in the Netherlands to 113, in Denmark to 126 and in Germany to 145 (OECD, 2020b). For this reason, too, the Italian research system has to face many serious obstacles, including brain drain, over-bureaucratization, under-staffing, obsolescence of scientific equipment and often opaque hiring and promotion practices. In spite of these structural problems Italian researchers maintain high levels of scientific productivity (Nascia and Pianta, 2018).

Italian politics has also been facing serious problems. It suffered from a rapid and uncontrolled self-renewal process between 1992 and 1997, due to a series of scandals affecting many politicians, businessmen and administrators (Vannucci, 2016). Some historical parties collapsed and people's trust in politics faded away in a few years. Then a complex period followed, marked by an extremely divisive bipolarity of the political framework, which ended with the 2018 general elections when a new political party – the Five Star Movement – took the scene, profoundly modifying the political landscape. This complex path has been characterized by unsuccessful attempts to implement constitutional reforms, a long-lasting economic crisis and problematic relations between politics and the judiciary. All that did not help restore citizens' trust in the political system – gauged by a decrease in election participation rates of roughly 20 percent from 2001 onward (Istat, 2018) – and led to an increase in populism and far-right extremism. A compounding factor is the chronic ineffectiveness of public administrations that seriously limits any public policy and generates citizens' disaffection towards political leaderships. It is worth noting that the success of the Five Star Movement was largely due to its anti-establishment approach, which also affected the research system (the movement supported positions contrary to mainstream science on, e.g., vaccines and some diagnostic tests).

This complex situation impeded the development of consolidated mechanisms allowing scientists to regularly contribute to policymaking, including the establishment of procedures aimed at developing evidence-based policies or the creation of hybrid institutions at the intersection of university and government (Ranga and Etzkowitz, 2013).

Tentative phenomenology of science-government relations in the Covid-19 crisis

It is too early to draw a consolidated picture of science-government relations in the Covid-19 crisis and even more to define reliable future scenarios. However, a tentative phenomenology can be defined.

Lack of institutional and technical preparedness

To start with, it is worth noticing that the Italian Constitution – differently from many European countries – *does not contemplate a state of emergency* other than the 'state of war'. This does not mean that there are no procedures to manage emergency cases. When 'extraordinary cases of necessity and urgency' occur, the government is allowed to issue 'decrees-law' which should be presented on the same day to the Chambers for approval (Massa Pinto, 2020). However, the Italian Constitution does not provide for any kind of reorganization of powers between, for example, the Parliament and the executive or this latter and the regional administrations. This entails that this reorganization, when needed, can be ensured only through a negotiation among the many institutional actors involved.

In the case of the Covid-19 outbreak, with clear procedural guidelines lacking, the government opted to largely use an administrative tool (the Prime Minister's decree) which allowed 'bypassing' the Chambers (Lupo, 2020). This approach elicited much criticism since it created a strong concentration of power in the executive branch without a solid constitutional ground.

The lack of institutional preparedness was coupled with a *low technical preparedness* for what concerns the management of pandemics (differently from other types of emergency situations Italy is more recurrently exposed to, like earthquakes): no plans were available when the crisis started and, in the regions where they existed, they were not implemented (Capano, 2020). This is probably at the same time the cause and the effect of some of the most striking aspects of the phenomenology of the crisis.

The ambiguous role of experts

With the start of the crisis, different committees and task forces have been activated. The most important one is the ad-hoc Technical-scientific Committee of the Civil Protection Department. Established on February 3, it came to include 20 members (plus an unknown number of consultants). Comparing this committee with a similar one established in France, Giacomo Mingardo (2020) highlights some features which are particularly relevant for our analysis:

- Experts were presented (and probably selected) based on their positions in the administration rather than their qualifications.
- There were no experts with competences in social sciences.
- The consultation procedures of the Committee were not explicit, so that, although it was expected to support the Civil Protection Department, it directly provided its advice to the government.
- The opinions expressed by the Committee were not made public (for example, through their publication online, like occurred in France) and only short excerpts reported by the mass media were available.

Only four members out of 20 were representatives of scientific institutions (universities and national scientific societies) and, in its original composition, there were no women in the Committee membership (a circumstance strongly discussed in the media; Openpolis, 2020a).

These features seem to be mainly due to the 'extemporaneous' nature of the Committee and reflect the dominant procedures of the Italian Public Administrations which make them convoluted, non-transparent, ineffective and closed to the contribution of external actors (scientists, in this case).

The excessive visibility of science in the public arena

This unclear and marginal role of scientists contrasts with their overabundant presence as experts in the public debate and media during the Covid-19 crisis. According to Alessia Farano (2020), this is due to the 'exceptional role of the scientific community' in the formation of public opinion, which reflects 'the unprecedented proximity' of scientists with the public decision-makers, while other authors (Campati, 2020; Tonelli, 2020; Vaudo, 2020) interpreted such a presence as a 'return of expertise' in public decisions, seen as one of the few positive effects of the pandemic. In the lockdown phase, people's trust in both scientists and the government was extremely high (Battiston, Kashyap and Rotondi, 2020) and the visibility of science in the media was somewhat amplified by the press conference of the experts of the Civil Protection Department on the Covid-19 diffusion, broadcast daily at 18:00 (the 'ritual of 18:00', as Aldo Grasso pointed out, 2020).

This sudden visibility of scientists in the public sphere can hardly be considered in positive terms as a sign of a real change in science-government relations, precisely because of the limited weight of scientists in the institutional emergency structures highlighted above.

The deterioration of the image of science during the crisis

Yet this particular situation did not last long. In a few weeks, a progressive deterioration occurred in the image of science in public opinion and especially in the media. This was due to several factors. Three of them are worth mentioning here.

The first factor was the *instrumental use of science* by the government and political leaders. The ambiguous relationship between government and experts described above allowed the former to adopt different tactics depending on its needs (Mingardo, 2020), such as 'hiding' behind the experts (as happened elsewhere; Besley and Velasco, 2020), supporting the indications of the experts or openly ignoring them.

When in late May the loosening of lockdown was decided, the President of the Council of Ministers Giuseppe Conte expressly highlighted how such a decision had been taken against the experts' opinion, stating that 'the theory of professors must deal with reality' (Lombardo, 2020a). Two days later, he defended his choice not to apply lockdown measures in two municipalities in Lombardy (Alzano and Nembro) at the beginning of the pandemic, stating to have taken that decision on the basis of the 'opinion of the scientists' of the Technical-scientific Committee (Lombardo, 2020b).

The two sentences clearly reveal their instrumental nature. In the first one, an opposition is made between the abstractness of theory and the supposed problem-solving ability of politics. The hidden assumption is that theory is abstract and useless for solving practical problems. Moreover, in the first sentence, the term 'professor' (sometimes used in the public debate in a derogatory way) is chosen while in the second one the more high-profile term 'scientist' is preferred.

It is notable that scientists have been engaged as advisors of both the central government and regional administrations (overall, at least 1,466 experts were mobilized by the central and regional governments; Openpolis, 2020b), often harshly conflicting each other. In this way, political conflicts have been instrumentally turned into conflicts between 'scientific truths'.

The second factor which led to a deterioration of the image of science was what we could refer to as a *perception shift*. Lockdown time was the time of the emergency, dominated by fear of the pandemic and characterized by a sense of community and equality. This allowed the government to assume exceptional powers in setting priorities, allocating financial resources and imposing restrictions. The progressive decrease in the contagion led to a different public perception of the situation, dominated by concerns about the differentiated social and economic consequences of the pandemic. The feeling of commonality and equality rapidly faded away and the people's conflicting interests re-emerged. Scientists' indications, mainly dictated by the precautionary principle and based on uncertain forecasts, started to be perceived as unjustified limitations to people's freedom. From virologists, public attention moved to economists.

The third factor was the rapid *changes that occurred in scientific production and science communication.*

As for scientific production, an acceleration of the research processes occurred which led to a rapid surge in the number of preprints (preliminary versions of research articles that the authors share before peer-review) on Covid-19 (Ciani, 2020). This acceleration is risky, since it occurs in research systems already globally affected by a pressure to produce more in less time and with fewer resources (Müller, 2014).

More interesting here are the changes which affected science communication. Driven to produce new knowledge about Covid-19 in a short time, scientists began to confront each other, no longer in the context of research, but directly in the media. In this way scientists, rather than communicating already consolidated scientific facts, have been forced, to some extent, to communicate with each other in public while science was still in the making (Latour, 1987). Media practitioners played a role in that, for example using individual articles, still in their provisional form, as if they reflected the scientific knowledge as a whole or amplifying conflicts among scientists to 'build the news'. It is worth also noticing, in this regard, that scientists showed, on average, a limited capacity to master media language.

As Anna Sfardini notes (2020, p. 67), all that 'created a crack in the credibility of scientific competence'. Therefore, it is no surprise that, according to a survey carried out in the midst of the crisis, 48 percent of respondents declared themselves confused because of the diversity of opinions expressed by scientists (Bucchi and Saracino, 2020).

This situation made more visible those (and there are many in Italy) who consider science subservient to the interests of economic and political powers, unreliable or involved in plots of all kinds, favoring what the journalist Giuliano Ferrara called 'the childish hunt for the scientist' (2020). As a by-product, the perceived unreliability of scientists also paved the way to increased circulation of fake news of a scientific nature (ADN Kronos, 2020).

The poor understanding of science by political leaders

Another aspect that emerged in the context of the Covid-19 crisis is the political leaders' poor understanding of how science works, what can be legitimately expected of it and how to translate the indications that emerge from it.

With respect to the *functioning of science*, there has been the tendency of politicians – shared by many laypeople – to discuss scientific contents and to question science procedures. An example is provided by the President of the Veneto Region, Luca Zaia, who wanted to have his say on the artificial nature of the virus, stating that 'the fact that it is losing strength means that the virus is artificial. A virus in nature does not lose strength with this speed' (La Repubblica, 2020).

These forays of political leaders into the contents of science become possible since scientists – once placed outside the institutions of science – are perceived as bearers of opinions and no longer of certified knowledge. Similar forays have also been reported in other national contexts (see, in this regard, the statements of the President of the United States Donald Trump on the injection of disinfectants as a possible treatment against the virus; BBC News Online, 2020).

The poor understanding of science on the part of political leaders also concerns the *expectations about the outputs of science*. A good example of it is the statement that the Minister of Regional Affairs and Autonomies, Francesco Boccia, addressed to scientists: 'I ask the scientific community ... to give us irrefutable certainties and not three or four options for each issue ....We demand clarity, otherwise there is no science. We, politicians, take responsibility for making decisions, but scientists have to put us in a position to do so' (Il Post, 2020). This statement provoked a harsh reaction from the Italian Federation of Life Sciences (FISV, 2020), who highlighted that 'no serious scientist' is able to give certainties to the Minister 'in the absence of sufficient data to analyze' and evoked 'the crazy policy' adopted by the governments over the past 20 years aimed at reducing funds precisely to that research system which is now being asked to provide certainties.

It is easy to observe that this idea of science as a provider of certainties is incredibly obsolete and positivistic, although it is relaunched by many societal actors (e.g., populist movements, radical religious groups) to 'construct' science as their own enemy so to better challenge its authority.

Finally, also the attempts by political leaderships to *translate experts' orientations into political measures* were revealed to be largely inadequate and ineffective. The lack of consolidated relations with science and the limited capacity to develop well-grounded policies forced the government to directly translate them into the only language it knows, that is, the language of laws. This led to paradoxes, ambiguities and uncertainties.

Numerous controversies, for example, arose around the government decree authorizing citizens 'to meet relatives', leaving unspecified which group of relatives were being contemplated (this was an important aspect for citizens since a fine had been established in case of unauthorized visits). The subsequent attempt by the government to better specify this sentence resulted in an even more obscure interpretation, which was also the subject of many satirical comments. According to it, the term 'relatives' had to refer to 'relatives and relatives in law, spouses, cohabiting partners, stable partners and stable affective relationships'. In this way, a common concept has been transformed in an impracticable legislative measure (Busani, 2020).

Interpreting science-government relations in the light of the Covid-19 crisis

Although this chapter is not based on a comparative analysis, it is quite easy to observe, on the interpretive side, that what happened in Italy during the Covid-19 crisis reflects at least two general tendencies which can be detected across many, if not the majority of, national contexts.

The declining capacity of governance systems

The first general tendency can be referred to as the 'declining capacity of governance systems'. Political institutions are proving to be less and less capable of governing societies which are increasingly diversified, weakened in their structures, hierarchies and authority and exposed to widespread emotional and cognitive dynamics. The overall effect is that of a quite rapid transformation and fragmentation of political structures (Marsh, 2011) which can also undermine the solidity of democratic institutions, as witnessed by the widening literature on the 'crisis of democracy', revolving around concepts like 'post-democracy', 'democracy backsliding' and 'legitimation crisis' (see, for example, Fraser, 2015; Facchini and Melki, 2019), ultimately leading to the proliferation of hybrid regimes (illiberal democracies, competitive autocracies) (Gilbert and Mohseni, 2011; Mufti, 2018) and dangerous transformations in liberal democracies.

The Covid-19 crisis has made the difficulties of governments to guide social processes more evident. In Italy, this decreasing capacity of governance led to the instrumental use of the emergency we described above. Indeed, emergency or 'exceptional' situations (e.g., the 2015 World Expo, the 1990 World Football Championships, the 2000 Holy Jubilee, even the formation of a new government in 2011 explicitly defined as an 'emergency government' to manage the public financial and political crisis) have been used several times to reduce the frictions hampering the political process and to derogate from the ordinary rules (for example, those relating to public procurement). The Covid-19 outbreak has been also used in this way. It has generated a 'suspended time' (Turner, 1970) which allows the government to introduce policy measures otherwise impossible to implement, even at the cost of reducing the space for democratic debate, in order to bypass its lack of mastery of long-term processes.

A striking example of this general attitude has been the attempt by the government to use the emergency to address the chronic slowness of the public administration – that is crucial to stimulate economic recovery after the emergency and to face the old Italian problem of stagnating productivity – simply adopting a decree aimed at simplifying administrative procedures, with the paradox of introducing further complexity (Boeri and Perotti, 2020).

This tendency to use an emergency strategy to face long-term problems appears to be even more simplistic considering that no one can precisely say how the 'normal times' will be. For example, in 2020 newborn babies in Italy are expected to decrease by 10,000 units (Istat, 2020). This tendency, while showing how much Italians' trust in the future has already been reduced because of the Covid-19 crisis, also suggests that changes in contemporary societies are becoming so rapid and so strongly connected to collective risks that approaching long-term future issues as if they were emergencies could be revealed to be increasingly misleading.

This orientation to exploit the emergency situation, coupled with a simplified view of social and political processes, also contributes to explaining some of the tendencies highlighted in the previous section. Science has been instrumentally used by political leaders to influence public perception of the crisis and, when needed, to protect themselves and their political action. This has been done despite having little knowledge of how science works and what it can do.

As Capano (2020) highlights, ultimately, the response of the government to the crisis has been in continuity with the erratic and conflicting ways of designing and implementing policies characterizing the Italian politics, notwithstanding 'the massive involvement of experts'.

The under-socialization of science

A second interpretive framework to account for the difficulties met in managing the Covid-19 crisis can be referred to as the 'under-socialization of science' (Bijker and d'Andrea, 2009). Throughout the 19th and 20th century, science was organized as a relatively self-directed and autonomous institution, quite separate from society, not directly involved in the implications and use of its outputs, if not in specific situations and contexts (for example, in the case of military research). This social model of science has been often expressed with the image of the 'ivory tower'.

With the shift to late modernity, this model started collapsing, under the pressure of a diversified set of social, economic and political forces, overall related to globalization. This is leading science and scientists to be more focused on the production of 'useful knowledge' in economic, technological and social terms, more transparent and accountable, more explicitly and directly steered by governments and policymakers and more open to the contribution of other actors (businesses, local authorities, civil society organization and the general public) (Ziman, 2000; Nowotny, Scott and Gibbons, 2001).

Scientific institutions are still under-socialized with respect to this new social context, that is, they are not prepared to adequately cope with these transformations and to take the lead in the process. Consequently, in a paradoxical way, while science is becoming more relevant in every aspect of society, it is also becoming socially weaker and more exposed to risks. Its authority is declining, its results are challenged by laypeople, in both their validity and usefulness, and its boundaries are continuously trespassed by policymakers and economic actors.

These changes also affect the role of science and scientists in decision-making processes (Collins and Evans, 2002). In the past, the involvement of scientists in the definition and implementation of policies was quite regulated. Now they are often 'launched' into the policy arena, with little support, authority and legitimation. As experts, they can no longer rely upon the scientific community (which serves to generate scientific facts, not to take public decisions). At the same time, in many cases, they cannot rely on an established institutional system connecting science and policymaking able to provide them with clearly defined roles, authority, autonomy and recognition. In this way, scientists, as experts, are exposed to criticisms and judgments coming from journalists, decision-makers and laypeople and their knowledge becomes suspected as being instrumentally used for any short-term political objective.

In such a context, the same boundaries between science and science-based advice become increasingly blurred. The result is that science itself can be forced to develop not only through its internal, protected channels, but more and more in the public arena and in the media, where scientific debate turns into political conflict. In Italy, this has been clearly seen: there has not been an ecosystem protecting and supporting experts, who have thus been thrown into public debate playing roles (bearers of truth, prophets, scapegoats, entertainers) which are not theirs. However, similar situations of mistreatment of science and scientists have been observed in many national contexts during the Covid-19 crisis.

Managing the double weakness of governance and science

Overall, the crisis made more visible the existence of a double weakness – of the political governance systems, on the one hand, and of science, on the other – that had a reciprocal compounding effect.

These trends manifest themselves in different ways and intensity across national cultures and political systems. In Italy, for example, the political crisis of the 1990s paved the way for widespread populist attitudes centered on a systematic attack of any existing authorities, including science. Similar tendencies can be found in political regimes led by rightwing governments, such as in the United Kingdom, United States and Brazil, but less in more cohesive and hierarchical political and social cultures, such as in some Asian democracies. Nonetheless, the transformations occurring in both science and political systems are global in nature and, in different ways, affect all national systems, whatever be their political regime and political orientation. This also helps to explain the lack of preparedness to face the crisis observed everywhere, which is not solely the outcome of increasingly fragile democratic systems but also the consequence of a low level of socialization of science.

Preparedness requires forms of power redistribution also involving scientists: power to raise the alarm, to take guiding decisions, to establish priorities or to impose given behaviors. In many national contexts, these mechanisms are revealed to be feeble, questionable or ineffective (Renda and Castro, 2020), regardless of even the technical capacity of the State to face the outbreak (Capano et al., 2020).

This is not, of course, a responsibility to attribute to scientific institutions and even less so to individual scientists. Rather, what that the Covid-19 pandemic, acting as *contrast liquid*, eventually revealed is precisely the limited capacity of science and government to cooperate in establishing forms of governance based on *anticipatory systems*, that is, predictive models allowing social actors to adopt appropriate anticipatory behaviors before that the predicted events actually occur (d'Andrea, Declich and Caiati, 2020). Such an incapacity may prove to be particularly serious, if not fatal, in a stage of the evolution of society – that of so-called late modernity – characterized by increasing complexity, mounting uncertainties, rapid and profound changes and wider exposure to risks of different kind.

(Note: The quotations/phrases in Italian have been translated into English by the authors.)

References

ADN Kronos (2020). *Con emergenza coronavirus impennata 'fake news', esperti le svelano.* April 29.

Allan, J., Donovan, C., Ekins, P., Gambhir, A., Hepburn, C., Reay, D., Robins, N., Shuckburgh, E. and Zenghelis, D. (2020). A net-zero emissions economic recovery from Covid-19. *COP26 Universities Network Briefing.* April.

Battiston, P., Kashyap, R. and Rotondi, V. (2020). *Trust in science and experts during the Covid-19 outbreak in Italy.* SocArXiv, 11 May.

BBC News (2020). *Coronavirus: Outcry after Trump suggests injecting disinfectant as treatment.* 24 April. (www.bbc.com/news/world-us-canada-52407177). Retrieved on June 10, 2020.

Besley, T. and Velasco, A. (2020). *Politicians can't hide behind scientists forever – even in a pandemic.* LSE Covid-19 Blog. 6 May.

Bijker, W. E. and d'Andrea, L. (2009). *Handbook on the socialisation of scientific and technological research.* Rome: River Press Group.

Boeri, T. and Perotti, R. (2020). Semplificare, non basta la parola. *La Repubblica.* 7 July.

Bucchi, M. and Saracino, B. (2020). *Italian citizens and Covid-19: One month later – April 2020* (https://sagepus.blogspot.com/2020/04/italian-citizens-and-covid-19-one-month.html). Retrieved on June 10, 2020.

Busani, A. (2020). Coronavirus, ecco chi sono i congiunti che si potranno incontrare dal 4 maggio. *Il Sole 24 Ore.* April 27.

Campati, A. (2020). La rivincita delle competenze? In Raul Caruso and Damiano Palano (eds). *Il mondo fragile. Scenari globali dopo la pandemia.* Milan: Vita e Pensiero.

Capano, G. (2020). Policy design and state capacity in the Covid-19 emergency in Italy: if you are not prepared for the (un)expected, you can be only what you already are. *Policy and Society. States and Covid-19 Policy-making, 39*(3): 326–344.

Capano, G., Howlett, M., Jarvis, D. S., Ramesh, M. and Goyal, N. (2020). Mobilizing policy (in)capacity to fight Covid-19: Understanding variations in state responses. *Policy and Society. States and Covid-19 Policy-making, 39*(3): 285–308.

Ciani, O. (2020). *Comunicare la ricerca scientifica ai tempi del coronavirus.* SDA Bocconi School of Management. (www.cergas.unibocconi.eu/wps/wcm/ connect/abc758f5-e8c0-4ce8-a48e-2a37cccb26a3/Ciani_PreprintCOVID-19.pdf?MOD=AJPERES&CVID=n5AutAI). Retrieved on June 1, 2020.

Collins, H. M. and Evans, R. (2002). The third wave of science studies: Studies of expertise and experience. *Social Studies of Science, 32*(2): 235–296.

d'Andrea, L., Delich, A, and Caiati, G. (2020). Processi anticipatori e complessità sociale: per il superamento di una visione prescrittiva dell'anticipazione. *Futuri.* 13 Anno VII, luglio.

Euractive (2020). The Coming Revolution: Europe's Digital Transition in a Post-Covid World. Special report.

Facchini, F. and Melki, M. (2019). The Democratic Crisis and the Knowledge Problem. *Politics & Policy, 47*(6): 1022–1038.

Farano, A. (2020). La Repubblica degli scienziati? Saperi esperti e politica ai tempi del coronavirus. *Biodiritto.* March.

Ferrara, G. (2020). L'infantile caccia allo scienziato. Competenti e dotati di stile. I nuovi esperti non meritano disprezzo. *Il Foglio.* 5 May.

FISV (2020). *Replica di FISV al Ministro Boccia per le sue dichiarazioni sulla Scienza* (www.fisv.org/documenti-e-position-papers/441-replica-di-fisv-al-ministro-boccia-per-le-sue-dichiarazioni-sulla-scienza.html). Retrieved on June 10, 2020.

Fraser, N. (2015). Legitimation crisis? On the political contradictions of financialized capitalism. *Critical Historical Studies, 2*(2): 157–189.

Freedman, L. (2020). Strategy for a pandemic: The UK and Covid-19. *Survival, 62*(3): 25–76.

Gilbert, L. and Mohseni, P. (2011). Beyond authoritarianism: The conceptualization of hybrid regimes. *Studies in Comparative International Development, 46*(3), 270.

Grasso, A. (2020). In casa, mani lavate: tutto qui? *Corriere della Sera – Sette.* April 24.

Hamilton, L. C. and Safford, T. G. (2020). Ideology affects trust in science agencies during a pandemic. *Carsey Perspective*, March.

Il Post (2020). Il ministro Boccia vuole dalla scienza 'certezze inconfutabili'. April 13.

Istat (2018). *Annuario Statistico Italiano 2018.* Capitolo 11, 'Elezioni e attività politica e sociale' (www.istat.it/it/files//2018/12/C11.pdf) Retrieved July 8, 2020.

Istat (2020). *Rapporto Annuale 2020. La situazione del Paese.* Istituto Nazionale di Statistica.

La Repubblica (2020). Zaia: 'Se virus perde forza, è artificiale'. E Pregliasco: 'Non si può escludere in maniera totale, ma dati indicano che è naturale,' May 8.

Latour, B. (1987). *Science in action: How to follow scientists and engineers through society*. Cambridge, MA: Harvard University Press.

Lombardo, I. (2020a). Ho preso io la decisione contro il parere degli esperti. *La Stampa*. May 28.

Lombardo, I. (2020b). La difesa di Conte contro le parole della pm: la decisione di non chiudere Alzano e Nembro dopo il parere degli scienziati. *La Stampa*. May 30.

Lupo, N. (2020). L'attività parlamentare in tempi di coronavirus. *Il Forum di Quaderni costituzionali*, n. 2, 121–142, April.

Marsh, D. (2011). Late modernity and the changing nature of politics: Two cheers for Henrik Bang. *Critical Policy Studies*, *5*(1): 73–89.

Massa Pinto, I. (2020). La tremendissima lezione del Covid-19 (anche) ai giuristi. Fiat iustitia et pereat mundus oppure Fiat iustitia ne pereat mundus? *Questione Giustizia* (www.questionegiustizia.it/articolo/la-tremendissima-lezione-del-covid-19-anche-ai-giuristi_18-03-2020.php). Retrieved on June 6, 2020.

Mingardo, G. (2020). Il ruolo del comitato tecnico-scientifico in Italia e Francia nell'emergenza Covid-19. *Biodiritto*, March.

Moatti, J. P. (2020). The French response to Covid-19: Intrinsic difficulties at the interface of science, public health, and policy. *The Lancet Public Health*, *5*(5): e255.

Mufti, M. (2018). What do we know about hybrid regimes after two decades of scholarship? *Politics and Governance*, *6*(2): 112–119.

Müller, R. (2014). Racing for what? Anticipation and acceleration in the work and career practices of academic life science postdocs. *Forum Qualitative Sozialforschung/Forum: Qualitative Social Research*, 15(3) Art. 15, September 2014.

Nascia, L. and Pianta, M. (2018). *Research and Innovation Policy in Italy*. MPRA Paper No. 89510.

Nowotny, H., Scott, P. and Gibbons, M. (2001). *Re-thinking Science: Knowledge and the Public in the Age of Uncertainty*. Cambridge, UK: Polity Press.

OECD (2020a). *OECD Employment Outlook 2020: Worker Security and the Covid-19 crisis*. Paris: OECD Publishing.

OECD (2020b). *Main Science and Technology Indicators* (www.oecd.org /sti/msti.htm). Retrieved on June 1, 2020.

Openpolis (2020a). *Coronavirus: Chi decide durante lo stato di emergenza* (www.openpolis.it/esercizi/una-ricostruzione-degli-eventi/). Retrieved on June 10, 2020.

Openpolis (2020b). *Gestione Covid19, poche donne e non nei ruoli chiave*. 29 aprile 2020 (www.openpolis.it/gestione-covid19-poche-donne-e-non-nei-ruoli-chiave/). Retrieved on June 1, 2020.

Ranga, M. and Etzkowitz, H. (2013). Triple Helix systems: An analytical framework for innovation policy and practice in the Knowledge Society. *Industry and Higher Education*, *27*(4): 237–262.

Renda, A. and Castro, R. (2020). Towards stronger EU governance of health threats after the Covid-19 pandemic. *European Journal of Risk Regulation*, 11, Special Issue 2: Taming Covid-19 by Regulation, June 2020: 273–282.

Scally, G., Jacobson, B. and Abbasi, K. (2020). The UK's public health response to Covid-19. *BMJ* 2020: 369.

Sfardini, A. (2020). Come comunicare la pandemia? Credibilità e fiducia delle fonti istituzionali nell'informazione italiana sul Covid-19. In Marianna Sala e Massimo Scaglioni (eds). *L'altro virus. Comunicazione e disinformazione ai tempi del Covid-19*. Milan: Vita e Pensiero.

Tesar, M. (2020). Towards a Post-Covid-19 'new normality?' physical and social distancing, the move to online and higher education, *Policy Futures in Education*, 18(5): 556–559.

Tonelli, G. (2020). Il peso della responsabilità per scienziati e ricercatori, *Corriere della Sera*, May 3.

Turner, V. W. (1970). *The Forest of Symbols: Aspects of Ndembu ritual* (Vol. 101). Ithaca, NY: Cornell University Press.

Vannucci, A. (2016). The 'clean hands' (mani pulite) inquiry on corruption and its effects on the Italian Political System, *Em Debate*, 8(2): 62–68.

Vaudo, E. (2020). La scienza come esercizio della democrazia, *Il Sole 24 Ore*. May 17.

Ziman, J. (2000). *Real Science: What it is, and what it means*. Cambridge: Cambridge University Press.

24

GLOBAL INFODEMIC

Covid-19 and the organization of disinformation

Wasim Khaled and Naushad UzZaman

Blackbird.AI provides *Disinformation Defense and Response* to national security and enterprise customers. Our AI Platform empowers organizations to defend and respond to a new class of *cyberattacks on human perception* and the manipulation mechanisms that drive them. During the last several years Blackbird.AI has observed a sharp rise in the speed and scale of harmful influence campaigns designed to manipulate public opinion, policy making and the very cohesion of our societies; a trend that continues to grow as these operations become more automated and sophisticated. During any major event, we have found that disinformation actors, conspiracy theorists and other harmful factions rapidly mobilize to hijack attention around emerging world events to amplify their goals by promoting and twisting certain narratives in efforts to polarize and control perceptions. The 2020 Covid-19 pandemic is the most prominent example of these trends to date. The widespread uncertainty and dislocation that the virus has precipitated has proven fertile ground for exploitation of information and opinions: Covid-19 is described as the 'Disinformation Olympics' (Khaled, quoted in O'Brien, 2020), denoting the sheer breadth, depth and complexity of manipulation generated by this global event.

Across the world the pandemic has been perceived, interpreted and mitigated in different ways by national governments, local communities and individuals. Numerous variable social, economic, political and cultural factors determine what form specific pandemic responses have taken in their jurisdictions. Blackbird.AI proposes that disinformation is one of these factors in its own right, but given its qualities as a non-geographically bound phenomenon able to adapt itself to local and specific dynamics, it also holds the potential to affect these other contextual considerations. In recognizing this, Blackbird.AI aims to broaden and deepen the World Health Organization's description of the pandemic as 'an infodemic of misinformation and disinformation' (WHO et al., 2020) beyond an interpretation around purely health and medical-related topics. Based on Blackbird.AI's original social media analysis and investigation conducted in the first half of 2020, this chapter will examine critical ways in which synthetically amplified manipulated content has affected perceptions and responses to the Covid-19 pandemic. In our discussion we draw on some of the relevant cross-cutting social, political and cultural themes referenced in the introduction of this volume to illustrate the permeation of disinformation around different factors that have contributed to the non-containment of the virus.

Methods

Blackbird.AI defines disinformation as false information that is spread with the intent to cause harm. This differs from misinformation, when false information is spread unintentionally. For the purposes of this investigation, we refer to both under the term 'disinformation'.

Blackbird.AI's methodology is based on man-machine cooperative intelligence. Our proprietary AI toolsets screen large volumes of digital content to surface high disinformation threat risks. We use algorithmic processing to identify subtle data patterns that suggest deliberate manipulation, focusing on:

- Suspicious patterns of propagation and sharing.
- Manipulated messaging around specific content including hashtags, URLs and images.
- Evidence of falsification introduced via technical means.
- Traffic inorganically generated via bots or coordinated user campaigns.
- Cohort analysis: identifying specific users and communities engaged in manipulation.

Once surfaced by our system, human intelligence is brought to bear on salient items, identifying focused conversations or evolving 'storylines' known as narratives. Our process of analysis also produces a Blackbird Manipulation Index (BBMI) score reflecting the predicted percentage of total inorganic content in a given feed, based on the above characteristics. Scores between 0 to 10 percent indicate a low-risk threat; 11 to 40 percent medium; 41 to 70 percent high; and 71 to 100 percent critical.

Blackbird.AI analyzed three periods of Twitter activity related to the Covid-19 pandemic comprising 175,748,538 tweets in total, of which 30.6 percent were assessed to have been synthetically manipulated (Blackbird.AI, 2020c; 2020d; 2020e). Using a generic, primarily English-language wordpack we captured data across more than 63 languages which surfaced a large volume of specific disinformation narratives, out of which we mainly focused on content of relevance to our readership in the United States. Those narratives discussed below should be considered a representative sample of relevant themes given the sheer volume of disinformation examined and expositional limitations of this chapter. (See Table 24.1)

TABLE 24.1 Blackbird.AI results of Covid-19 social media manipulation analysis

	Reporting period	*Tweets analyzed*	*Manipulated tweets identified*	*BBMI score*	*Risk rating*
1	February 2 to February 14, 2020	6,923,257	2,679,300	38.7%	Medium
2	February 27 to March 12, 2020	49,755,722	18,889,396	37.95%	Medium
3	May 2 to May 20, 2020	119,069,559	32,148,780	27%	Medium
	Total	175,748,538	53,717,476	30.6%	Medium

Source: Blackbird.AI, 2020c; 2020d; 2020e.

Discussion

Trust in government

Cultures of societal trust in the institution of government can affect the way a national or local pandemic response is received by subject populations. If disinformation can exploit levels of public trust, it holds the power to radically alter the effectiveness of measures put in place by governmental authorities. Blackbird.AI noted the emergence of prominent disinformation narratives flourishing among certain demographics of the US population where Big Government is traditionally mistrusted. The American Right has historically stood for small government and strong individualism; opposition to pandemic control measures introduced in US states from mid-March onwards has therefore unsurprisingly tended to split along partisan lines of Democratic (broadly pro-lockdown) and Republican (broadly anti-lockdown).

Calls to *Re-Open the Economy* following the closure of nonessential businesses contained organic sentiments that the 'cure is worse than the disease' and dislike of perceived government overreach. However, we also noted high levels of manipulation within these *Re-Open* narratives with a BBMI score of 44.73 percent during our third reporting period, coalescing around notions that the Democratic Party has pushed lockdowns as a smokescreen for population control or government takeover. This builds on previous disinformation campaigns around the denigration of Democratic politicians' calls for precautionary anti-virus measures. The *Dem Panic* narrative (BBMI 33.1 percent, second reporting period) amplified depictions of the Democrats as purposefully overreacting to the dangers posed by Covid-19, bolstered by Donald Trump's reference to Democrat criticism of his handling of the pandemic as 'their [the Democratic Party's] new hoax' at his February 28, 2020 rally in Charleston, South Carolina.

Linked to this is the emergence of *Pro-Militia* disinformation campaigns that merge extant pro-Second Amendment, libertarian sentiments with distrust of lockdown. Blackbird.AI observed *Pro-Militia* narratives with a BBMI score of 58 percent in our third reporting period. Groups such as the *Boogaloo* movement (a right-wing militia group seeking the incitement of a second US civil war) appear to have capitalized on organic frustration within *Re-Open* and *Dem Panic* narratives as an opportunity to expand their visibility and popularity.

In the short term, the exploitation of anti-government sentiment via targeted disinformation campaigns can have a detrimental effect on state-led efforts to curb the spread of Covid-19. It can also lead to incidences of real-life violence occurring as a consequence of synthetically amplified anti-government or hyper-partisan radicalization. For example, the summer of 2020 witnessed numerous rallies held at state capitol buildings across the US where self-identified militias and other armed individuals gathered to protest lockdown measures, as well as incidences of violence at anti-racism protests broadly split along left-right political lines (Beckett, 2020; Beutel and Johnson, 2020). In October 2020 the FBI revealed a thwarted plot to kidnap Democratic Michigan Governor Gretchen Whitmer over her pro-lockdown stance, hatched by militia members who also conspired to attack law enforcement, overthrow the government and eventually ignite civil war (Zapotosky, Barrett and Hauslohner, 2020).

In the longer term, manipulated narratives that incite and exploit anti-government sentiment run the risk of exacerbating long-lasting cultures of distrust in government and its institutions. This includes influencing the voting public to elect political candidates into office that disinformation actors hope will further their own agendas; Russian online interference into the 2016 US presidential election in favor of Donald Trump proves the past effectiveness of such techniques. As the US prepares to return to the polls in 2020 at the time of writing, the effect of sustained disinformation campaigns aimed at fomenting political fissures could greatly hamper the possibility of enacting a sustained and effective Covid-19 response.

Institutions

Just as institutions of government have been affected by disinformation during the Covid-19 pandemic, so too have other key institutions that provide guidance, resources and information to the public. For example, the *Dem Panic* and *Re-Open* narratives displayed significant overlap with an emergent narrative of *Media Delegitimization* (BBMI 42 percent) during the second reporting period. Blackbird. AI uncovered widespread accusations that the Democratic Party controls US media and leverages it to criticize Republican responses to the Covid-19 pandemic. All mainstream media (colloquially referred to as 'MSM') becomes 'fake news', designed to create widespread panic by sensationalizing the threat posed by the virus and undermining genuine public health messaging.

Other credible, accepted voices of authority have also been targeted by manipulation campaigns, most notably those based around scientific expertise. This includes the World Health Organization, the US National Institute of Allergy and Infectious Diseases (NIAID) and its director Dr Anthony Fauci, the latter of whom requires security protection following repeated death threats and harassment towards himself and his family provoked by his public health guidance (Newburger, 2020). Medical misinformation and hoaxes have been in abundance since the beginning of the pandemic, with false medical advice circulated on social media responsible for thousands of deaths worldwide as sufferers attempt dangerous home remedies or refuse to seek hospital treatment (Satariano, 2020).

One prominent disinformation example is the *Plandemic* documentary hoax posted to YouTube on May 4, 2020. The video—titled *Plandemic: The Hidden Agenda Behind Covid-19*—featured discredited American scientist Judy Mikovits, who claimed her research around coronaviruses and immunization had been purposefully buried by a cabal of global elites (including Fauci and NIAID) using the pandemic as a pretext for population control. Within a week the hoax had gone viral, making *Plandemic* one of the most successful and highly manipulated pieces of digital content disseminated during the pandemic at this time. By platforming Mikovitz under the guise of 'fighting censorship', the documentary created shared discourse between disparate elements of disinformation and fringe communities where their ideologies intersected. This includes traction of #plandemic and #scandemic hashtags within *anti-vax*, *anti-mask*, *anti-5G*, *anti-lockdown*, *QAnon* and other online disinformation-centric communities.

Global cooperation

The Covid-19 pandemic proposes the need for greater global cooperation in which resources, medical expertise and data are shared. Disinformation poses a real risk in undermining processes of multilateral action and partnership and entrenching geopolitical divides. For example, Blackbird.AI noted several disinformation campaigns vilifying China as the source of the virus, particularly during our first reporting period. This includes the *delegitimization of Chinese culture* (promoting racial stereotypes—'Coronavirus came from Chinese people eating bats'), conspiracies around *Covid-19 as a bioweapon* (many countries such as the US, Canada, Iran and Israel have been accused of manufacturing the virus, with China and the Wuhan Institute of Virology receiving a large proportion of this speculation), or the *Tencent/Chinese Government cover-up* (falsified screenshots of Tencent's 'Epidemic Situation Tracker' showed a virus death toll almost 80 times higher than official Chinese government figures, provoking claims of a Beijing cover-up).

The success of these disinformation campaigns is no doubt in part to their offline amplification, as well as online. Given that an aggressive posture towards China has been a hallmark of the Trump administration and his two election campaigns, it is unsurprising that a number of prominent Republican Party figures have repeatedly echoed claims that Covid-19 is a manufactured Chinese *bioweapon*, despite the thorough debunking of the theory from multiple credible sources (BBC News, 2020; Sabbagh, 2020; Stevenson, 2020). This is a keystone example of a conspiracy being pushed into the mainstream by persons of influence, thus dramatically expanding its reach and apparent legitimacy. This exacerbates existing geopolitical tensions and reduces the possibility for constructive international dialogue, as well as emboldening xenophobic anti-Asian stigmatization and abuse on an individual level (Karalis Noel, 2020).

Speed

Timely action taken to control the spread of coronavirus can have a huge impact on mitigating its reach and impact. Situations in which authorities react quickly or preemptively to the virus fare better than those who delay. Disinformation can be conceived of in a similar way—if synthetic content is able to disseminate to wide audiences without intervention, this can only have a greater negative impact on pandemic control responses, medical advice, public reception and so on. Given that digital connectivity permits instantaneous global communication, a real-world event can permutate into online disinformation almost immediately. For instance, the *Dem Panic* narrative witnessed large spikes in manipulated messaging after the February 28, 2020 Trump Charleston rally, and again on March 9, 2020 following the Italian government's imposition of a nationwide quarantine, which triggered heightened concern around the virus and calls for action within the US met with a parallel increase in disinformation.

The *Plandemic* hoax documentary is also a useful example: posted on May 4, 2020 and taken down three days later for its promotion of false medical information, the video was viewed more than eight million times on YouTube alone and cross-posted to numerous social media platforms, making it the most significant piece of Covid-19 disinformation at this point in time. This is partially a result of poor regulatory mechanisms for detection and removal of manipulated messaging, but also due to factors inherent to the content itself. According to a 2018 MIT study, fake news travels six times faster than its truthful counterparts due to its often heightened emotive and novel value that drives higher levels of human engagement (Vosoughi, Roy and Aral, 2018). Fake news is also disproportionately recommended to platform users on this basis—disinformation spurs higher levels of user engagement, which allows greater opportunities for collection of users' data, which can then be sold by tech companies for profit. Algorithms which seek to promote high-engagement content will therefore incline to push disinformation over a truthful counterpart (Blackbird.AI, 2020a). This has serious consequences for both Covid-19 disinformation and our digital ecosystems in general—slowing the speed in which fake news is transmitted online will not be achievable without a wholesale dismantlement of the current structures of profit and control upheld by Big Tech and permitted by a dearth of regulatory oversight.

Uncertainty

The Covid-19 pandemic has produced unprecedented disruption into every level of human life, from the global economy, international travel and national governance, down to the everyday realities of individual daily routines. This dislocation from established habits and ways of understanding the world naturally produces the desire to reground and navigate oneself through this period of uncertainty. When face-to-face contact has been inhibited by quarantines and lockdowns, turning to the Internet for human connection and information is a logical outcome.

Accordingly, the Covid-19 pandemic has precipitated dramatic increases in Internet usage as working or studying from home, video calls with loved ones and online entertainment stand in for offline activities. In March and April 2020 global online traffic increased by up to 40 percent as many countries experienced their first months of lockdown (Sandvine, 2020).

Conspiracy and disinformation thrive in these unfamiliar realities, presenting answers to confusion and unpredictability, or purporting to show a reality which has been hitherto obscured. A conspiracy theory such as *QAnon* is demonstrative of this appeal. *QAnon* first surfaced online in 2017 as a fringe phenomenon that celebrates Donald Trump as the singular champion of freedom and justice, waging righteous war on a shadowy deep-state of Democratic politicians and Hollywood celebrities embroiled in a global pedophilia ring. In March 2020—the beginning of pandemic lockdown for many—online QAnon traction jumped exponentially; on Facebook alone, membership of *QAnon* groups increased by 120 percent and engagement rates by 91 percent during this month (Gallagher, Davey and Hart, 2020). *QAnon* capitalizes on the human desire for answers in uncertainty by encouraging followers to 'do the research for themselves' by interpreting world events in relation to its claims of secret cabals and Leftist cover-ups (its take on Covid-19 is largely as a hoax or cover for Democratic overreach). This gamification of conspiracy is a perverse empowerment that self-affirms and perpetuates the movement as new followers find recourse for their own worldviews and experiences within the dislocation of lockdown and the *QAnon* mythos (Blackbird.AI, 2020b). Conspiracy theories by definition, however, will never offer closure; they feed off antagonism and subversion. For Covid-19 and beyond, this means the exacerbation of pandemic-induced uncertainty into entrenched misrepresentations of the external world.

Truth

Truth matters to the Covid-19 pandemic in the sense that falsified information holds the very real potential to precipitate offline harm, from the promotion of medical misinformation (*Plandemic*), racial stigmatization (*delegitimization of Chinese culture*) or incitement to violence (*Militias*). Disinformation campaigns may seek to disguise their synthetic origins in order to convince audiences of their legitimacy and thus drive higher engagement.

For example, our first reporting period revealed widespread use of high-volume accounts and bots promoting consistent hashtag-driven campaigns. This creates a highly centralized and well-organized disinformation ecosystem. One such example is the *Anti-Meat* narrative promoted by Indian spiritual guru Saint Rampal Ji Maharaj under the hashtag #NoMeat_NoCoronaVirus. Rampal used his significant cross-platform presence to launch a massive spam campaign alleging that meat eaters were responsible for bringing Covid-19 to India and vegetarianism inoculates against infection, reflecting his teachings that eating meat is a sin. The narrative exhibited a huge spike on February 2, 2020 which quickly tailed off, and a BBMI score of 99.4 percent, suggesting a deliberate push to disseminate heavily manipulated content with little organic engagement.

Large-volume, manipulative actors were still apparent during our later reporting periods, but gave way in precedence to huge numbers of low-volume accounts pushing given narratives from slightly different angles. The disinformation space became muddied by vast amounts of decentralized manipulation gaining organic traction across diverse communities and subjects. For example, Blackbird.AI identified the practice of astroturfing within the *Re-Open* narrative. Astroturfing artificially orchestrates an illusion of grassroots support for a message, product or entity, thus masking the original sponsor and concealing wider networks of manipulation. A number of privately-owned media organizations (such as Salem Media Group, Media Research Centre, Heritage Foundation and Rick Dees) were identified as pushing *Re-Open*-based talking points across a vast back-linked architecture of websites, outwardly appearing as disconnected publication ventures. This rendered it extremely difficult for audiences to recognize that seemingly disparate media outlets were operating as a singular interest group intent on disguising their share of voice.

We also noted the co-option of organic public interest pieces around American business owners suffering from lockdowns by influencers and manipulation campaigns. These focused around local personas such as a 'Dallas salon owner', 'Michigan barber' or 'New York tailor' presented as faux-viral stories pushed to several authentic communities which became synthetically galvanized under the memetic *Re-Open America* banner. Although *Re-Open* holds a much lower BBMI score than a highly manipulated narrative such as *Anti-Meat* for example, its strength lies in its ability to absorb organic engagement by masquerading as genuine, thus drawing in wider, diverse audiences.

However, simply exposing the falsehood or synthetic origin of a news story or conspiracy is not enough to stem its spread or dull its message. Disinformation's tenacity lies in its ability to tap into extant sentiments and appear to corroborate them. Truth is a relative construct that resonates with audiences based on their preconceived beliefs. *Boogaloo* ideology is unlikely to convince a pro-gun control Democrat voter to incite for civil war; the Second Amendment anti-masker, however, may prove more sympathetic. Simply, if someone *wants* something to be true, *it will be true to them*, regardless of its credibility. Or, to take this a step further, even if the false origin of disinformation is acknowledged, if its message produces a desired outcome then this takes precedence over its veracity. The repetition of the *coronavirus-bioweapon* conspiracy by senior Republican politicians outlined above is a case in point. This has worrying consequences for the Covid-19 pandemic; the potential for disinformation to galvanize public opinion and influence ideas and behavior runs far deeper than a 'fake news' label on social media can hope to prevent.

Conclusion

What our research reveals is that perceptions of the Covid-19 pandemic have been consistently manipulated *from the very start* to create and exacerbate widespread partisan divides, social unrest and anti-science attitudes to public health and societal cohesion. Disinformation actors and the online platforms that have permitted their activity are thus key antagonists in the outcome of the severity of this pandemic, particularly within the US where many of our most prominent narratives have surfaced. The new disinformation ecosystem has transformed a health crisis into one that is increasingly more to do with a transformed media landscape and toxic political discourse upheld by indifferent digital infrastructures and technology corporations.

Disinformation narratives around the Covid-19 pandemic demonstrate a wide-ranging ability to exploit factors that inhibit successful institutional responses to the virus and exploit social antagonisms. The efficacy of established authorities such as local and national government, scientific establishments and reputable media agencies is vital to ensuring a robust plan of action to contain the pandemic. A responsive public with high levels of trust in such institutions is also crucial to ensure containment measures are upheld. Blackbird.AI's investigation demonstrates that disinformation has proven a key factor in undermining public trust and polarizing the political spectrum, most notably in the US where a pre-existing culture of anti-Big Government and bipartisan politics provided fertile ground for manipulation campaigns attacking lockdown measures as a Democratic Party-sponsored hoax or overreach. This has already contributed to acts of real-life violence witnessed during the summer of 2020 and beyond.

The exposure of disinformation as false is by no means a panacea. False information thrives precisely because it resounds with preconceived ideas and human desires, whether unknowingly consumed or deliberately deployed as a political stunt. The ability of disinformation to produce compelling, emotionally relatable frameworks for understanding the world therefore moves our challenge beyond merely providing a True or False value for online content. Rather, it is a constant battle to understand how to inoculate against manipulative infodemics that influence almost every major and rising information warfare arms race. Governments and societies worldwide must prepare to defend against these types of attacks with the same urgency and attention as they would any other type of attack from threat actors that aim to harm their citizens, economies and way of life.

References

BBC News. (2020, May 1). Coronavirus: Trump Stands by China Lab Origin Theory for Virus. *BBC News*. Retrieved from www.bbc.co.uk/news/world-us-canada-52496098 (accessed October 13, 2020).

Beckett, L. (2020, April 30). Armed Protesters Demonstrate Against Covid-19 Lockdown at Michigan Capitol. *The Guardian*.

Beutel, A. and Johnson, D. (2020, August 3). Far-Right Extremist Mobilization Surges During U.S. Unrest. *Center for Global Policy*. Retrieved from https://cgpolicy.org/articles/recent-protests-and-civil-unrest-highlight-challenges-of-far-right-extremism-to-american-democracy-and-security (accessed October 14, 2020).

Blackbird.AI. (2020a, October 13). The Global Disinformation Cycle: Surveillance Capitalism and Reality. *Blackbird.AI*. Retrieved from www.blackbird.ai/blog/2020/10/13/the-global-disinformation-cycle (accessed October 12, 2020).

Blackbird.AI. (2020b, October 3). The Global QAnon Phenomenon. *Blackbird.AI.* Retrieved from www.blackbird.ai/blog/2020/10/03/the-global-qanon-phenomenon (accessed October 12, 2020).

Blackbird.AI. (2020c, June 10). Covid-19 Disinformation Report—VOL. 3. *Blackbird.AI.* Retrieved from www.blackbird.ai/wp-content/uploads/2020/06/Blackbird.AI-Disinformation-Report-Covid19-Volume-3-2.pdf (accessed October 12, 2020).

Blackbird.AI. (2020d, March 17). Covid-19 Disinformation Report—VOL. 2. *Blackbird.AI.* Retrieved from www.blackbird.ai/wp-content/uploads/2020/03/Blackbird.AI-Disinformation-Report-Covid19-Volume-2.pdf (accessed October 12, 2020).

Blackbird.AI. (2020e, February 19). Covid-19 Disinformation Report—VOL. 1. *Blackbird.AI.* Retrieved from www.blackbird.ai/wp-content/uploads/2020/02/Blackbird.AI-Disinformation-Report-Covid-19.pdf (accessed October 12, 2020).

Gallagher, A., Davey, J. and Hart, M. (2020). Key Trends in QAnon Activity Since 2017. *Institute for Strategic Dialogue.* Retrieved from www.isdglobal.org/wp-content/uploads/2020/07/The-Genesis-of-a-Conspiracy-Theory.pdf (accessed October 12, 2020).

Karalis Noel, T. (2020). Conflating Culture with Covid-19: Xenophobic Repercussions of a Global Pandemic, *Social Sciences & Humanities Open, 2*(1), 1–7.

Newburger, E. (2020, August 5). Dr. Fauci Says His Daughters Need Security as Family Continues to Get Death Threats. *CNBC.* Retrieved from www.cnbc.com/2020/08/05/dr-fauci-says-his-daughters-need-security-as-family-continues-to-get-death-threats.html (accessed October 15, 2020).

O'Brien, C. (2020, April 3). Blackbird.AI CEO: 'Covid-19 is the Olympics of Disinformation'. *VentureBeat.* Retrieved from https://venturebeat.com/2020/04/03/blackbird-ai-ceo-covid-19-is-the-olympics-of-disinformation/ (accessed October 12, 2020).

Sabbagh, D. (2020, May 4). Five Eyes Network Contradicts Theory Covid-19 Leaked from Lab. *The Guardian.*

Sandvine. (2020, May). The Global Internet Phenomena Report Covid-19 Spotlight. *Sandvine.* Retrieved from www.sandvine.com/covid-internet-spotlight-report (accessed October 13, 2020).

Satariano, A. (2020, August 17). Coronavirus Doctors Battle Another Scourge: Misinformation. *The New York Times.* Retrieved from www.nytimes.com/2020/08/17/technology/coronavirus-disinformation-doctors.html (accessed October 12, 2020).

Stevenson, A. (2020, February 17). Senator Tom Cotton Repeats Fringe Theory of Coronavirus Origins. *The New York Times.*

WHO, UN, UNICEF, UNDP, UNESCO, UNAIDS, ITU, UN Global Pulse & IFRC. (2020, September 23). Managing the Covid-19 Infodemic: Promoting Healthy Behaviours and Mitigating the Harm from Misinformation and Disinformation. *World Health Organization.* Retrieved from www.who.int/news/item/23-09-2020-managing-the-covid-19-infodemic-promoting-healthy-behaviours-and-mitigating-the-harm-from-misinformation-and-disinformation (accessed October 12, 2020).

Vosoughi, S., Roy, D. and Aral, S. (2018, March 9). The Spread of True and False News Online. *Science, 259*(6380), 11146–1151.

Zapotosky, M, Barrett, D. and Hauslohner, A. (2020, October 9). FBI Charges Six Who It Says Plotted to Kidnap Michigan Gov. Gretchen Whitmer, as Seven More Who Wanted to Ignite Civil War Face State Charges. *The Washington Post.*

CONCLUSION

Habibul Khondker and Jan Nederveen Pieterse

This book focuses on the relationship between governance institutions and public health, approaches to Covid-19 and health outcomes. It doesn't dwell on chronicles of unfolding government responses such as lockdown, curfew and other restrictions or stimulus packages to rebuild economies. Such chronicles date quickly. Detailed country by country reports and narratives are available elsewhere (IMF 2020).

Among general questions that arise from the Covid-19 pandemic are the following. Does a high GDP per capita yield good public health and low Covid-19 mortality? Studies in the book show this is not the case (Chapters 10, 14, 15). Do rich countries do better than poor countries? Not necessarily, the United States isn't short in resources and scientific capacity, but poorer countries such as Rwanda did a far better job in suppressing the virus (Chapter 19). Cuba, for 60 years the target of US hostility and disdain, derided for socialist governance, delivers exemplary public health performance and in addition contributes to international health care aid (Chapter 17). Do advanced societies show quality public health and low Covid-19 mortality? Studies in this book don't confirm this. Rich OECD countries show uneven responses. While the UK, Italy, Spain, Belgium and the Czech Republic buckled, Northeast Asian countries, Germany and Nordic countries in general were able to lessen the impact of the crisis and avoid tragedy.

Do democracies provide quality public health and low Covid-19 mortality? Studies in the book don't confirm this. Francis Fukuyama observes: 'some democracies have performed well, but others have not, and the same is true for autocracies' (2020). Democracy doesn't guarantee an efficient response as the US, Brazil and South Africa show. Compare India and China. Organization and social protection are decisive factors. India, a democracy, cared little about the rights of informal sector workers who, upon a total lockdown imposed with four hours' notice, were forced to trek to their villages, traversing a vast land on feet or bicycle. Such pandemonium did not take place in China. An efficient administration implemented the lockdown of large cities (Wuhan 11 million, Beijing 20 million) and carried out testing 11 million people in Wuhan in less than a week. In the US, after eight months facing the pandemic, testing capacities still don't come close to matching the demand.

Are western societies more individualistic and therefore less willing or able to comply with social distancing, wearing masks and other restrictions than Asian societies? The categories east and west are old-fashioned and studies in this book don't confirm this (such as Germany, Chapter 12).

Varieties of market economies probe further than these general queries. The Introduction asks a leading question: do coordinated market economies and developmental state-led market economies perform better in the Covid-19 pandemic than other market economies? The studies indicate that this holds true for *developmental state-led market economies*; discussed in the book are China, Singapore, Cuba and Rwanda. Another instance is Vietnam. It also holds true for *coordinated market economies*, although here outcomes show a wide spread. Quality public healthcare and low Covid-19 mortality occur in Northeast Asia (Taiwan, Korea, Japan) and Nordic Europe (Germany and Scandinavia, with higher mortality in Sweden), but Belgium, the Netherlands and France show higher mortality. Spain and Italy have fared worse still, while Greece has performed better (289 deaths per million).

Most chapters in the book refer to the political economy character of the societies they examine, but not all use varieties of market economies or institutional categories because this isn't part of authors' vocabulary or toolkit.

Varieties of market economies provide guideposts of probabilities. They provide estimates but they are not exhaustive nor should we expect them to be exhaustive. Of course, a host of other variables come in, in diverse combinations—the quality of governance, political organization, geography, demography (composition and age of population), experience with infectious diseases, the status of the economy, and so forth (Introduction). Some countries can rely on institutional synergies (such as Iran, Chapter 8) while others experience clashes between institutions and politics (such as Brazil, Chapter 16).

Thailand's score (0.9 per million) is remarkably low, lower than one would expect of a country led by a conservative military-monarchy alliance. Close-up study shows a public health system that functions effectively in a crisis thanks to popular support (Chapter 7); thus, Thailand taps on resources of social cohesion that run deeper than governance institutions (in spite of struggles of red shirts/yellow shirts and Muslims in southern Thailand). Also, Malaysia's Covid-19 score (12 per million) is lower than one would expect of a state-led market economy governed by ruling party cronies and traditional elites (the sultans). Thus, in each country not just pattern matches, but also pattern deviations are revealing.

When things fall apart, what do we learn about how things fit together? A key variable, of course, is the public health system. Public health systems in Korea and Canada helped them to deal with the crisis better than the US private health care system (Chapter 14). No surprise either is that small government (the preferred size in liberal market economies) is of little help in a public health crisis while capacious, capable government is an asset. These variables are included in the framework of varieties of market economies, however, the varieties of market economies schema do not include what is probably a profound underlying resource in a pandemic—*social cohesion* (Chapter 15). Social cohesion enables trust, so 'trust in government' may imply this dimension. Social cohesion accounts for Covid-19 success in Thailand, Malaysia and many other countries while its absence accounts for tragic failures in the US, India and Brazil. While many people blame failure in India, Brazil and the US on rightwing populist governments, the underlying variable that accounts for weak or inept governance in the first place is weak social cohesion. The best ways to *build* social cohesion are measures that mitigate inequality (such as progressive taxation, spending on services and education and social spending).

Editors of the *New England Journal of Medicine* observe that Covid-19 put the world to a test and in the United States, 'leaders have failed that test. They have taken a crisis and turned it into a tragedy' (Editors, 2020). Not just the US, which saw the largest share of deaths, caseloads and economic loss, but also many other countries could have minimized the losses and the scale of human tragedy had they been more organized in their response.

The US government was quick to pass the blame to China, misrepresenting facts and making false claims. China promptly alerted the World Health Organization of the virus danger. China conducted gene-sequencing of coronavirus 2 (SARS-CoV-2) and shared its gene sequence with the world scientific community by publishing it on virological.org, a professional website on January 11, 2020, only days after the discovery of the disease (CIDRAP 2020). This gene sequence has been the basis of all vaccines in the making the world over.

The pandemic started as a disrupter of public health and economies and may end as a disruptor of global geopolitics, as the US has been unable to take leadership in fighting the pandemic globally. 'Pandemics and plagues have a way of shifting the course of history', notes Wade Davis, and Covid-19 'has reduced to tatters the illusion of American exceptionalism'; the US behaved like a 'failed state' 'ruled by a dysfunctional and incompetent government' (Davis 2020). The US Covid death rate (870 per million) is more than double than that of Canada (334 per million), exceeds that of Japan (18), a country with a vulnerable elderly population, by a factor of almost 50, and exceeds the mortality in low-middle income countries such as Vietnam (0.4) by a factor of almost 2000. Compare China's death rate of 3 per million to 870 per million in the United States (Editors, 2020).

Does a public health crisis magnify existing strengths and weaknesses? Is global risk society as strong as the weakest link? How risk cuts multiple ways is a collective learning experience. The world hegemon turns out to be a weak link in global pandemic cooperation. Leaving the WHO during a global pandemic is a crime against humanity. The US is one of the founders of the G20 that was created to deal with the financial-economic crisis of 2008; however, the US president did not attend the part of the virtual G20 meeting, chaired by Saudi Arabia (November 21–22, 2020), that addressed the ramifications of Covid-19 and opted for a game of golf instead.

The crisis brought home the lesson that a pandemic calls for a global approach to handle a global crisis. Global cooperation and coordination—in sharing knowledge, technology, resources or vaccines—are requirements for overcoming the public health crisis. In an integrated world, pathogens in one region or country are a threat to all, hence a global approach to deal with this crisis is not a choice but an imperative. Networks of relationships occur at much higher levels of population, as population densities and connectivity grow hand in hand. Globally, 7.5 billion people are connected 24/7 in many ways. Connectivity does not guarantee a free-flow of evidence-based information: alongside scientific knowledge, an infodemic of misinformation and disinformation poses challenges to the globally networked society (Chapter 24). Does the Covid-19 pandemic signal deglobalization, as in reviewing global supply chains? It may rather signal a new phase of globalization with greater collective awareness of the risks as well as the necessity of connectivity and cooperation, a more reflexive globalization.

The Covid-19 pandemic occurs with a larger world population, at much higher levels of population density and connectivity than past pandemics. Compared to past pandemics, the impact of Covid-19 is more serious, its economic impact is far more wide-ranging (in economies shrinking, in global supply networks and the travel sector) and so is its political impact because Covid-19 is test of governance and leadership.

Covid-19 is part of the Anthropocene. HIV/Aids, Ebola, SARS, MERS and Covid-19 are all part of humans encroaching on nature and wildlife. Which isn't new because there are four times more viruses in our human genome (8 percent, nonactive remains of past infections) than our actual genes (2 percent). But most past plagues were regional and Covid-19 is global. Climate change is part of the same challenge as Covid-19 and, likewise, requires global cooperation.

References

CIDRAP 2020 China releases genetic data on new coronavirus, now deadly, January 11.

Davis, Wade 2020 The unraveling of America, *Rolling Stone*, August 6.

Editors 2020 Dying in a leadership vacuum, *The New England Journal of Medicine*, October 8, 385 (15).

Fukuyama, Francis 2020 The pandemic and political order: It takes a state, *Foreign Affairs*, July/August.

IMF 2020 Policy Responses to COVID-19: Policy Tracker, www.imf.org/en/Topics/imf-and-covid19/Policy-Responses-to-COVID-19.

AFTERWORD

The material in this volume was submitted before or in November 2020. After almost six months have passed data show several trends. The table below shows all countries with Covid-19 deaths *over a thousand* per million of population, by region.

Eastern Europe		*Western Europe*		*Americas*	
Czechia	2586	Belgium	2011	US	1731
Hungary	2407	Italy	1886	Brazil	1644
Bosnia/Herzegovina	2235	UK	1864	Peru	1629
Montenegro	2173	Portugal	1662	Mexico	1593
Bulgaria	2071	Spain	1632	Panama	1410
North Macedonia	2007	France	1505	Colombia	1273
Slovenia	1978	Sweden	1342	Chile	1258
Slovakia	1920	Luxembourg	1212	Argentina	1241
Poland	1538	Switzerland	1201	Bolivia	1054
Croatia	1534	Austria	1068		
Lithuania	1363				
Moldova	1333				
Romania	1307				
Armenia	1254				

(Worldometer data per 4/10/2021)

Several points stand out in this review of data. There are *no* countries in Asia, the Middle East and Africa with Covid deaths over a thousand per million of population. In Asia, the highest is India (122 per million, probably an undercount, now experiencing a surge). In the Middle East, the highest are Lebanon (975 per million) and Iran (757). In Africa, the highest is South Africa (889).

In addition, over the last six months Covid-19 deaths have risen significantly and continue to rise by the day in the United States, much of Latin America and Europe, but have not risen or only marginally in most of Asia, Australasia, the Middle East and Africa. Covid deaths in the US are over half a million (575,545) and deaths per million of population (1731) are the highest in the Americas. With the world's highest spending on healthcare, US Covid deaths are closer to Brazil, Peru and Mexico than to Canada (612 per million).

Contrary to expectations, in low-income countries virus cases and mortality are, so far, generally low. Several considerations apply: in many developing countries there is less throughflow while several countries with experience of infectious disease are well organized. Also mentioned in relation to Africa are young populations, a warm climate with ample ventilation, an outdoors lifestyle, highly diverse DNA and strong immune systems. 'African DNA is the world's most diverse, because 99 percent of our evolutionary history occurred on the continent' (Christian Happy, 'With pathogens we need to play offence', Financial Times, February 20–21, 2021). There may also be undercounts. In war-torn counties reported mortality is low (Syria 77 per million, Afghanistan 64, Yemen 34), but data are unreliable.

Since the 1960s infectious diseases have mostly affected developing countries (with deaths of 4 million per year, including malaria 2 million; Delanty 2021: 13). With Covid-19 it is other way round; its greatest impact is in high-income countries (but not in all high-income countries). Thus, the list of high-risk countries that some governments (such as Ireland) keep is way off.

Considerations for high deaths in Central and Eastern Europe are late action, neglect of controls, multi-generation households and much work is not remote (J. Shotter and V. Hopkins, Central and Eastern Europe ravaged by virus, Financial Times, March 25, 2021). Among Nordic European countries, only Sweden shows over a thousand deaths per million (1334). An outlier in Scandinavia, Sweden adopted a no restrictions and mask-less approach to the virus. Compare Finland 156, Norway 125. European city states with much throughflow and tourism also show high mortality (Gibraltar 2791 deaths per million, San Marino 2501, Andorra 1551, Liechtenstein 1465).

Northeast Asia, China, New Zealand and Australia applied the hammer, the control of movement of people, swiftly and decisively and the dance of testing and tracing competently. They stopped the virus. Social life resumed and their economies are growing while international travel is still banned or controlled. Also, much of Southeast Asia has managed well with low deaths per million in Vietnam (0.4), Thailand (1), Singapore (5) and Malaysia (40). Over six months time the needle has barely moved.

In April 2021 we are well into the vaccine phase, a race between vaccines and variants, mutations that emerge as the virus spreads (such as UK, P.1 Brazil, South Africa, California and India variants). This phase comes with vaccine silos, vaccine hoarding, vaccine nationalism, vaccine diplomacy, vaccine inequality, vaccine apartheid (Palestinians), vaccine tourism (UAE), vaccine corruption, vaccine price gouging and profiteering. The landscape is multicentric with US, UK, Russian, Chinese and Indian vaccines and production in several countries (AstraZeneca is also produced in Belgium, the Netherlands, Italy, India and the US).

Problems that affect virus control also play a part in the vaccine phase, with differences. In countries where the public sector held a backseat, government is back. Government is key to pandemic response, healthcare, vaccine funding and distribution and economic recovery. Liberal market economies shift gear to the government side. Vaccines belong to the corporate sphere, with public funding; the purchase, distribution and application of vaccines are government responsibilities. The UK manages vaccine distribution well thanks to the NHS. The Biden administration has activated the Defense Production Act and the National Guard in vaccine production and distribution. In governance, competence outflanks charisma.

The UK and US bungled the virus control phase but are doing well in the vaccine phase. The question is, is it possible to skip the hammer and the dance and be saved by vaccines? Is it possible to ignore restrictions and regain ground with vaccines? This is what the US is finding out when Republican-led states reopen for business and travel, vaccines are on the rise and cases and deaths are on the rise as well.

The EU lags in the vaccine phase. The EU Commission took acquiring vaccines for 27 countries in its own hands but had no experience in handling this, waited for full test results ('an abundance of caution') and haggled over prices and conditions. There is also a whiff of Brexit. AstraZeneca provided a weak contract (supply and timing are subject to 'best efforts') at a time when in Britain there is satisfaction of being outside the EU in this phase.

Low-income countries lag in both virus control and vaccines. If we consider the world, as the WHO does, vaccines are a public good. Intellectual property should be lifted so Covid-19 vaccines can be produced as generic drugs (the 'parallel importation' that South Africa achieved, overcoming huge resistance of big pharma, with HIV drugs in the 1990s). Despite broad government support for the COVAX program to help countries of the global South with vaccines, at least 85 poor countries will not have significant access to coronavirus vaccines before 2023 (Chowdhury and Jomo 2021). India's spike in cases in April means that vaccines produced in India's Serum Institute, the world's largest vaccine manufacturer, that were earmarked for developing countries now go to domestic use first. A wider problem is that while government donors provide 78% of funding of the COVAX program and corporations just 1.2%, yet the governance of COVAX grants stakeholder status to Big Pharma. Thus, COVAX protects commercial markets and in effect, 'COVAX is more like a merchant bank or an international financing institution than a health care organization' (Gleckman 2021).

Comparative history in the tradition of McNeill (1977) provides lessons: with a virus no country is an island. Eradicating Covid-19 is not yet on the horizon but the virus is over when excess deaths, more than normal rates of mortality cease.

References

Chowdhury, A. and Jomo K.S. 2021 End vaccine apartheid before millions more die, *IPS*, March 23.

Delanty, G. ed. 2021 *Pandemics, politics, and society: Critical perspectives on the Covid-19 crisis*. Berlin: De Gruyter.

Gleckman, H. 2021 *COVID, global governance, and COVAX*. Amsterdam: Friends of the Earth International and Transnational Institute.

McNeill, W. H. 1977 *Plagues and peoples*. Oxford: Basil Blackwell.

INDEX

Note: Page numbers in **bold** refer to tables and those in *italic* refer to figures.